Endovascular Surgery for Aortic Aneurysms

Endovascular Surgery for Aortic Aneurysms

Brian Hopkinson FRCS, MCh
Professor of Vascular Surgery, Queen's Medical Centre,
Nottingham, UK.

Waquar Yusuf FRCS
Research Fellow, Queen's Medical Centre,
Nottingham, UK

Simon Whitaker MRCP FRCR
Consultant Radiologist, Queen's Medical Centre,
Nottingham, UK

Frank Veith MD
Professor of Vascular Surgery, Montefiore Medical Center,
New York, USA

W. B. Saunders Company Ltd
London Philadelphia Toronto Sydney Tokyo

W. B. Saunders Company Ltd

24–28 Oval Road
London NW71 7DX

The Curtis Center
Independence Square West
Philadelphia, PA 19106-3399, USA

Harcourt Brace & Company
55 Horner Avenue
Toronto, Ontario, M8Z 4X6, Canada

Harcourt Brace & Company, Australia
30–52 Smidmore Street
Marrickville
NSW 2204, Australia

Harcourt Brace & Company, Japan
Ichibancho Central Building
22-1 Ichibancho
Chiyoda-ku, Tokyo 102, Japan

This book is printed on acid-free paper

A catalogue record for this book is available from the British Library

ISBN 0-7020-2148-2

Typeset by Paston Press Ltd, Loddon, Norfolk
Printed in Great Britain by Cambridge University Press, Cambridge

Contents

Contributors

Matthew P. Armon FRCS (ED)
Department of Vascular Surgery, University Hospital, Queen's Medical Centre, Nottingham NG7 2UH, UK

Daryll M. Baker FRCS
Department of Vascular Surgery, Royal Free Hospital, London, UK

Bryn R. Baxendale FRCA
Department of Anaesthesia, University Hospital, Queen's Medical Centre, Nottingham NG7 2UH, UK

Peter R.F. Bell MD FRCS
Department of Surgery, Clinical Sciences Building, Leicester Royal Infirmary, Leicester LE2 7LX, UK

Ulrich Blum MD
Department of Diagnostic Radiology, University Hospital Freiburg, Germany

Jan D. Blankensteijn MD
Department of Vascular Surgery, Academic Hospital Utrecht, Heidelberglaan 100, 3584 CX Utrecht, The Netherlands

Ivo A.M.J. Broeders MD
Department of Vascular Surgery, Academic Hospital Utrecht, Heidelberglaan 100, 3584 CX Utrecht, The Netherlands

Timothy A.M. Chuter MD
Department of Surgery, University of California, San Francisco, USA

Michael D. Dake MD
Section of Cardiovascular and Interventional Radiology, Department of Radiology, Stanford University Medical Center, Stanford, CA 94305, USA

Jean Pierre E. Dereume MD
Department of Vascular Pathology, Erasmus University Hospital (ULB), 808 Route de Lennik, 1070 Brussels, Belgium

Carlos E. Donayre MD
Division of Vascular Surgery, Department of Surgery, Harbor/UCLA Medical Center, Box 2910, 1000 West Carson Street, Torrance, CA 90509, USA

Bert C. Eikelboom MD
Department of Vascular Surgery, Academic Hospital Utrecht, Heidelberglaan 100, 3584 CX Utrecht, The Netherlands

Nabil M. Elmarasy MS
Department of Vascular Surgery, University Hospital, Queen's Medical Centre, Nottingham NG7 2UH, UK

Jose Ferreira MD
Department of Vascular Pathology, Erasmus University Hospital (ULB), 808 Route de Lennik, 1070 Brussels, Belgium

Brian R. Hopkinson FRCS MCh
Department of Vascular Surgery, University Hospital, Queen's Medical Centre, Nottingham NG7 2UH, UK

Krasnodar Ivancev MD
Department of Radiology, Malmö University Hospital, Malmö, S-21401, Sweden

Ricardo La Mura MD
Department of Vascular Surgery, Instituto Cardiovascular de Buenos Aires, Mercedes 4255, Cap. Fed., Buenos Aires, Argentina

Michael M.D. Lawrence-Brown FRACS
Department of Vascular Surgery, Royal Perth Hospital GPO 2213, Perth 6001, Australia

Shane T.R. MacSweeney MA MChir, FRCS
Department of Vascular Surgery, University Hospital, Queen's Medical Centre, Nottingham, NG7 2UH, UK

Michael L. Marin MD
Division of Vascular Surgery, Department of Surgery, Montefiore Medical Center, The University Hospital for the Albert Einstein College of Medicine, 111 East 210th Street, New York, NY 10467, USA

James May MS FRACS FACS
Department of Vascular Surgery, Royal Prince Alfred Hospital and Department of Surgery, University of Sydney, Australia

Ahktar Nasim MB CHB FRCS
Department of Surgery, Clinical Sciences Building, Leicester Royal Infirmary, Leicester LE2 7LX, UK

Juan Carlos Parodi MD
Department of Vascular Surgery, Instituto Cardiovascular de Buenos Aires, Mercedes 4255, Cap. Fed., Buenos Aires, Argentina

Bo Risberg MD
Department of Surgery, Malmö University Hospital, Malmö, S-21401, Sweden

Robert D. Sayers MD FRCS
Department of Surgery, Clinical Sciences Building, Leicester Royal Infirmary, Leicester LE2 7LX, UK

Charles P. Semba MD
Section of Cardiovascular and Interventional Radiology, Department of Radiology, Stanford University Medical Center, Room H-3647, 300 Pasteur Drive, Stanford, CA 94305, USA

Claudio Schonholz MD
Department of Vascular Surgery, Instituto Cardiovascular de Buenos Aires, Mercedes 4255, Cap. Fed., Buenos Aires, Argentina

Matthew M. Thompson MD FRCS
Department of Surgery, Clinical Sciences Building, Leicester Royal Infirmary, Leicester LE2 7LX, UK

Frank J. Veith MD
Division of Vascular Surgery, Department of Surgery, Montefiore Medical Center, The University Hospital for the Albert Einstein College of Medicine, 111 East 210th Street, New York, NY 10467, USA

Peter W. Wenham FRCS MD
Department of Vascular Surgery, University Hospital, Queen's Medical Centre, Nottingham NG7 2UH, UK

Simon C. Whitaker MRCP FRCR
Department of Radiology, Queen's Medical Centre, University Hospital, Nottingham NG7 2UH, UK

Geoffrey H. White FRACS
Department of Vascular Surgery, Royal Prince Alfred Hospital and Department of Surgery, University of Sydney, Australia

Rodney A. White MD
Division of Vascular Surgery, Department of Surgery, Harbor/UCLA Medical Center, Box 2910, 1000 West Carson Street, Torrance, CA 90509, USA

Weiyun Yu MB BS
Department of Vascular Surgery, Royal Prince Alfred Hospital and Department of Surgery, University of Sydney, Australia

Waquar Yusuf FRCS
Department of Vascular Surgery, University Hospital, Queen's Medical Centre, Nottingham NG7 2UH, UK

Preface

Endovascular aortic aneurysm repair has increased in popularity since Parodi demonstrated its technical feasibility in a patient nearly six years ago. Despite improvements in peri-operative management, the morbidity and mortality following conventional aortic aneurysm surgery remains considerable, particularly, in cases of leaking aneurysms, thoracic aneurysms and in the sub group of patients with significant co-morbidity. The concept of aneurysm repair without surgical exposure and aortic clamping is, therefore, attractive as it has the potential for reducing morbidity and mortality. Endovascular techniques are evolving rapidly and several different systems are currently undergoing development and evaluation. While the general principles are similar, each endoprosthesis and delivery system has certain unique features. Endovascular Surgery for Aortic Aneurysms brings together up-to-date information on the design and results of most of the systems currently in clinical use. At this stage, most of the systems appear to be effective in achieving satisfactory exclusion of the aneurysm from the circulation. However, many hurdles remain to be crossed before this procedure become technically feasible for the majority of patients. Endovascular techniques must be compared with the conventional approach in terms of morbidity, mortality, cost, patient acceptability and post operative recovery. More importantly data on long term safety and efficacy are needed before wide-spread use can be justified. There is no doubt that many technical changes will be necessary to overcome the problems and limitations of the first-generation systems, but it can be said with cautious optimism that endovascular aneurysm repair holds considerable promise for the future.

S.W.Y.
B.R.H.
S.C.W.
F.J.V.

1

Guidelines for the development of transluminally placed endovascular graft devices for aortic aneurysm repair

Frank J. Veith and Michael L. Marin

Division of Vascular Surgery, Department of Surgery, Montefiore Medical Center, The University Hospital for the Albert Einstein College of Medicine, 111 East 210th Street, New York, NY 10 467, USA

It is feasible to place prosthetic grafts within the arterial tree by inserting them via a remote site, guiding them intraluminally to the appropriate location, and fixing them there with attachment systems, such as a variety of expandable stents. Accordingly, there is a potential for these transluminally placed endovascular grafts (TPEGs) to provide improved treatment for a variety of arterial lesions, including aortic and aortoiliac aneurysms. Because TPEG repairs can be performed less invasively, their risks and costs may be lower than those of standard vascular graft operations. They are, therefore, extremely attractive to both patients and physicians, and consequently there is enormous pressure to develop and use these devices rapidly.

However, in the interests of patients and their well-being, it is appropriate to further the development of safe, effective devices for performing TPEG repairs of various arterial lesions at all levels of the arterial tree. To this end a combined committee of vascular surgeons, interventional radiologists and other interested scientists prepared a document of guidelines to help with the 'careful and structured evaluation and monitoring ... necessary to document the safety, efficacy and effectiveness of these (TPEG) devices in various settings before they undergo widespread clinical use'.[1] The purpose of this document was to 'help avoid premature and potentially harmful usage of TPEGs'.[1]

The present chapter will abstract portions of the original 'Guidelines' document that are particularly relevant to endovascular aneurysm surgery with particular emphasis on infrarenal aortic aneurysms.

Generalities

Types of TPEG

TPEGs can be divided into *covered single stent devices* and *end fixation devices*, which comprise a prosthetic graft fixed with a stent or other attachment system at both ends. Variants of the latter are bifurcated Y grafts or branched grafts with attachment devices at all three ends and long grafts stented at one end and with no stent or a suture anastomosis at the other end. Further division of TPEGs can be based on the *characteristics of the device*, specifically the nature of the *delivery system* (e.g. sheath or no sheath, over a wire or not over a wire, etc.), the nature of the *attachment or fixation system and method* (balloon-expandable, spring-expandable, or mechanically expandable stent or other device, with or without hooks for fixation to the vessel wall), and the nature of the *graft or covering material component.*

Comparison between TPEGs and standard arterial grafts and stents

It should be recognized that some properties of TPEGs may differ from those required of standard grafts or stents used to treat similar lesions in similar locations. Because TPEGs will be inserted from a remote site and guided into position, there are clear advantages to reducing their unexpanded cross-sectional diameter or 'profile' as much as possible. In this way the requirement that they be introduced through an open arteriotomy in a large-caliber artery will be minimized. Thus devices with a low profile offer clear advantages in terms of feasibility and applicability. However, making the TPEG thin and flexible to achieve a low, unexpanded profile may require a thinner graft with reduced strength.

At present it is not known whether TPEGs need the same burst strength or porosity characteristics as a standard arterial graft. A TPEG that will be placed within the unsupported lumen of an aortic aneurysm must have adequate strength and durability to withstand aortic pressures and flows, although it may not have to meet the same safety factors required of standard aortic grafts with regard to these parameters. In addition, a TPEG intended for use in the treatment of unruptured aneurysms may not require the same porosity specifications as a standard graft used to treat the same condition. Because the endoluminally inserted device will be contained within the intact aneurysm sac, greater porosity may be tolerable because transinterstitial bleeding will be contained by the aneurysm wall until fibrin deposition occludes the pores. Moreover, a TPEG placed within a stenotic or occluded artery may receive structural support from the surrounding arterial wall, thereby allowing the use of grafts with different physical properties (e.g. decreased wall thickness and strength). Long-term experimental and clinical studies will be required to settle these issues. In contrast, some endoluminally placed grafts may require unusual characteristics not needed with standard grafts. Examples include physical properties that contribute to an intact and fixed friction seal at junction points with host arteries, to the development of rapid and secure impermeability to blood in ruptured aneurysms and traumatic arteriovenous fistulas, or to resistance to compression when a TPEG is placed within occluded arteries.

Developmental study protocols

When TPEGs and appropriate systems for their insertion are developed and are believed to be suitable for treatment of specific lesions in specified locations, the following general guidelines are recommended for preclinical and clinical testing *before* the devices are brought into widespread usage. For any device, the evaluation must consist of four phases: bench testing (structural and mechanical), preclinical (animal) testing, clinical testing – feasibility, and clinical testing – comparative performance. However, in identifying appropriate testing for any device, consideration must be given to the mode(s) of failure and its effect on the performance of the device.

Bench testing

For the *graft portion* of the device, bench testing should consist of essentially the same tests of physical properties, such as strength, durability, porosity, kink resistance, suture holding ability, flexibility, and longitudinal and radial stretchability, as are required for a currently standard or proposed new arterial prosthesis.[2–4] The possibility also exists that modified requirements may need to be developed for new graft materials that may be developed and used for TPEGs. In addition, the *stent portion or attachment system* of a TPEG device will have to be evaluated for the various characteristics important to its function, such as inertness in blood, lack of toxicity, absence of metal fatigue, flexibility, compression resistance, and other physical properties that contribute to a leak-proof seal and secure fixation at junction points with arteries.[5] Finally, the *delivery system* of a device will require bench testing to demonstrate appropriate manoeuvrability, kink resistance, radiopacity, and marker visibility to be effective in the clinical setting in which it will be used.

Animal testing

Successful animal implantation of all TPEG devices, by use of the same introduction systems and localization and deployment methods that will be used in patients, should be required before clinical trials can be undertaken. Successful implantation includes the ability to visualize and deploy the device by techniques similar to those that will be required in patients; the firm fixation of the device at the site of original implantation; and acceptable freedom from leakage, migration, vessel wall erosion, thrombosis, excessive intimal hyperplasia with luminal narrowing, and distal embolization. There should also be acceptable freedom from other complications related to the fixation component or stent, particularly those with hooks or spikes. The duration of observation in animal testing should be for a minimum of *6 months* before clinical tests can be undertaken. Longer studies may be needed if synthetic materials not currently in use in the vascular system are involved.

The TPEG should be inserted in animal models at similar, although not necessarily identical, anatomic locations to those intended for use in patients. Every effort should be made to use animal models that mimic as closely as possible the clinical problem being addressed. Device insertion techniques and endpoints studied should parallel those that will apply in the clinical setting as much as possible. Imaging techniques, such as angiography or intravascular ultrasonography (IVUS), that provide visualization and localization of the fixation device and the graft are important parameters to evaluate in these studies.

It is recognized, however, that animal models have several limitations in evaluating TPEGs. First, the commonly available large animal models (dogs, pigs, or sheep) have arteries that are smaller than comparable arteries in human beings. Calves are larger, and their arteries better approximate the size of human arteries, but their rapid growth limits their utility for anything other than short-term studies. Second, it is not possible to produce in animals arterial lesions that are comparable to those in patients, with the possible exceptions of traumatic arteriovenous fistulas, false aneurysms, and aortic dissections. Although animal models with fusiform polyester cloth aneurysms have been described[6–9] and have some limited applicability, good models of true aneurysms and arteriosclerotic occlusive disease do not exist. Accordingly, animal studies have limited applicability in predicting the outcome of TPEGs in treating some human arterial lesions. Furthermore, it may be necessary to test some devices in more than one animal model to address all concerns (e.g. long-term implants in dogs, with acute studies in calves to study clinically sized devices). All animal studies should include gross and histologic evaluation and, if possible, angiographic evaluation, computed tomography (CT) with contrast, magnetic resonance imaging (MRI), and/or IVUS to document device, luminal, and arterial wall structure and relationships.

Clinical testing

Clinical testing must demonstrate the safety, efficacy, and effectiveness of TPEGs in the treatment of human arterial diseases. Separate studies may be needed for each usage category. However, it is possible that some devices will be suitable for treating multiple categories of lesions. Therefore it may be appropriate to combine lesion sites and pathologic categories for clinical testing when this can be supported and justified. This is particularly likely when treatment of uncommon lesions is being considered. Clinical testing will be divided into two phases: feasibility testing and comparative performance testing.

Feasibility testing

This should demonstrate that insertion of a TPEG device is possible in a given disease state in a given location and that the device functions safely and effectively for at least *6 months*. These tests must include comparative preprocedural and postprocedural noninvasive measurements of the distal circulation and, in the case of aneurysms, their size before and 3 and 6 months after TPEG placement. These measurements include lower extremity segmental systolic pressures and pulse volume recordings (or Doppler waveform measurements) and ultrasonography, contrast-enhanced CT, MRI, and/or IVUS measurements of aneurysm size.* They must be available in at least *ten patients* and should be supplemented by appropriate imaging studies to demonstrate device patency, confinement of flowing blood to the graft lumen, and freedom from leakage, migration, and aneurysm enlargement. Preplacement, completion, and 6 months postplacement arteriographic confirmation should be provided in at least one half of the patients, preferably in all. However, if other less invasive modalities can provide accurate equivalent information, arteriographic study may be unnecessary.

There are two types of *feasibility study*. In the first, *standard usage*, the TPEG treatment is offered to patients who are candidates for standard operative abdominal aneurysm repair.[10] In this setting, the patient must be prepared for and willing to undergo the standard procedure if the TPEG placement is impossible or unsuccessful or has a complication. In general, if the aorta or iliac arteries are involved, patients having these initial TPEG procedures should have them performed in a location that is equipped and staffed for emergency operative repair.

In the second form of feasibility study, *high-risk usage*, patients who are unsuitable or at high risk for the standard treatment may be offered the new TPEG treatment as an option. In the case of abdominal aneurysm repair, these can be patients with large threatening aneurysms whose operative risk is excessive, for example in excess of three to four times normal, on the basis of heart, lung, or liver disease, or previous abdominal scarring or infection.[10]

Comparative performance testing: clinical trials

This phase of evaluation is designed to show that the TPEG device will perform essentially equivalent to or significantly better than standard treatment. There are several ways to test safety, efficacy, and effectiveness and to show equivalence or superiority. However, such trials

*These measurements should permit accurate definition of wall, clot, and lumen (flowing blood) dimensions.

should be conducted in a fashion that is scientifically sound and that provides statistically valid data relating to the important criteria to be described below for the various usage categories. When it is feasible and appropriate, these studies should be designed to permit a valid comparison of the safety, efficacy, and effectiveness of a new TPEG device and current standard treatment(s) of similar arterial lesions in similar patients. In other circumstances, when it may not be feasible or in the interests of patients to obtain such valid comparative performance data, the clinical trial study protocol should clearly indicate the reasons for this and provide an acceptable alternative method for testing the hypotheses posed in the study and documenting the new TPEG device's safety, efficacy, and effectiveness. In general, *comparative performance studies* should include an adequate number of patients in the device test group monitored after the procedure to allow statistically valid comparisons after 1–2 years with similar patients with similar stages of the disease process. Comparative performance studies should include the primary criteria listed in Table 1.1 with regard to procedural (30-day) morbidity and mortality rates and 1–2-year device safety and efficacy. The results should allow statistically valid and biologically meaningful conclusions, indicating whether a given device provides results that are better than, worse than, or equivalent to standard treatment as measured by these criteria. Demonstration of statistically significant equivalence between two treatment groups may require unacceptably large numbers of patients so that comparative studies should be designed to show statistically significant differences between the TPEG and standard treatment or *essential equivalence*, that is, no grossly apparent difference.

Every effort must be made in all clinical stages of testing to carry out postmortem examination of patients who die from any cause to determine the cause of death, and to perform a complete explant analysis including gross and microscopic examination of the device and the sites of device implantation and fixation to determine the structure and histologic condition of the proximal and distal vessel and of the aneurysm or other arterial lesion being treated.

Other data that should be collected and analysed in addition to those listed in Table 1.1 are duration of the procedure, time in an intensive care unit, length of hospital stay, and the number of units of homologous blood transfused. Systemic complications of these procedures (defined in Table 1.2) and device-related failures or complications (defined in Table 1.3) must also be documented and analysed.

Table 1.1 Important study criteria.

Criteria	*Infrarenal and thoracic aorta tubular device*	*Infrarenal AAA with iliac aneurysm bifurcated device*
Procedural death	++	++
Complication*		
Myocardial infarction	++	++
Other cardiac	++	++
Pulmonary	++	++
Renal failure	++	++
Bowel ischaemia	++	++
Bowel obstruction	++	++
Procedural failure†	+	+
Leak	++	++
Device migration	++	++
Embolism	++	++
Thrombosis	++	++
Inadequate function‡	++	++
Limb loss	+	+
Paraplegia or paraparesis	+	+
Other§	++	++
Death from rupture	++	++
Conversion to standard open operation	++	++
Increase in aneurysm size	++	++
Lack of increase in aneurysm size	++	++
Graft patency	++	++
Graft enlargement (>25%)	++	++
Persistent flow in sac or branch artery	++	++
Normal flow without leak, twist, or migration	++	++

AAA, abdominal aortic aneurysm; ++, primary criterion; +, secondary criterion.
*Definitions provided in Tables 2 and 3.
†Inability to insert device.
‡Flow reduction without thrombosis.
§Infection, bleeding. Infection involving an endoluminal device is ++ in all categories.

Table 1.2 Definitions of systemic or organ-related complications.

Complication	*Definition*
Myocardial infarction	Significant elevation of CPK-MB; appearance of new significant Q wave or loss of R waves
Other cardiac complications	
Arrhythmia	Requiring treatment with drugs, cardioversion, or pacemaker
Congestive heart failure	Requiring tracheal intubation or ICU care
Pulmonary complication	Requiring tracheal reintubation, extension of ventilator support beyond 48 hours, ICU care beyond 3 days or return to ICU
Renal failure	Creatinine rise >30% or requiring dialysis
Bowel ischaemia	Mucosal haemorrhage or requiring bowel resection or colostomy
Bowel obstruction	Requiring extended (>4 days) nasogastric intubation or laparotomy
Neurologic complications	
Stroke	New neurologic event lasting >24 hours
Transient ischaemic attack	Neurologic event lasting < 24 hours
Paraplegia or paraparesis	Lasting >24 hours
Limb loss	Major amputation at level of ankle or above

CPK-MB, creatinine phosphokinase myocardial band; ICU, intensive care unit.

Table 1.3 Definition of device failures or complications.

Complication	*Definition*
Device occlusion	Absence of flow through the device with or without intraluminal thrombosis
Stenosis	Device-related lumen reduction in, proximal to, or distal to the device associated with a reduction in flow or pressure
Leak	Flow of blood outside the lumen of a device when all such flows should be contained within its lumen
Migration	Displacement of the device sufficient to be associated with another complication (e.g. occlusion, stenosis or leak)
Embolism	Formation of thrombosis within the device with migration to a distal artery

Abdominal aortic aneurysm (infrarenal): tubular devices

Adequate data must be collected so that, after a group of patients* has been treated with the TPEG device and compared with standard operative repair with a prosthetic graft, it can be determined that the groups being compared are similar except for the form of treatment.

Preprocedural data should be collected on age, sex, ethnic origin, height, weight, diabetic status, cardiac function and risk factors, pulmonary function and risk factors, hepatic and renal function, haematologic values, lower extremity pulse status and ankle : brachial indices (ABIs), and previous abdominal operations and scars (Table 1.4). CT, MRI, ultrasonography, and/or arteriography should be performed and data acquired with regard to aneurysm length, transverse and anteroposterior diameters; the extent and dimensions of intraluminal clot and flowing blood; the diameter, length, and degree of calcification of the normal infrarenal aortic segment (i.e. the proximal and distal aortic 'neck' or 'cuff'); the diameter and tortuosity of the common and external iliac arteries (supplement with diagram); and the location and relationship to the aneurysm of patent renal arteries, lumbar arteries, and the superior and inferior mesenteric arteries. These data may be supplemented by MRI or CT three-dimensional aortic reconstructions showing aneurysm, neck, and branch structure, including a definition of the areas occupied by intraluminal clot and flowing blood.

Intraprocedural data should be collected regarding the site of device placement, including that of the proximal and distal attachment, if appropriate, relative to the aorta and aneurysm; the relationship of the device, its stented and unstented portions, and its covered and uncovered portions to patent arteries; and the diameter and length of the stent(s) (when applicable) after deployment. Data should also include the length and diameter of the graft, the site and route of introduction, sheath configuration and diameters, blood loss, total fluoroscopy time, hematoma formation, and any problems associated with device insertion.

If balloons or stents other than those designated in the experimental protocol are used, the length, diameter, specifications, and manufacturer should be recorded along with inflation volume, time, and

*Patient selection criteria will be based on device characteristics. However, all patients must be suitable candidates for standard operative repair of the aneurysm and must have appropriate indications for such repair.

Table 1.4 Prerequisite information regarding risk factors.

Risk factor	*Information*
Cardiac function	Left ventricular ejection fraction History of myocardial infarction Presence of significant Q waves Arrhythmias Thallium persantine stress test abnormalities History of angina pectoris History of congestive failure History of diastolic blood pressure >90 mmHg or systolic pressure >160 mmHg History of diabetes
Renal function	Serum blood urea nitrogen level Serum creatinine level
Pulmonary function	Arterial blood gases on room air FEV_1 Chest radiograph abnormalities Decreased exercise tolerance
Haematologic profile	Complete blood count, platelet count, prothrombin time, partial thromboplastin time
Liver function	Serum albumin, bilirubin, SGOT and SGPT levels Prothrombin time History of cirrhosis, hepatitis
Local risk factors	History of previous operations Description of scarring and infections (past, present)

FEV_1, forced expiratory volume in 1 second; SGOT, serum glutamic–oxaloacetic transaminase; SGPT, serum glutamic–pyruvic transaminase.

pressure. Data on any associated procedure that is required, such as transluminal balloon angioplasty of the iliac arteries, placement of additional stents, covered stents, stented grafts, or arterial repair or thrombectomy, should also be recorded. The type of anaesthesia, medication required, the duration of the procedure, and a description or diagram of the procedure should be recorded, and a hard copy of the completion arteriogram should be kept on file.

Any procedural complications such as device twisting, leakage, misplacement, migration, or failure should be recorded along with the endovascular or operative manoeuvres required to manage the complication. If device removal is required, the steps involved should be detailed together with the outcome of these corrective efforts. Complications involving the native arterial tree and their management should also be documented.

Early postprocedural data (7–10 days) should include the duration of hospitalization, a description of wound healing, an evaluation of device position, luminal patency, and complications (e.g. leakage, migration, kinking, twisting, or obstruction). These device-related evaluations should be based on conventional radiographic, CT, MRI, IVUS, or colour-flow duplex imaging studies. Further evaluation by arteriography may be needed to exclude or assess leakage further, and ultrasonography may be used to demonstrate shrinkage and pulsatility of the aneurysm wall.

Complications from the procedure or the device should be described along with the steps taken to manage them and the outcome. During this early postprocedural period, all preprocedural data relative to renal and haematologic function, noninvasive evaluation of the peripheral circulation, aneurysm, and aortic structure should be repeated. This will permit an early assessment of device safety and efficacy.

Early midterm (6 months) postprocedural data should include all the parameters evaluated in the first 7–10 days after device insertion and *must* include at least one adequate imaging technique (CT, IVUS, MRI, duplex ultrasonography, or arteriography) to evaluate luminal patency, device integrity and localization, aneurysm size and pulsatility, and freedom from leakage. All these parameters plus a haematologic and biochemical evaluation of organ function should be studied approximately *6 months* after device insertion, although it is understood that many of these tests, particularly those that can be performed noninvasively or by blood sampling, may be performed at more frequent intervals, specifically between 2 and 3 months after device insertion.

Late midterm (1 year) postprocedural data, including all the parameters outlined for early midterm evaluation, should be collected *1 year* after device insertion. If a new device is as effective and as safe as standard operative aneurysm repair, according to the primary criteria in Table 1, for *1 year*, the manufacturer of that device may seek clearance to market and sell it for specific indications.

The same data, including adequate imaging, should be collected at 6- to 12-month intervals thereafter for the life of all patients receiving these devices. In that way, a determination can be made of long-term or *late postprocedural* (3–5 years) safety, efficacy, and effectiveness; and comparative performance of the device in relation to standard aneurysm repair can be determined. With this information and the data regarding adverse effects of the device, it will be possible to determine whether the TPEG device should be used as preferential treatment for selected patients at high risk, for patients now subjected to standard surgical repair, or even for some smaller aneurysms not currently being treated. In addition, information will be obtained that will help to determine when the device should not be used or its use should be restricted to certain anatomic situations, and whether it should be considered for use in circumstances other than those provided by an unruptured infrarenal aortic aneurysm, such as anastomotic aneurysms, aortic aneurysm proximal to a previous aneurysm repair, ruptured aneurysms or infected aneurysms.

Abdominal aortic aneurysm (infrarenal) with iliac involvement or aneurysm(s): bifurcated devices

TPEG repair of these aneurysms will require a bifurcated or branched device, although it is possible for some aortoiliac aneurysms to be repaired by a tubular TPEG device to revascularize one limb supplemented by femorofemoral bypass and occlusion of the opposite common iliac artery by some means. (This type of procedure is considered to be a subgroup of the aneurysms in the previous section.)

In general the feasibility testing, the preprocedural, intraprocedural, early postprocedural, midterm postprocedural, and late postprocedural data, and the design of comparative performance clinical trials will be similar to those outlined in the previous section addressing tubular devices for abdominal aortic aneurysms. The use of a bifurcated device may be more complicated and possess specific additional risks during device insertion and in the postprocedural period. With bifurcated devices specific information regarding the status and maintenance of perfusion in the internal and external iliac arteries should be recorded before and at the various intervals after device insertion. Information regarding possible continued flow into the aneurysm from the internal iliac arteries and the status of the colonic circulation after the procedure should also be obtained.

Descending thoracic aorta

The TPEG devices that will be used to treat lesions in this location will have expanded external diameters up to 45 mm or more. They may be comprised of a single or multiple contiguous stents covered by a graft, two separate stents or attachment systems at each end of a tubular graft, or have some other design. They may be used to treat acute or chronic aortic dissections, degenerative atherosclerotic aneurysms, traumatic or postoperative false aneurysms, ulcerating mural lesions, intramural haematomas, and possibly other lesions. They will probably be inserted in a fashion similar to that employed for devices used to treat infrarenal aortic aneurysms.

The requirements for bench and animal testing, as well as feasibility and comparative performance trials, will be similar to those already described for abdominal aortic aneurysm devices. However, because several pathologic processes will be treated in the thoracic aorta, it will probably not be feasible to perform separate trials on each before marketing approval for general clinical usage is requested.

Imaging of thoracic lesions with transoesophageal echo and with Doppler colour-flow studies may be used to supplement the preprocedural and postprocedural evaluations recommended for abdominal aortic aneurysms. Experience to date dictates that TPEG procedures on the thoracic aorta be performed in a procedural room in which the following techniques are available: general anaesthesia with endobronchial intubation, pulmonary artery catheterization, and, in some instances, the equipment and staff to perform emergency operation with complete cardiopulmonary bypass. When the latter may be required, the participation of a cardiothoracic surgeon is mandatory.

Training requirements for usage of TPEGs

For initial clinical studies with each device, principal investigators will need to work with the manufacturer to develop appropriate training programmes for all investigators. The teams that will be involved in the use of a given TPEG device must include an experienced vascular surgeon (or cardiothoracic surgeon for procedures on the thoracic aorta) and interventional radiologist, both of whom devote a major portion (more than 50%) of their activity to the management of noncardiac vascular disease. The training programme must include adequate experience with large animals (or mock circulatory model experience) to ensure technical proficiency with the usage of the device being evaluated. Although it is recognized that good animal models for human aneurysmal and occlusive disease do not exist, animal (or model) experience should be obtained by placing the device under fluoroscopic control in an anaesthetized animal (or model) in arteries large enough to approximate those that will be encountered in human patients.

When individuals or teams have had this initial animal or model experience and have then implanted the TPEG device in at least *three patients* with acceptable results, they may qualify as *instructors* for other individuals who desire to perform investigational procedures with the device in question. The individuals or teams being qualified in this way must possess the full knowledge of vascular disease and all its treatment methods and the requisite surgical and catheter-guidewire skills and experience, as already outlined. They must participate as assistants in at least *three procedures* that use the device and that are being carried out by the individual or group serving as instructor. These background and training requirements apply to individuals or teams at other centres wishing to join an ongoing comparative clinical testing protocol.

Modifications of the guidelines

The developmental paths of TPEGs, the optimal technology, their ultimate value, the complications of their insertion, their impact on various arterial disease processes, and the various modifications that may be introduced are presently unknown. It is therefore probable that these guidelines will evolve and change to encompass new treatment developments.

Acknowledgements

Supported by grants from the US Public Health Service (HL02990–01), the James Hilton Manning and Emma Austin Manning Foundation, the Anna S. Brown Trust, and the New York Institute for Vascular Studies.

Portions of this chapter are reproduced from Veith *et al.* Guidelines for development and use of transluminally placed endovascular prosthetic grafts in the arterial system. *J Vasc Surg* 1995; **21**: 670–85 and *JVIR* 1995; **6**: 477–92, with permission.

References

1. Veith FJ, Abbott WM, Yao JST *et al.* Guidelines for development and use of transluminally placed endovascular prosthetic grafts in the arterial system. *J Vasc Surg* 1995; **21**: 670–85 and *JVIR* 1995; **6**: 477–92.

2. *Standards for Vascular Graft Prostheses.* ANSI/AAMI VP20. Arlington, VA: Association for the Advancement of Medical Instrumentation, 1986.
3. Abbott WM, Callow A, Moore W, Rutherford R, Veith FJ, Weinberg S. Evaluation and performance standards for arterial prostheses. *J Vasc Surg* 1993; **17**: 746–56.
4. US Dept HHS, Public Health Service, Food and Drug Administration, Center for Devices and Radiological Health. *Guidance for the Preparation of Research and Marketing Applications for Vascular Graft Prostheses* (draft). Rockville, MD: Prosthetic Devices Branch, Division of Cardiovascular, Respiratory and Neurological Devices, Office of Device Evaluation, 1993.
5. US Dept HHS, Public Health Service, Food and Drug Administration, Center for Devices and Radiological Health. *Guidance for the Submission of Research and Marketing Applications for Interventional Cardiology Devices: PTCA Catheters, Atherectomy Catheters, Lasers, Intravascular Stents* (draft). Rockville, MD: Interventional Cardiology Devices Branch, Division of Cardiovascular Respiratory and Neurology Devices, Office of Device Evaluation, 1993.
6. Laborde JC, Parodi JC, Clem MF *et al.* Intraluminal bypass of abdominal aortic aneurysm: feasibility study. *Radiology* 1992; **184**: 185–90.
7. Chuter TAM, Green RM, Ouriel K, Fiore W, DeWeese JA. Transfemoral endovascular aortic graft placement. *J Vasc Surg* 1993; **18**: 185–97.
8. Balko A, Piascek GS, Shah DM, Carney WI, Hopkins RW, Jackson BT. Transfemoral placement of intraluminal polyurethane prosthesis for abdominal aortic aneurysm. *J Surg Res* 1986; **40**: 305–9.
9. Mirich D, Wright KC, Wallace S *et al.* Percutaneously placed endovascular grafts for aortic aneurysms: feasibility study. *Radiology* 1989; **170**: 1033–7.
10. Hollier LH, Taylor LM, Ochsner J. Recommended indications for operative treatment of abdominal aortic aneurysms. *J Vasc Surg* 1992; **15**: 1046–56.

2

Preoperative imaging

Simon C. Whitaker

Department of Radiology, Queen's Medical Centre, University Hospital, Nottingham NG7 2UH, UK

Introduction

As endovascular techniques have developed in scope and complexity, so accurate and comprehensive imaging has become an essential component of preoperative planning. For endovascular aneurysm repair to be successful, the morphology of the aorta and iliac arteries must be shown to be suitable for the system being used and the size of the prosthesis must be correct in every detail.

There are three aspects to preoperative imaging: selection of suitable patients, determination of appropriate measurements for sizing of the graft and detection of additional features that may affect the outcome in individual patients. The discussion that follows is based on the preoperative imaging of infrarenal aortic aneurysms as undertaken at Nottingham, where the Chuter–Gianturco and Ivancev–Malmo systems have been used. The same general principles apply to any aneurysm that is being considered for endovascular repair. Details for specific graft systems and aneurysm types are covered in greater detail in the respective chapters.

Case selection

Suitability for endovascular graft insertion is dependent on the presence of vessels above and below the aneurysm to which the stent–graft can attach securely and which do not exhibit gross tortuosity. For abdominal aortic aneurysms the important sites to consider are the aneurysm neck, the abdominal aorta below the aneurysm, the common iliac and the external iliac arteries.

Aneurysm neck

The single most important criterion for assessment of suitability is that there should be a satisfactory neck to the aneurysm – the cuff of undilated aorta between the lowermost renal artery and the start of the aneurysm itself. The attachment of the proximal part of the graft to the aortic neck must be secure to prevent displacement during deployment of the rest of the prosthesis and to produce an efficient seal that excludes the aneurysm sac from the circulation. This portion of aorta should be free from significant atheroma or thrombus, should have walls that are parallel, and should not show marked tortuosity (Fig. 2.1). The length should be sufficiently long to accommodate the

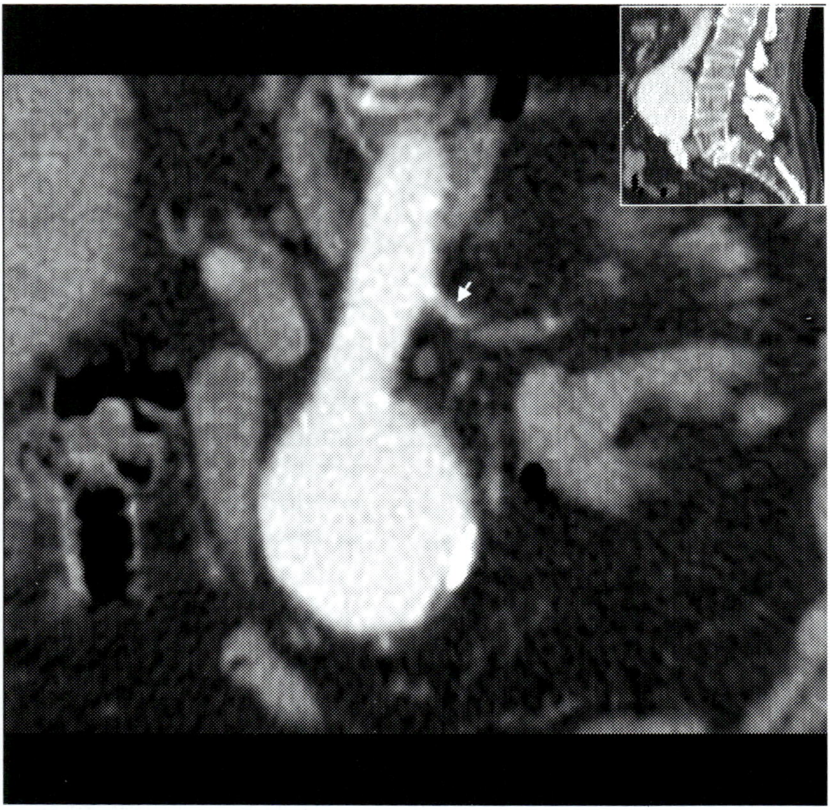

Fig. 2.1 Spiral CT reconstruction showing ideal aneurysm neck for stent–graft placement. The neck is long and straight with no atheroma or thrombus lining it. The arrow shows the left renal artery.

attachment mechanism at the top of the graft and its diameter must not exceed the limit for the device being used. Most systems require the neck to be at least 1.0 cm in length, some 1.5 cm. The maximum diameter depends on the largest diameter of graft that can be accommodated by the chosen delivery system but is generally in the range of 2.5–3.0 cm. Grafts with self-expanding proximal stents are usually oversized by 1–2 mm to ensure a tight fit. Individual system requirements are described in detail in subsequent chapters.

Infra-aneurysmal abdominal aorta

In our experience most abdominal aortic aneurysms extend to the bifurcation and there are very few that are suitable for straight aortoaortic grafts. If such a system is to be employed, there must be a suitable length (greater than 1.5 cm) of normal aorta below the aneurysm.

Iliac arteries

For aortoiliac grafts, a suitable site for implantation of the distal end of the prosthesis must be identified which is of appropriate length (at least 2.5 cm) and diameter (usually 1.0–1.5 cm) and is free from significant atheroma or thrombus. Vessels that are 1.5–2.0 cm in diameter can also be accommodated, depending on the delivery system, but vessels with a greater diameter are not usually considered suitable. The common iliac artery is the ideal site for distal placement as this preserves the internal iliac artery supply to the pelvis. External iliac placement on one side may be an option in a small number of patients with very short or aneurysmal common iliac vessels, provided the external iliac is sufficiently wide to accommodate the graft and the contralateral internal iliac is of good quality and patent. Occlusion of the ipsilateral internal iliac artery may be carried out with embolization coils to prevent retrograde perigraft perfusion of the aneurysm.

The calibre of the external iliac arteries should be known for every patient in order to be certain that the delivery system can be inserted without damage to the vessel wall. The appendix gives a conversion table for French sizes to diameter in millimetres. As a guide, the outside diameter of a catheter in millimetres is one third of its stated French size. Thus a 24-Fr delivery system has an external diameter of 8 mm and would require an external iliac artery diameter of 9 mm or more for easy insertion.

Measurements

The calibre of the graft is determined from the diameter of the vessels to which it will attach. The longitudinal measurements of the graft are determined from the distance between the lowest renal artery (or proximal limit of the upper implantation site) and the distal limit of the lower implantation site as measured along the path the graft is expected to take. The measurements that are usually required are shown in Fig. 2.2.

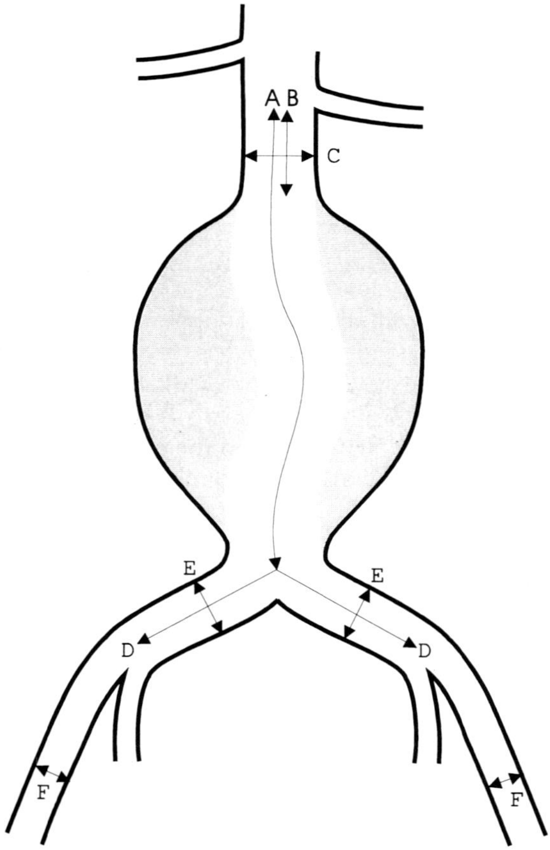

Fig. 2.2 Diagram showing the basic set of measurements required to plan endovascular repair of an abdominal aortic aneurysm. A, renal artery to aortic bifurcation; B, length of aortic neck; C, diameter of aortic neck; D, length of common iliac arteries; E, diameter of common iliac arteries; F, diameter of external iliac arteries.

Additional features that may affect deployment

Vessel tortuosity is almost always present to some degree in patients with abdominal aortic aneurysms. Marked tortuosity in the region of the aortic neck can prove to be a major obstacle to the successful endovascular deployment of a graft (Fig. 2.3). Even if the stiff delivery unit can be manipulated into the correct position (perhaps over a guidewire passed from brachial artery to femoral artery), the curvature of the aortic neck makes accurate positioning of the top of the graft difficult and is apt to cause an unsupported graft to kink once the delivery sheath is withdrawn. Tortuosity of the iliac arteries or at the aortic bifurcation is also of importance but is more amenable to correction by external manipulation of the vessel.

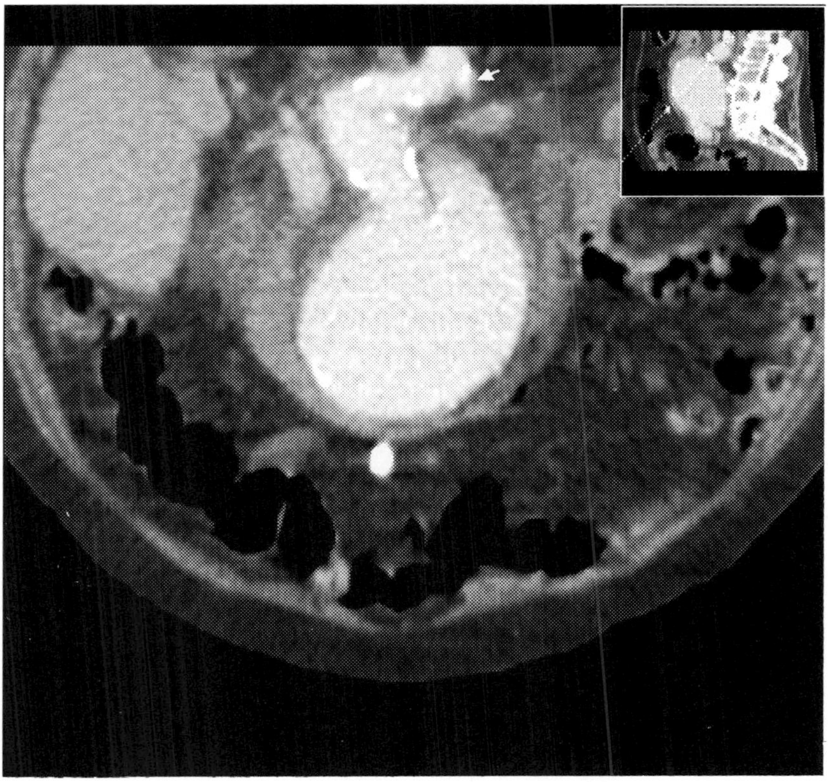

Fig. 2.3 Spiral CT reconstruction showing marked tortuosity of the aneurysm neck, which is a major obstacle to successful stent–graft placement. The arrow indicates the renal artery level.

Iliac stenosis may be present and may prevent insertion of the delivery system unless iliac angioplasty is performed as the first stage.

Imaging modalities

The four imaging modalities that may be used for preoperative assessment of aortic aneurysms are ultrasonography, computed tomography (CT), magnetic resonance imaging (MRI) and angiography.

Ultrasonography

Ultrasonography is cheap, readily available and painless but unfortunately cannot reliably provide all the information required for case selection. It is, however, a useful means of confirming the presence and size of an aortic aneurysm before proceeding to more invasive tests. Beyond determination of these parameters, ultrasonography is often limited by the presence of bowel gas and by difficulty in providing accurate longitudinal measurements.

Contrast-enhanced CT

Spiral CT is at the core of the preoperative assessment routine in most units. Spiral scanners combine fast data acquisition and processing with the ability to scan continuously for 20–40 s as the patient moves through the scanner, features that allow for the scanning of a large section of the patient in one breath-hold. Because of the short duration of the scan, vascular contrast opacification can be maximal throughout. The data are reformatted into large numbers of finely spaced, truly contiguous, axial slices which are an ideal base from which to make the multiplanar sections and three-dimensional images required for aneurysm assessment. In the absence of a spiral CT facility, conventional CT may be used, although it has been found to be a less satisfactory modality.[1] Whenever possible, spiral CT should be used in preference to conventional CT for preoperative aneurysm assessment.

Spiral CT

Our protocol for spiral CT of the abdominal aorta is given in Table 2.1 and is based on the maximum duration of 24 s for an individual spiral scan using our scanner (Seimens Somatom Plus). A pitch of 2 (table

Table 2.1 Example protocol for spiral CT.

Collimation	5 mm
Table speed	10 mm/s
Pitch (scanner rotation 1 per second)	2
Contrast	Iopamidol 370 (or similar) 100 ml
Contrast injection rate (pump injection)	2 ml/s
Delay to start of scan (from start of contrast injection)	30 s
Start level	Midpoint of L1 (i.e. above level of renal arteries)
Finish level	Mid-pelvis (minimum)
Reformatting interval	2 mm

This example spiral CT protocol has been found to be practical on a Seimens Somatom Plus with a maximum spiral scan time of 24 s. Scanner makes and models with different limitations will allow or require modification to this protocol. For instance, a longer maximum scan time could allow the complete aortoiliac segment (to the level of the symphysis) to be scanned in one pass.

speed 1 cm/s, spiral speed 1 rotation per second, collimation 5 mm) is used to give a workable scan length of 22 cm. Longer scan durations and lengths are available on newer equipment and would allow narrower collimation (e.g. 3 mm) and better coverage of the iliac arteries. Similarly, the spacing of 2 mm between axial images is a compromise between the desire for the highest reconstruction quality possible and the practicalities of generating and handling the large amount of data required for a narrower interval. Scanning is commenced just above the level of the renal arteries at the level of the midpoint of the L1 vertebral body (Fig. 2.4) and continued to the pubic symphysis (or for the maximum scan length of the scanner). A preliminary reference scan serves to confirm that the renal arteries will be included in the scan.

Oral contrast is not required and indeed would interfere with the generation of three-dimensional surface-rendered images. These, although not useful for measurement, help to give an overview of the aorta and iliac arteries (Fig. 2.5). Intravenous contrast enhancement is essential, making CT unsuitable for patients with a clear history of a previous contrast reaction. The injection of contrast is timed such that the aorta is imaged when it is maximally opacified. The exact timing for each patient could be ascertained with a preliminary dynamic scan at the upper margin of the region of interest but in practice the scheme

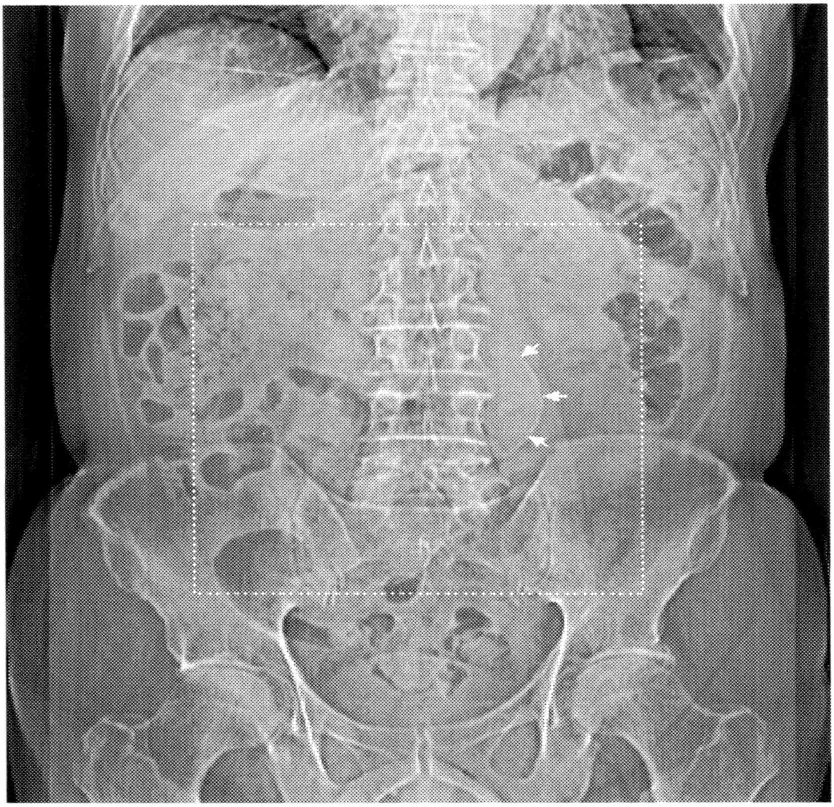

Fig. 2.4 Pilot scan for spiral CT to assess an abdominal aortic aneurysm. The white dotted line shows the extent of the region that will be scanned. The upper limit is mid L1. The lower limit is at the lower margins of the sacroiliac joints but could usefully be lower if the scanner permits. The edge of the aneurysm can just be seen (arrows).

given in Table 2.1 provides good results in almost all patients. The delay of 30 s before scanning commences is sufficient in most patients to allow full vascular opacification before scanning starts, and the duration of the injection (50 s) ensures that contrast is still being injected as the scan is performed, helping to maintain opacification throughout. Appropriate cardiac monitoring is advisable for patients considered at risk of cardiac arrhythmias.

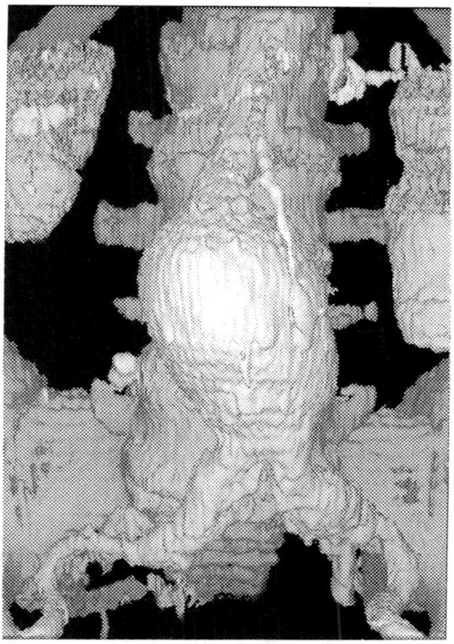

(a)

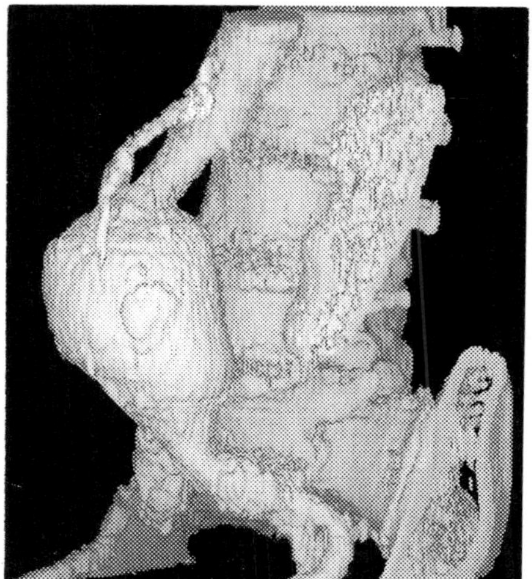

(b)

Fig. 2.5 Three-dimensional surface reconstruction of aortic aneurysm (same patient as in Figs 2.1 and 2.6). (a) Anteroposterior view; (b) oblique view.

Non-spiral CT

The protocol for imaging with a scanner without spiral capability (Table 2.2) depends to some extent on the speed of the scanner. The region of the aortic neck must be examined in detail with contiguous slices not more than 5 mm thick to allow for reconstruction along the axis of the aorta. As for spiral CT, oral contrast is not required but intravenous contrast enhancement is essential to demonstrate the lumen boundary. Some 100 ml iopamidol (370 mg/ml) is given in a manner similar to the spiral CT protocol. If the scanner is reasonably quick, the remainder of the aneurysm and iliac arteries may then be scanned with thicker (e.g. 10 mm) contiguous slices. The residual opacification from the original contrast injection will probably be sufficient for most of these remaining scans but a further 50 ml injected as the iliac arteries are scanned is helpful. On older scanners with longer inter-scan delays, it is not practical to try to obtain contiguous slices throughout the aorta with dense intravenous opacification. It is preferable to perform a smaller number of non-contiguous slices with adequate contrast enhancement to allow for iliac diameter measurements and to rely more on angiography for longitudinal measurements.

Table 2.2 Example protocol for non-spiral CT

Aortic neck	
Collimation	5 mm
Table increment	5 mm
Contrast	Iopamidol 370 (or similar) 100 ml
Contrast injection rate (pump injection)	2 ml/s
Delay to start of scan (from start of contrast injection)	30 s approximately
Start level (check with reference scan)	Midpoint of L1 (i.e. above level of renal arteries)
Finish level	5 cm below start (10 slices)
Remainder of aorta and iliacs	
Collimation	5–10 mm
Table increment	5–10 mm
Contrast	Iopamidol 370 (or similar) 50 ml as pelvis scanned
Contrast injection rate (pump injection)	2 ml/s
Start level	Contiguous with first series
Finish level	Symphysis pubis

This protocol for non-spiral CT scanners is an example only; the exact parameters that are chosen will depend on the capabilities of the equipment being used.

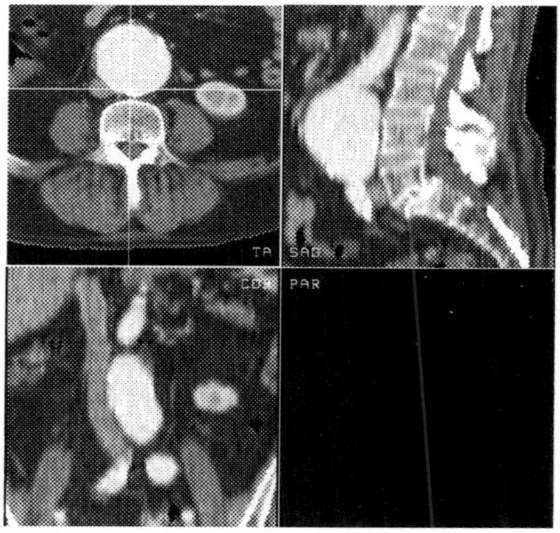

(a)

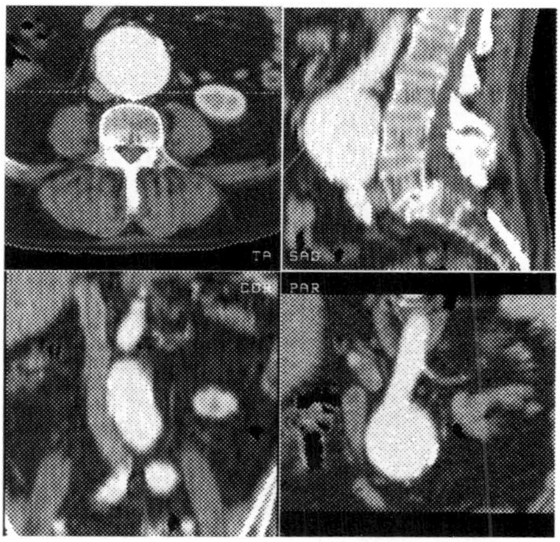

(b)

Fig. 2.6 Performing a coronal section of the neck of the aneurysm. (a) Initial screen; the top left image is the mid-slice of the axial images. The crossed lines show the planes for the straight coronal (bottom left) and straight sagittal (top right) images. (b) The straight sagittal view has been used as the pilot for placement of an oblique coronal reconstruction plane through the aortic neck. (Same patient as in Fig. 2.1.)

Processing and measurement

Diameter and length measurements of the aortic neck are best obtained from reconstructions that are coronal or sagittal to the axis of the neck. Software will vary from scanner to scanner but this task usually requires the ability to use a sagittal reconstruction as the pilot slice upon which the plane of the new oblique coronal slice is selected (Fig. 2.6). The diameter of the neck may also be measured from ordinary axial CT slices if allowance is made for tortuosity of the aorta. If the aneurysm neck deviates from the axial line, it will appear elliptical in section and the shortest diameter of this ellipse should be taken as the lumen diameter.

Measurement of the distance between the renal arteries and the aortic bifurcation requires a reconstruction in the same plane as the major curvature of the abdominal aorta: a sagittal view if the aorta shows marked curvature in the anteroposterior plane or coronal if the major curvature is from side to side (Fig. 2.7). Similarly, measurement of the length of the common iliac arteries requires a suitable reconstruction along the length of the vessel. The configuration and curvature of the iliac arteries varies enormously and the ideal plane for measurement in an individual patient is usually found by trial and error. Some scanners provide the facility for a curved plane of reconstruction which can be set to follow the axis of the vessel to provide a more accurate sectional view of the vessel lumen.

(a)

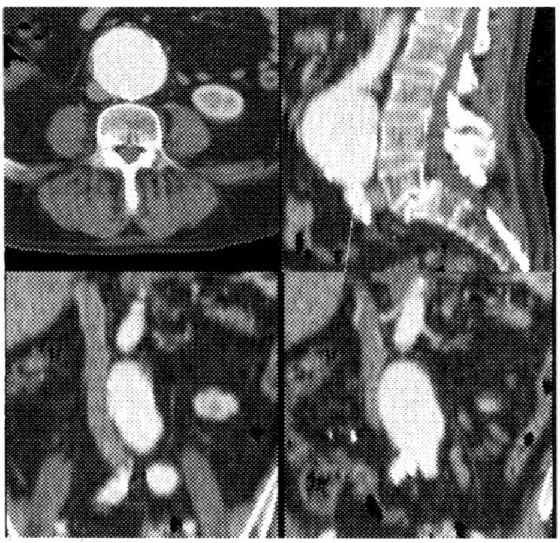

Fig. 2.7

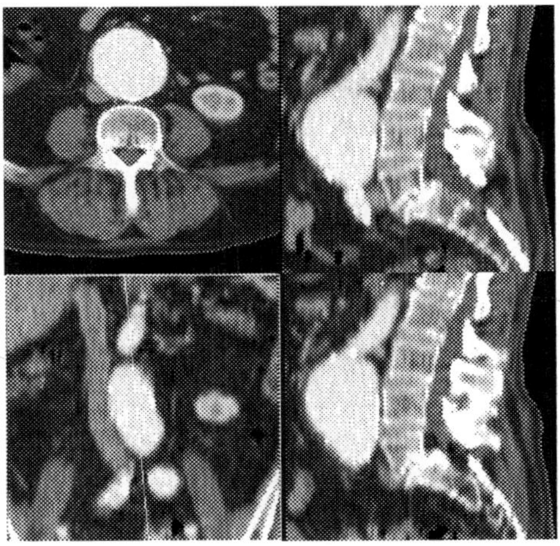

(b)

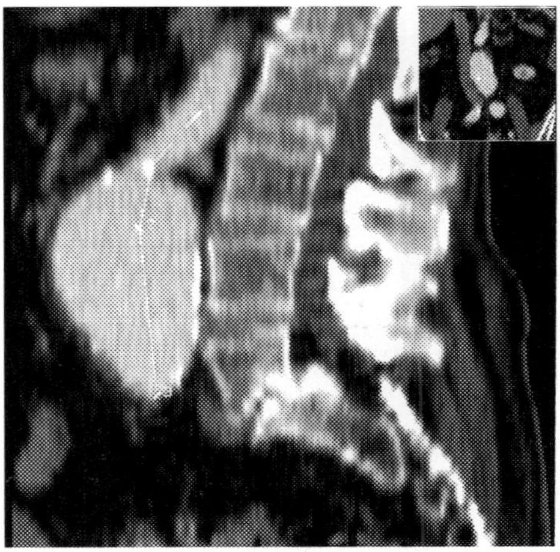

(c)

Fig. 2.7 Measurement of the longitudinal length of the aortic aneurysm from renal artery to bifurcation on a system that does not have the capability of curved reconstruction planes. (a) Initial selection of oblique coronal plane (top right of image) will give shortened measurement that will not account for anterior curve of aorta (bottom right). (b) Selection of oblique sagittal plane (bottom left) to account for anterior curve of aorta. (c) Final image showing line of measurement. This follows the expected line of the graft lumen rather than the centre line of the aneurysm.

The ease with which these reconstructions and measurements are made is dependent on the level of sophistication of the processing software. There are a number of graphics workstations available with software designed specifically for the complex analysis of three-dimensional medical images. These provide a greater level of functionality than most integral scanner software and may be a worthwhile investment for a busy department. Even with such equipment, however, image processing and reconstruction can be a time-consuming and specialized task. Where the number of patients examined does not justify the expense of an on-site workstation and trained staff, the idea of a third-party image processing facility that processes the raw CT data on a cost-per-patient basis is attractive. As an example of this concept, Figure 2.8 shows still images from AAA Preview (Medical

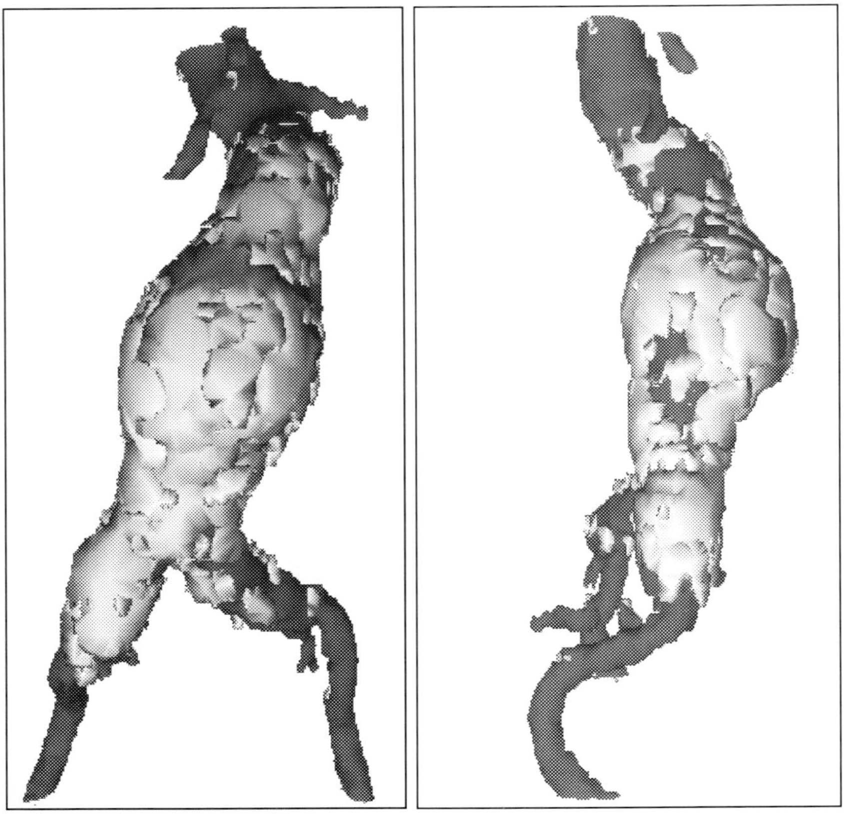

Fig. 2.8 Anteroposterior and lateral view of the three-dimensional model produced from spiral CT data by AAA Preview.

Media Systems, West Lebanon, NH, USA), a modelling system designed specifically for the assessment and measurement of the aorta. Axial images from a contrast-enhanced spiral CT scan are processed by the company, who return a three-dimensional model with appropriate viewing and measurement software on compact disk. This can be viewed and analysed on a relatively inexpensive desktop computer. As well as standard linear measurements, the system can also provide measurements of the aneurysm volume between selected points, which may be a more sensitive indicator of change in aneurysm size following aneurysm exclusion than simple postoperative diameter measurements.

An alternative approach, used by the Perth group, to determine longitudinal measurements is to plan the graft on a paper diagram of the aorta (copied from a MIP CT – reconstruction or from an angiogram). The longitudinal interval between fixed reference points (such as the renal arteries and the aortic bifurcation) are determined from the table positions of axial CT slices that show these structures. This interval and a measurement of the equivalent distance on the diagram are used to determine the scaling factor necessary to enlarge or reduce the diagram to true lifesize (using a photocopier) and lateral diagrams are prepared in this way and then used in planning the graft construction.

Magnetic resonance imaging

MRI has some advantages in that it can be performed with or without intravenous contrast and functional measurements (such as renal perfusion) can be made. Ionizing radiation is avoided, although this is a minor consideration in the age group of patients who have aortic aneurysms. Patients with cardiac pacemakers, intracranial metal surgical clips or metallic intraocular foreign bodies cannot be imaged with MRI. The disadvantages of MRI for the purposes of aneurysm assessment that we have encountered are that it is not well tolerated by claustrophobic patients and the boundaries of wall, thrombus and lumen are not as clearly delineated as they are with contrast-enhanced CT. Other workers, however, have had better success with MRI. For instance, the group in Leicester, UK, has found contrast-enhanced MRI to be superior to conventional CT for aneurysm assessment.[2] We have recently started using a T_1-weighted, contrast-enhanced, rapid gradient-echo sequence (TR ~ 7.7, TE ~ 4.2, FA 15, Seimens Vision 1.5T) as part of a protocol similar to that described by the Leicester

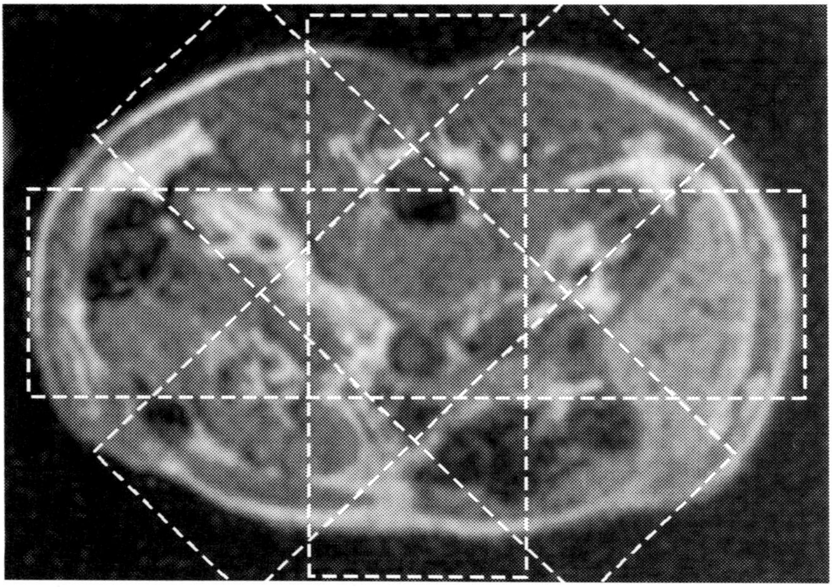

Fig. 2.9 Pilot scan for contrast-enhanced MRI showing planning of four image blocks at 45° to each other. Each block is acquired four times: precontrast, arterial phase, venous phase and steady state.

unit in which four separate, sequential, multiplanar acquisitions are made. The injection of contrast (dimeglumine gadopentetate 469 mg; Schering) is delayed until after imaging has commenced so that the four series correspond approximately to precontrast, arterial, venous and steady-state phases of contrast enhancement. Each series consists of four blocks (sagittal, coronal and two obliques), planned as shown in Figure 2.9. After image acquisition, the images that show optimum contrast enhancement can be viewed individually or can be combined using maximum intensity projection to give angiographic images that can be used for measurement (Fig. 2.10).

Angiography

The roles of preoperative angiography are to confirm or support the longitudinal measurements obtained from cross-sectional imaging and to provide a 'road-map' of the lower abdominal aorta and iliac vessels, which is invaluable at the time of surgery (Fig. 2.11). Angiography may

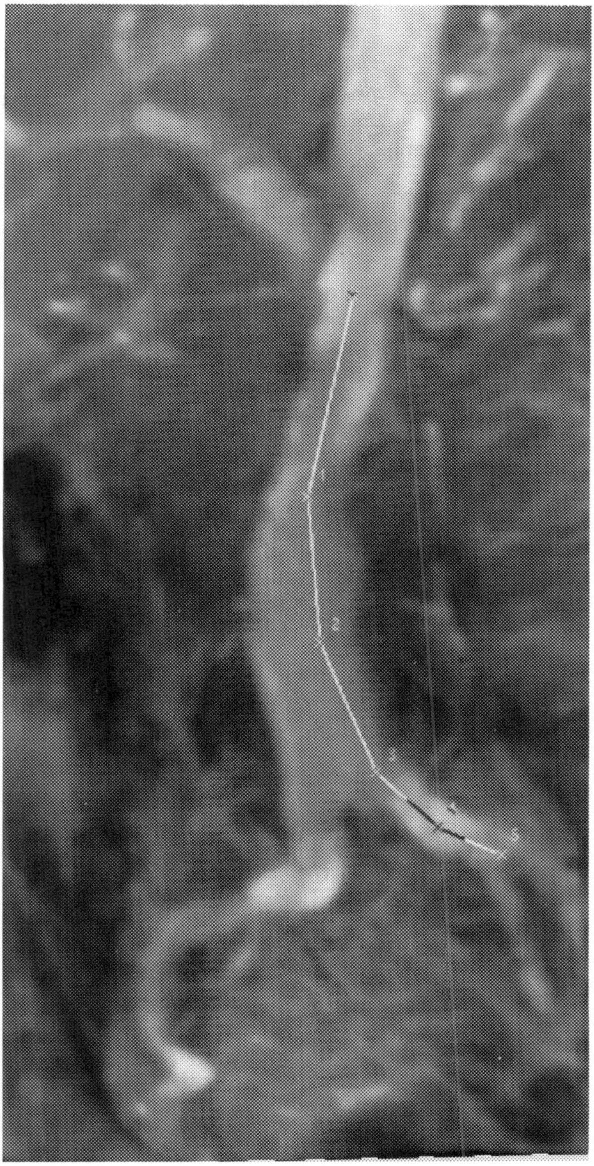

Fig. 2.10 Contrast-enhanced MRI of abdominal aortic aneurysm. Maximum Intensity Projection (MIP) reconstruction showing calliper placement for longitudinal measurements.

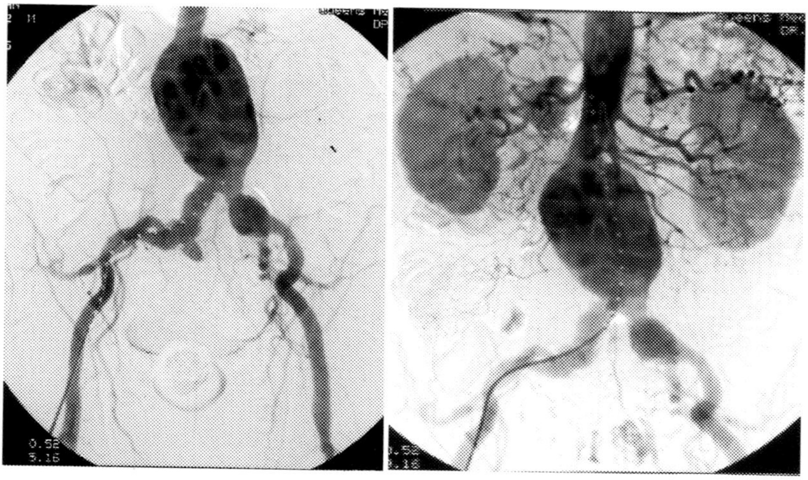

Fig. 2.11 Angiography with a calibrated catheter (same patient as in Figs 2.1 and 2.6).

also reveal additional relevant anatomical features, such as an accessory renal artery, or the need for specific preoperative manoeuvres, such as iliac angioplasty or vessel embolization. Angiography is invasive and carries a risk of embolization of material from within the aneurysm. It is best reserved for patients whose aortas have been declared suitable for endovascular repair by other methods such as CT or MRI. Catheters must be manipulated with great care within the aneurysm and the procedure should be performed by an experienced vascular radiologist.

Measurement of distances directly from angiographic images is made difficult by the inevitable magnification that is present. For an object that is straight and parallel to the film, reasonably accurate measurements may be made once a calibration factor has been calculated from an object of known dimensions. Longitudinal measurements of a tortuous structure such as the aorta and iliac arteries cannot readily be made by direct measurement from film or screen but require a calibrated catheter to overcome the errors of magnification and foreshortening where the vessel is oblique to the film. Calibrated catheters are available with markings every centimetre over 15 cm, and are ideal for aortic measurement (Cook, Bloomington, IL, USA) (Fig. 2.11). Available with the Endovascular Technologies (EVT) system is the Endoscale catheter, which is similar in design. If a suitable calibrated catheter system is not available, measurements can still be made with a guidewire and standard 4 or 5-Fr angiographic catheter. The wire is advanced in the catheter until its tip is at the renal arteries and then bent at the catheter hub. The wire is withdrawn until its tip is at the common iliac origin, and bent at the hub again. The distance between the two kinks can then be measured with a ruler and is a direct indication of the distance from renal artery to bifurcation. The same process is repeated for the common iliac arteries.

For preoperative imaging we perform angiographic runs in anteroposterior and lateral planes for the aorta, together with anteroposterior and oblique views for the iliac vessels. For the views of the aorta, the catheter is placed with the side-holes (or top marker) at the level of the lowest renal artery. The iliac arteries are usually inadequately opacified from a suprarenal aortic injection because contrast passes preferentially into the renal vessels and the remainder is diluted in the aneurysm. Views of the iliac vessels are best made with the catheter withdrawn until the side-holes are just above the bifurcation.

Specific points of difficulty

It is difficult enough to obtain accurate measurements of aortic aneurysms but this is only part of the task of preoperative assessment. Using the images and data obtained from CT or MRI, the questions of suitability and, in the patients selected, the dimensions of the graft to use must be addressed.

Suitability

Fortunately many patients are clearly suitable or unsuitable on the basis of measurements of the neck diameter and neck length. There remains, however, a group of patients in whom there is still uncertainty as to whether to proceed (and thereby risk procedural failure or complication requiring conversion to open repair) or decide that endovascular repair is unsafe and should not be offered (perhaps depriving a patient unsuitable for open surgery the chance of repair). A clear answer to this clinical challenge is not possible – much will depend on analysis of the individual case, the method of repair being used and the experience of the vascular team. A degree of caution is required in the application of endovascular methods that are still in

Table 2.3 Adverse features.

Neck diameter close to or at maximum for system	Leak may occur. Balloon dilatation of stent may be needed
Neck length at or below minimum	Leak may occur. Top stent may displace
Tortuous neck or upper abdominal aorta (bends $>60°$)	Placement of delivery system may be difficult. Brachiofemoral guidewire may be required
Conical neck – diameter increases progressively	Top stent may not be stable
Presence of clot or heavy atheroma lining otherwise suitable neck	Leak may occur. Top stent may not be stable. Balloon angioplasty may be needed
Marked angulation at aortoiliac junction	Placement of delivery system may be difficult
Short common iliacs (<2.5 cm)	No margin for error in graft length. Lower stent may not bed properly in common iliac artery if too short, or may occlude internal iliac origin if too long
Aneurysmal common iliac arteries	Placement of distal stent in external iliac may be needed
Narrow calibre to common or external iliac arteries ($\leqslant 8$ mm)	May be difficult to advance delivery unit. Direct approach via common iliac artery may be required
Prominent iliac calcification	CT diameter measurements may not be reliable. Underlying iliac narrowing may be present

their infancy. Adverse features that should be noted and brought into the equation are given in Table 2.3.

Graft dimensions

Selecting the graft diameter is not normally difficult once accurate measurements have been obtained. It is our policy to oversize the neck diameter of the graft by approximately 2 mm to ensure that it will form an efficient seal. A larger diameter margin than this is unlikely to improve the haemodynamic seal and may in fact decrease it.

Selection of the length of graft may be difficult. Features that make length determination difficult are a wide aneurysm sac with minimal mural thrombus and marked tortuosity of the expected graft line. The presence of a wide aneurysm sac generates uncertainty as to the line the graft will take during and after deployment. Unfortunately the line that a calibrated angiographic catheter takes is often rather different because of the relative stiffness of the delivery system compared with the flexible catheter. Satisfactory length determination is much easier when the aneurysm lumen is of similar calibre to the lumen of unaffected aorta above. The margin for error is reduced if the length of the distal implantation zone (i.e. the distal aorta below the aneurysm or the common iliac arteries) is short, and the combination of a wide aneurysm sac with a tortuous centre line and short implantation site demands very careful consideration indeed.

Differential renal function

If the renal arteries are at substantially different levels or there are multiple renal arteries on one side, the neck length measured from the lowest renal artery may be too short for stent placement, even though the higher renal artery is well clear of the aneurysm. If the patient is unfit for conventional open surgery, the question then arises as to whether it would be safe to sacrifice the lowermost renal artery to allow endovascular repair. Technetium-99m diethylenetriamine penta-acetate (DTPA) renography provides useful information in the form of differential renal function, which aids this decision.

Preoperative investigation of ruptured aneurysm

Ruptured abdominal aortic aneurysm is a difficult and dangerous condition to treat. The mortality rate in patients managed with conventional open repair in specialist vascular units is still 30–80%.[3] One of the more exciting possibilities for endovascular techniques for aortic repair is that they may be used in the management of ruptured aneurysms and help to reduce the mortality rate in patients with this condition. This will create a need for emergency preoperative CT to determine suitability and the size of the graft to be used. Ideally, the accident and emergency admissions unit should be equipped with a spiral CT scanner to allow rapid imaging of these patients close to full resuscitation facilities and personnel. At Nottingham we have used endovascular techniques in four patients with ruptured aortic aneurysms. In all four cases the patient had been stable for a number of hours before transfer to our unit and were considered to have been sufficiently stable for transfer to the radiology department for preoperative spiral CT. We did not perform preoperative angiography on these patients, however, preferring to rely on CT and intraoperative angiography.

Conclusions

Preoperative investigative pathway

Careful preoperative assessment and measurement of the aorta and iliac vessels is critical to the success of endovascular aneurysm repair. The presence and size of an abdominal aortic aneurysm may be detected or confirmed with a preliminary ultrasonographic scan.

All patients who may be suitable for endovascular repair should have a contrast-enhanced CT scan. In preference, this should be a spiral CT study, performed and analysed at the centre where repair will be carried out. MRI may be an acceptable alternative depending on the scanner that is used. The various parameters that should be measured and their acceptable ranges vary from system to system and are discussed in greater detail in the appropriate chapters.

The present recommendation is that all patients declared suitable for elective endovascular repair on the basis of contrast-enhanced CT findings should also undergo calibrated angiography for confirmation of measurements and to provide an anatomical road-map. Patients with suspected rupture of an aortic aneurysm in whom endovascular repair is being contemplated should have preoperative spiral CT as an emergency but calibrated angiography can be performed in the operating theatre. Hardware and software developments in CT image acquisition and processing may reduce the need for angiography in the future.

References

1. Beebe HG, Jackson T, Piggott JP. Aortic aneurysm morphology for planning endovascular aortic grafts: limitations of conventional imaging methods. *J Endovasc Surg* 1995; **2**: 139–48.
2. Cherryman GR, Moody AR, Rogers P. New imaging techniques and arterial disease. *Vasc Med Rev* 1994; **798**: 524–9.
3. Ernst CB. Abdominal aortic aneurysm. *N Engl J Med* 1993; **328**: 1167–72.

Appendix: Catheter size and diameter

Catheter size (Fr)	*Catheter diameter (mm)*
3	1.00
4	1.33
5	1.67
6	2.00
7	2.33
8	2.67
9	3.00
10	3.33
12	4.00
14	4.67
16	5.33
18	6.00
20	6.67
22	7.33
24	8.00
26	8.67
28	9.33
30	10.00

3

Intraoperative imaging in endovascular aortic aneurysm surgery

Matthew P. Armon and Brian R. Hopkinson

Department of Vascular Surgery, University Hospital, Queen's Medical Centre, Nottingham, NG7 2UH, UK

Introduction

High-quality radiographic imaging of the aortoiliac segment is an integral component of the management of patients undergoing endovascular repair of abdominal aortic aneurysms. Nowhere is this more critical than during the procedure itself. This chapter aims to discuss the purposes of intraoperative imaging, the ideal environment and equipment with which to carry it out, and the specific techniques involved.

Basic requirements

The basic requirements of an intraoperative imaging system are that it is able to:

- Provide high-quality screening/fluoroscopy throughout the aorto-iliac segment for passage of the delivery system.
- Demonstrate the exact location of the proximal and distal implantation sites.
- Visualize the deployment and subsequent position of the stents.
- Confirm blood flow through the graft and femorofemoral crossover if used.
- Assess the completeness of the seal between graft and vessel both proximally and distally.
- Ascertain postprocedural patency of the renal vessels and internal iliac artery.

- Provide imaging of sufficient quality, if required, for additional interventional procedures such as embolization, angioplasty, additional stent implantation and the introduction of guidewires and catheters via the upper limb vessels.

To meet these basic demands, the image intensifier must be able to screen over the abdomen and pelvis and preferably along the entire length of the patient. It must provide high-resolution images on a television monitor and be able to view the patient from different angles (anteroposterior, lateral, oblique). In addition, contrast doses and radiation exposure must be kept to safe levels.

Equipment

The ideal imaging system is a digital one with subtraction facilities. This will provide high-resolution, quality images that can be displayed and replayed on demand, allowing easy review of the angiographic data acquired. The ability to provide both hard copies and video recordings is useful as both a record of the procedure and for the subsequent review and audit of results. A road-mapping capacity can aid the passage of guidewires and catheters through tortuous iliac arteries without the need for additional contrast, but is hampered by the patient's breathing. Dual monitors are required for this process. A 21- or 23-cm image intensifier field size is ideal. A larger field size enables a greater portion of the operating site to be screened at any one time and this can be particularly helpful during deployment of the lower stent to allow simultaneous visualization of the proximal stent. A contrast injector is another useful aid, particularly when smaller catheters are being used.

A fluoroscopic system suspended from the ceiling and used in combination with a carbon fibre table allows both the best access to the patient and the flexibility to obtain images from any angle (Fig. 3.1). In conjunction with digital subtraction facilities this meets all the requirements for safe and accurate intraoperative imaging. However, it is expensive (in the region of £500 000).

A more affordable (approximately £100 000) and perfectly acceptable compromise is provided by an image intensifier with a mobile C-arm (Fig. 3.2). This must be used in conjunction with a radiolucent operating table which has sufficient travel to allow screening of the abdomen and pelvis. A number of machines are available with digital

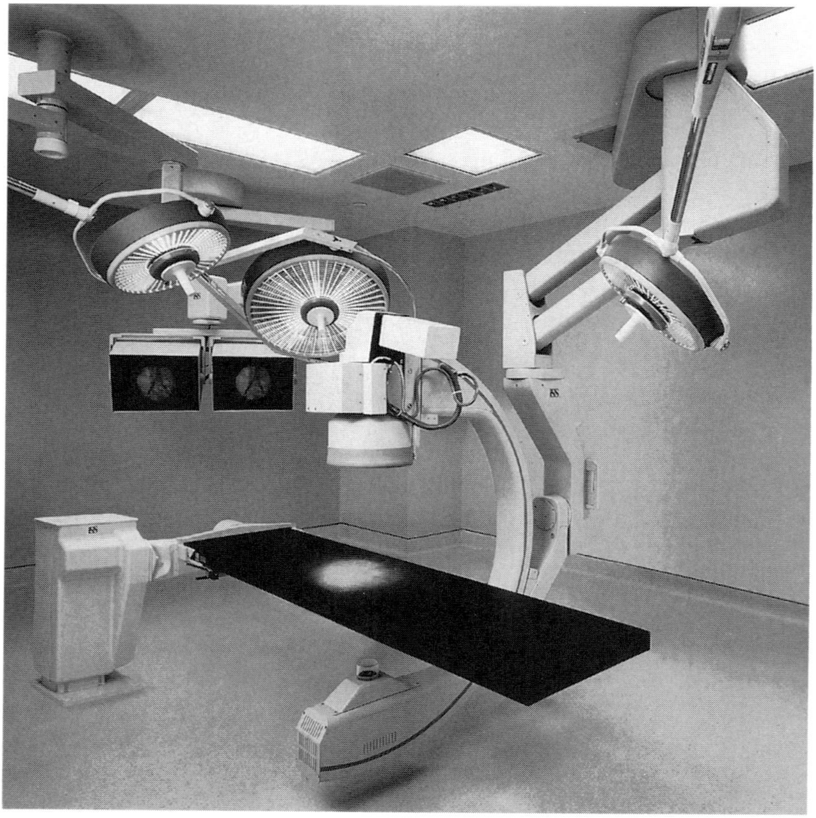

Fig. 3.1 A ceiling-suspended fluoroscopic system with a carbon fibre table (ISS-2000 Plus). Courtesy of International Surgical Systems, Phoenix, Arizona, USA.

subtraction facilities as well as dual monitors, road-mapping and the ability to display, replay and store images.

Many patients with abdominal aortic aneurysms have concomitant renal impairment (see Chapter 19), and it is therefore recommended that less nephrotoxic low osmolar non-ionic contrast media such as Iopamidol, Iohexol and Ioxaglate are used. A maximum dose of 70 g iodine per patient has been advised, even in those with good renal function[1] (approximately 200 ml Iopamidol 340). With the amount of screening required during an endovascular aneurysm repair, this is a difficult level to keep to but efforts must be made to keep doses to a minimum.

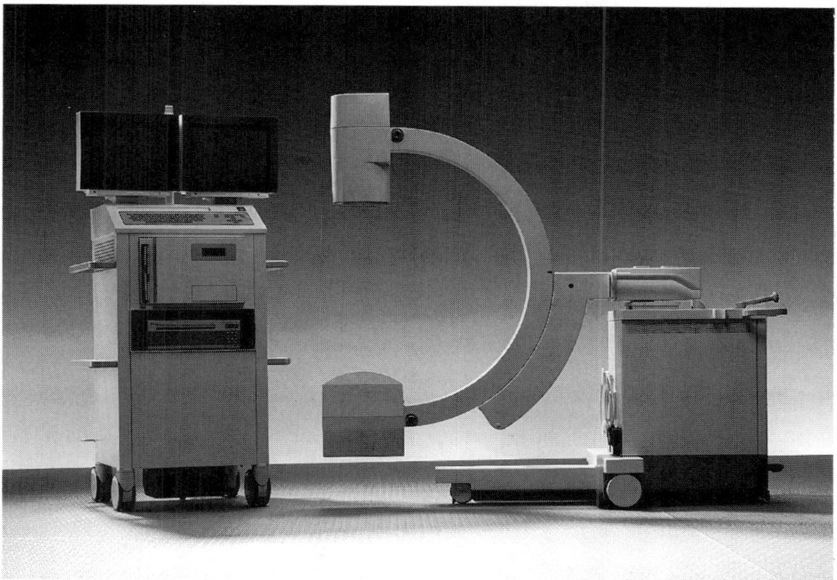

Fig. 3.2 An image intensifier with a mobile C-arm (Siremobil 2000). Courtesy of Siemens, Erlangen, Germany.

Screening is used for an average of 15–30 min per procedure, which should represent an acceptable risk in terms of radiation exposure for the patient when balanced against the overall risks of the aneurysm. For staff who are going to be exposed to this level of radiation on a recurrent basis, the wearing of radiation dose meters is advisable and 0.25–0.35-mm lead aprons mandatory.

Environment

Endovascular operations by their nature have placed a far greater emphasis on the need for high-quality intraoperative imaging than their traditional vascular predecessors. As the range of procedures carried out by vascular radiologists increases, the question as to which environment is best suited to the safe performance of endovascular aortic aneurysm repair is an important one.

Operating theatres are designed specifically with surgical staff and surgical procedures in mind. They provide a sterile environment with sophisticated ventilation systems and purpose-built scrub, preparation, anaesthetic and recovery rooms, usually with easy access to intensive care facilities. During endovascular aneurysm repair, at least the femoral arteries must be exposed surgically and, not infrequently, access to the iliac arteries may be required. Occasionally conversion to an open operation or at least abdominal exposure will be necessary. For all these eventualities, the ready access to surgical equipment and facilities found only in the theatre, as well as its familiarity, means that this is the preferred working environment of most vascular surgeons. However, an operating theatre is often not designed with high-quality angiography in mind. It may not be lined with lead or barium plaster, and the operating table may be radio-opaque and lack the required travel that allows adequate screening of the patient. The immobile anaesthetized patient may further hamper adequate visualization. To meet the basic needs outlined above, sophisticated radiographic equipment and its associated developing or processing requirements must be readily available and easily accessible, along with a well-stocked supply of guidewires, catheters, stents and balloons. It goes without saying that familiarity with this equipment is of fundamental importance to its efficient use, and that the best person to provide the necessary expertise, and therefore an essential member of the endovascular team, is the vascular radiologist.

A specifically designed endovascular theatre that meets the requirement of both surgeon and radiologist is undoubtedly ideal, but few centres in the UK have such facilities. At present, radiographic equipment and expertise is deemed more transportable than the surgical equivalent and for now these procedures are likely to continue taking place in operating theatres. However, as the evolution of the vascular specialist continues apace, this situation may change in the not too distant future.

Procedure

The procedure employed will vary with the particular system being used. This section therefore aims to discuss general principles based on, and with reference to, the aorto-uni-iliac device used in Nottingham.

As discussed in Chapter 2, accurate three-dimensional images delineating the anatomy of the aortic aneurysm and determining the patient's suitability for endovascular repair must be acquired before operation. These films should be available in theatre to provide the endovascular team with a mental picture of the anatomy of the aneurysm and for comparison with the images produced during surgery.

The first step in the procedure it to establish access for an initial angiogram, either via a percutaneous approach or by direct puncture of a surgically exposed artery. This is usually performed via the opposite common femoral artery to that being used for insertion of the delivery system. A 7-Fr introducer sheath with side-arm is inserted, and a guidewire passed to the suprarenal aorta followed by an angiographic catheter. As the angiographic catheter will be sandwiched between aortic wall and graft at deployment, and will then have to be pulled back past the stent, we prefer a 7-Fr straight flush angiographic catheter (Cook) to minimize the risk of snagging on the hooks and spikes of the proximal stent. Tortuosity of the iliac arteries or aneurysm makes the passage of catheters difficult and may require negotiation with a cobra catheter and guidewire. Alternatively, if access via the contralateral femoral artery is not available, the angiographic catheter can be positioned via the brachial artery. This has the potential disadvantage of using a smaller, more vulnerable, vessel and there is a risk of emboli being dislodged during manipulation of the catheter in a diseased aortic arch.

The initial angiogram must accurately delineate the proximal neck and position of the renal arteries, so the catheter is positioned at the origin of these vessels (Fig. 3.3). Lateral and oblique views may be necessary, particularly with an angled neck or aorta. A marker ruler taped to the patient or table can be placed to act as a reference point to the position of the renal vessels, but this is a potential source of error if the C-arm is moved in relation to the patient. The delivery system can also distort the relationship between marker and vessels as the latter may be moved in relation to the image intensifier during the delivery process. This is also a problem for markers placed on the screen. Anatomical landmarks such as the lumbar vertebrae are equally effective markers. Whilst determining the position of the renal arteries and during the subsequent stent deployment, the patient's ventilation must be temporarily halted to minimize respiratory motion artefacts. Immediately before and during deployment of the stent, repeated small boluses (3–4 ml) of contrast are given via the angiographic catheter to ensure that the stent is being placed accurately. Minor adjustments to the delivery system can then be made before final deployment from the sheath. Deployment of the distal stent is visualized with screening, preferably keeping the proximal stent in view to ensure that it is not dislodged during this stage.

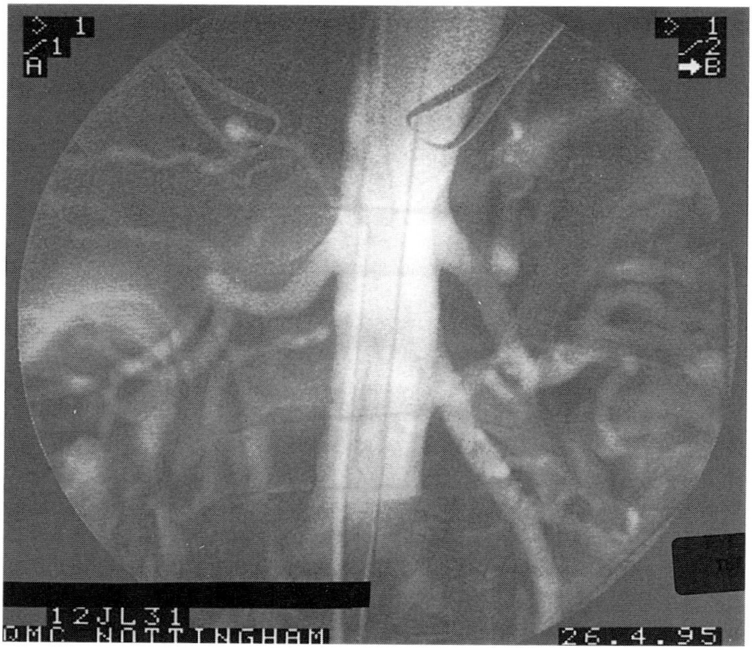

Fig. 3.3 Initial angiogram demonstrating the position of the renal arteries in relation to the proximal neck of the aneurysm.

After deployment, the delivery system is withdrawn over a guidewire and the initial angiographic catheter is removed to allow a complete seal of the proximal stent. A second angiographic catheter is then inserted over the remaining guidewire within the graft lumen and a further angiogram obtained to confirm the position of the stents in both posteroanterior and lateral views. Renal artery patency and perfusion must be checked as embolic material can be dislodged by the delivery system and this may be amenable to immediate correction (see Fig. 19.1). The adequacy of the seal between graft and vessel wall at both proximal and distal implantation sites is assessed by noting the presence or absence of contrast flow into the aneurysm sac (Fig. 3.4). Leaks can occur at either the proximal or distal stent sites or past the occluding device in the contralateral common iliac artery. These are not always clearly visible, particularly without digital subtraction. Those that are seen are more likely to be significant and must be dealt with by, for example, balloon dilatation. The perils of ignoring leaks have been well documented.[2] Twists or kinks in the graft may compro-

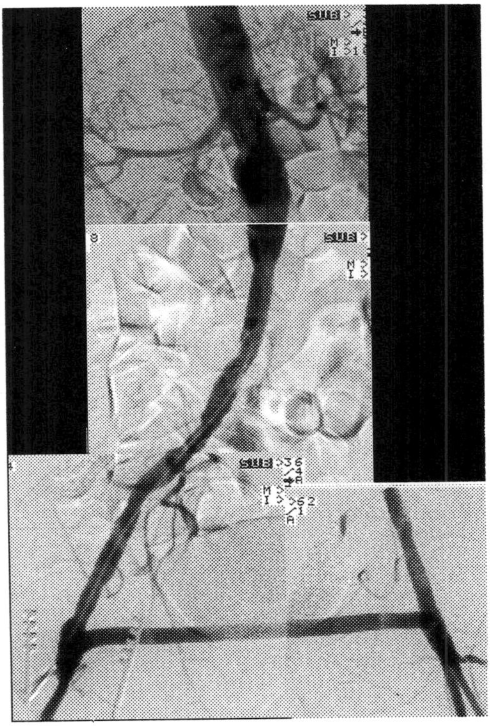

Fig. 3.4 Completion angiogram demonstrating flow through an aorto-uni-iliac graft and femorofemoral crossover graft.

mise blood flow with a subsequent risk of thrombosis, and these must also be looked for and treated if appropriate with, for example, a Wallstent. Adjunctive manoeuvres are discussed in more detail in Chapter 5.

Finally, the occluding device is screened whilst being positioned in the contralateral common iliac artery, and the patency of at least one internal iliac artery helping to maintain colonic perfusion is checked. Good flow through the graft and femorofemoral crossover are confirmed with a completion angiogram (Fig. 3.4).

References

1. Grainger RG. Intravascular contrast media. In: Grainger RG, Allison DJ, eds. *Diagnostic Radiology*. New York: Churchill Livingstone 1986; 11–22.
2. Lumsden AB, Allen RC, Chaikof EL *et al.* Delayed rupture of aortic aneurysms following endovascular stent grafting. *Am J Surg* 1995; 170: 174–8.

4

Application and use of intravascular ultrasonography in the placement of endovascular prostheses

Carlos E. Donayre and Rodney A. White

Division of Vascular Surgery, Department of Surgery, Harbor/UCLA Medical Center, Box 2910, 1000 West Carson Street, Torrance, CA 90 509, USA

Recently developed endovascular technologies have successfully demonstrated catheter-based exclusion of aortic aneurysms through the deployment of intraluminal vascular prostheses. These experimental endovascular prostheses generally consist of graft material affixed to a stent system. The imaging modalities to be utilized for the precise planning, guidance and assessment of healing of these prostheses have yet to be evaluated fully. The unique features of endovascular repair make accurate sizing of the graft, as well as its deployment, extremely important.

Development of miniaturized piezoelectric transducers positioned at the end of intraluminal catheters has allowed high-resolution ultrasonographic imaging of vascular structures. Current intravascular ultrasonography (IVUS) catheters provide real-time, luminal and transmural cross-sectional imaging of vessels. IVUS can delineate wall morphology, lesion shape, volume and length, and branch configurations.[1,2] In addition to diagnostic information, IVUS enables choice of appropriate angioplasty technique, endovascular device guidance and controlled assessment of the efficacy of interventions. Real-time IVUS imaging can be utilized during invasive diagnostic and therapeutic procedures only once vascular access has been established. Further acceptance and implementation relies on the effectiveness of IVUS in improving endovascular outcome and minimizing periprocedural complications compared with alternative imaging modalities.

Comparison of computed tomography and IVUS

Using a canine model we have compared computed tomography (CT) and IVUS measurements of the aorta, aneurysm neck, and endoluminal graft (ELG) cross-sections before and after aortic ELG placement in normal aorta and in artificially constructed abdominal aortic aneurysms.[3] Measurement of the diameters revealed an average difference between imaging modalities of 0.17 mm. IVUS measurements were slightly larger than those of CT (8.84 versus 8.65 mm, $P < 0.03$), but correlated well by linear regression analysis. Cross-sectional area analysis revealed an average difference of 7.21 mm^2 between both modalities. Again, the value with IVUS was greater than with CT (65.0 versus 57.9 mm^2, $P < 0.001$). Qualitative assessment of the graft and stent characteristics were more precise with IVUS. Graft folding, stent–aortic interfaces and thrombus formation were easily identified with IVUS, whereas these more subtle characteristics were missed by CT and angiography (Fig. 4.1).

Clinical utility of various imaging modalities

Based on the above experimental information we are comparing the clinical utility and accuracy of various imaging modalities including angiography, cinefluoroscopy, CT, magnetic resonance imaging (MRI), IVUS and duplex scanning during treatment of arterial lesions with endoluminal grafts in a study approved by the Food and Drug Administration.[4] This study has two objectives. The first is to evaluate prospectively all patients who are candidates for endograft treatment (aneurysms, arteriovenous fistulas, and occlusive disease) and to assess the technical feasibility of endovascular placement of prostheses in vessels with different pathological lesions. The second objective is to determine the optimal imaging modalities for deployment of endovascular devices, in particular the role of IVUS as an alternative and/or complementary method to cinefluoroscopy.

Thirty-five patients have been evaluated for these procedures, with 19 being treated: 13 abdominal aortic aneurysms, two iliac artery aneurysms, three traumatic arteriovenous fistulas and one aortic occlusive lesion. Ten of the thirteen patients with aortic lesions and all of those with iliac artery aneurysm were at high risk. Aortoiliac endoluminal bypasses with contralateral iliac artery occlusion and

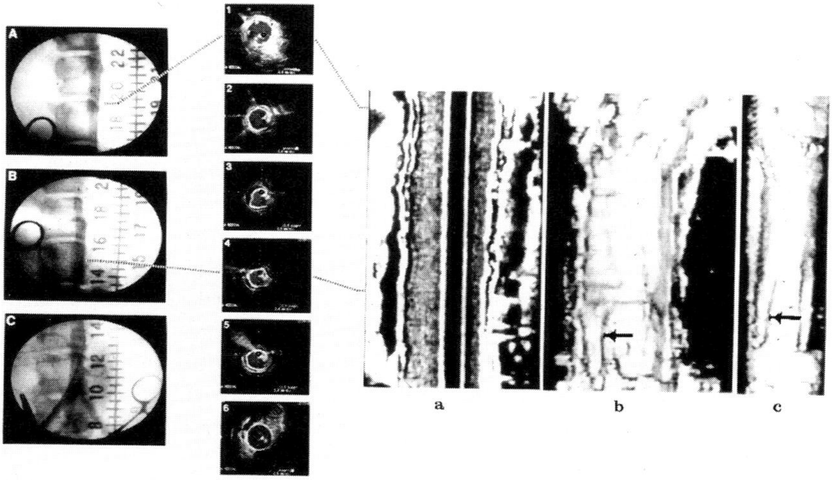

Fig. 4.1 Endovascular tube graft deployment in normal canine aorta without the use of a distal stent. *Left*: Cinefluoroscopy (A–C) reveals patent prosthesis with normal flow and no leaks, folds or kinks. *Centre*: Intravascular ultrasonography provides two-dimensional views of the stented graft at different levels. (1) Stent struts in good apposition with canine aorta. (3–5) Cross-sectional images reveal narrowing and separation from aortic wall at the midgraft level due to the lack of stent support. (6) Normal aorta. These findings were not seen on cinefluoroscopy. *Right*: Three-dimensional reconstruction of axial intravascular ultrasonographic images. Longitudinal grey scale shows separation of the graft from the aortic wall (a) confirming stent and graft aortic apposition and separation of graft from aortic wall. Surface reconstruction (b, c) identifies folds in a portion of the graft lacking stent support (arrows). Reproduced with permission from Donayre CE, White GH, White RA. Intraoperative imaging system requirements. In: Chuter TA, Donayre CE, White RA, eds. *Endoluminal Vascular Prostheses.* Boston, MA: Little, Brown, and Company, 1995: 302–4.

femoral–femoral bypass were employed because aortoaortic endoluminal interpositions were not possible in the majority of patients with abdominal aortic aneurysms.

Endovascular prostheses used in this study were fabricated by combining available vascular stents (Johnson & Johnson Interventional, Warren, NJ, USA) with standard grafts (Meadox Medical, Oakland, NJ, USA). The stent–graft prostheses were fabricated by securing stents to the grafts with sutures, using a technique similar to that described by Parodi.[5] Arterial traumatic lesions of smaller diameter were repaired by suturing the ends of an autologous vein to the ends of a 308 Palmaz stent.

Before deploying the endograft, contrast cinefluoroscopic images were acquired to confirm the location of proximal and distal fixation sites and branch vessels that had been identified previously by IVUS. The device was advanced to the desired position and the proximal stent deployed by balloon inflation. The distal end of the prosthesis was secured by inflating a second Palmaz stent, delivered by an appropriately sized balloon catheter. Following endoluminal deployment, the angiographic catheter was replaced by a guidewire and the IVUS catheter introduced; the length of the device was then assessed to determine the continuity of the prosthesis and to assure fixation of the proximal and distal sites and exclusion of the treated lesion. These findings were compared with images obtained by cineflouroscopy during operation and by spiral CT after surgery (Fig. 4.2).

For the smaller-diameter arterial lesions treated in this study, an alternate deployment technique utilizing real-time IVUS imaging was used. This method was used for deployment of the endografts for the three traumatic arteriovenous fistulas and the two iliac artery aneurysms. IVUS-guided deployment of the devices was accomplished by passing the appropriately sized balloon and delivery catheter containing the endoluminal graft to the chosen deployment site over a guidewire; the guidewire was then removed and a 0.035-inch 30-MHz ultrasound wire (WiseWire, Meditech, Natick, MA, USA) was passed through the balloon catheter guidewire lumen. The imaging element on the end of the wire was used to observe the placement of the proximal stent device in the desired location, and to ensure complete expansion of the prosthesis at the chosen location. The deployed device was assessed while the balloon was completely inflated and also following deflation of the balloon before it was removed. Further balloon inflations were performed as necessary to expand and secure the endograft completely. A final inspection along the length of the treated segment was made at the time of balloon withdrawal by inserting the WiseWire imaging element to a point beyond the end of balloon catheter; this allowed continuous axial imaging and three-dimensional reconstruction of these images during catheter withdrawal (Fig. 4.3).

In cases where real-time IVUS deployments were possible, contrast cinefluoroscopy was limited to images that were needed to confirm the anatomy of adjacent structures and to provide intraluminal contrast evaluation of the completed procedures. Using this technique, the

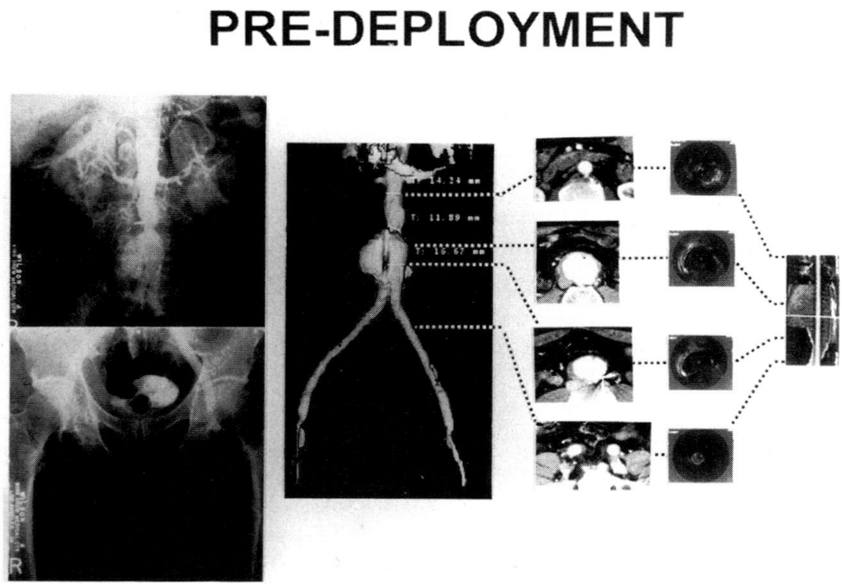

(a)

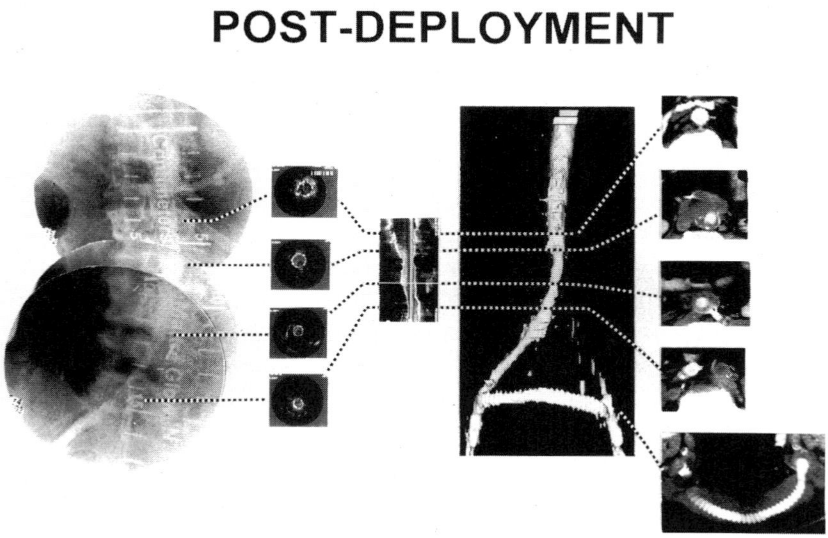

(b)

Fig. 4.2 (a) Predeployment images of a patient with aortic para-anastomotic aneurysm of a previously placed aortobifemoral graft. Preintervention angiogram and spiral CT demonstrate anastomotic stenosis with para-anastomotic aneurysm

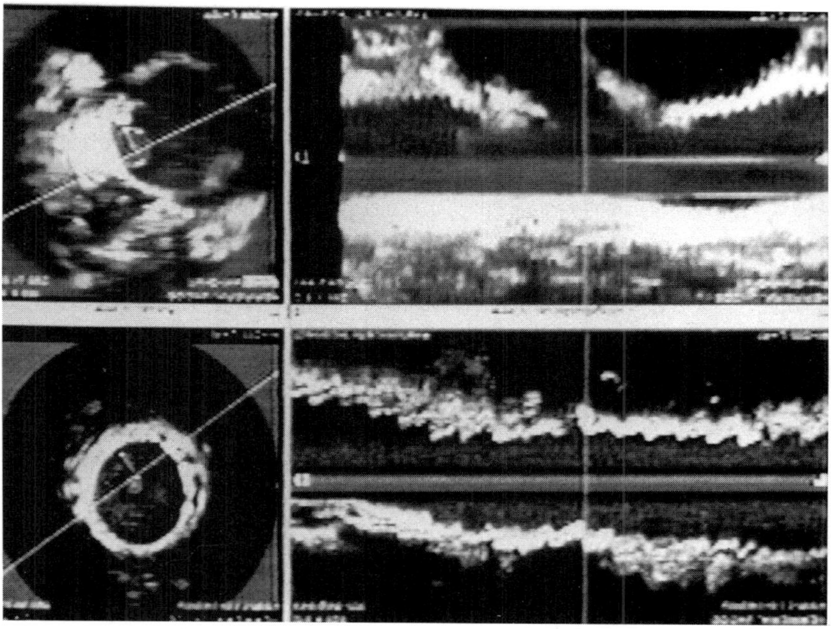

Fig. 4.3 Composite photograph of images before and after treatment acquired during IVUS-guided deployment of an endoluminal graft to treat an arteriovenous fistula of the right axillary artery following a gunshot injury. *Top panels*: IVUS images acquired at the beginning of the procedure revealed dimensions of the proximal and distal artery, and the length of the injury to the vessel. The corresponding duplex surface grey-scale surface ultrasonographic image of the lesion taken before beginning the intervention demonstrates the arteriovenous connection. *Bottom panels*: The postdeployment angiogram demonstrates complete isolation and exclusion of the arteriovenous fistula, which is confirmed by the IVUS inspection and postprocedure grey-scale surface duplex imaging of the device.

Fig. 4.2 *caption continued*
and patent iliac limbs. Dotted lines denote location of CT and intravascular ultrasonographic (IVUS) axial images from designated levels on the spiral CT and IVUS longitudinal grey-scale reconstructions. (b) Composite photograph of post-deployment images of aortic–right iliac endoluminal prosthesis and crossover femorofemoral graft. *Left to right*: Intraoperative cinefluoroscopy, IVUS axial images, longitudinal grey-scale IVUS reconstruction, spiral CT and axial contrast-enhanced images. Dotted lines denote location of axial images from designated levels on the cinefluoroscopy, IVUS and spiral CT images. Note good apposition of the stent at the aortic and iliac levels and lack of graft infolding on the IVUS images.

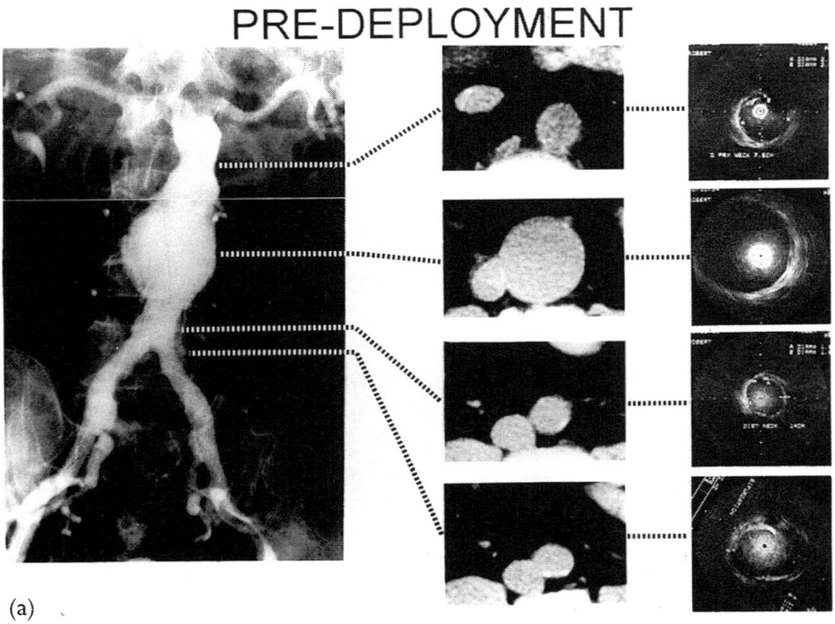

(a)

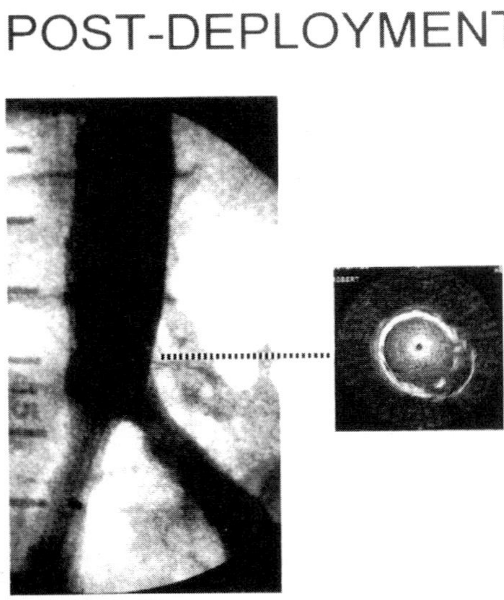

(b)

Fig. 4.4 (a) Composite photograph of predeployment images from an abdominal aortic aneurysm that appeared to have an ideal proximal neck and distal cuff for interposition aortoaortic endograft placement on the preintervention amount of contrast agent used during the procedures was limited to only essential images with the entire procedure, preintervention selection of deployment site, device deployment and postprocedure inspection being performed by IVUS.

Imaging and assessment of the distal neck of aortic aneurysms was found to be extremely treacherous. The third patient treated with an aortoaortic tube endograft was a patient who, on preintervention angiography, appeared to have a 3-cm length proximal and distal aneurysm neck. The distal neck was measured as 2.2 cm in length by axial CT images. At the time of the intervention, IVUS assessment of the distal neck revealed that the neck was only 1.4 cm in length. Following deployment of the device, cineangiography suggested complete exclusion of the aneurysm, while the IVUS demonstrated a leak (Fig. 4.4). During an attempt to dilate the stent further, to obliterate the endoleak, the iliac artery was lacerated and the patient required conversion to aortobifemoral bypass.

Conclusion

Contrast-enhanced CT (axial images and spiral reconstructions) were found to be the most accurate method for determining patient candidacy for the procedures and for choosing the site for deployment of devices. Angiography was misleading in several patients regarding critical determinants of patient candidacy and device deployment, particularly in the assessment of a distal aortic neck. Cinefluoroscopy was used in all cases and was particularly useful for determining the continuity of vascular structures and the anatomy of branch arteries, and for enabling precise positioning of stent devices. Cinefluoroscopy was limited when compared with IVUS for sizing the dimensions of fixation points. Dimensional information derived from both cinefluoroscopy and angiography was limited by inaccuracies produced by image magnification, parallax and uniplanar views. IVUS was used to

---

Fig. 4.3 *caption continued*
angiogram and CT scan (left and middle images). The axial IVUS images of the same levels shown on the CTs are displayed. IVUS evaluation demonstrated that the length of the neck was 1.4 cm rather than 3.0 or 2.2 as measured on the angiogram and CT respectively. (b) The postdeployment panels show a contrast cinefluoroscopy image that suggests complete sealing of the aneurysm from the lumen, but the IVUS image demonstrated a persistent endoleak.

determine the morphology of vascular structures (i.e. calcium, thrombus), to perform 'real-time' observation of the expansion of devices and to assure firm fixation of balloon-expanded stents before the procedures were completed. IVUS also reduced the amount of contrast dye used during interventions. Duplex scan was helpful in assessing and precisely identifying the location of arteriovenous fistulas before intervention, and provided assessment at follow-up intervals in all patients without requiring more costly and invasive imaging modalities. Three-dimensional reconstruction imaging technologies such as spiral CT were particularly helpful for assessing the morphology of vascular anatomy before the intervention and at follow-up intervals, while three-dimensional IVUS provided a similar real-time perspective during the procedure.

IVUS is an extremely useful adjunct to angiography and CT for determining parameters related to graft selection, device placement, deployment and assessment of graft infolding or stenosis. A combination of CT images (preferably spiral reconstruction) before and after intervention, and IVUS during procedures supplemented by contrast cinefluoroscopy, enables patient selection and precise balloon deployment of endograft devices. IVUS-monitored-positioning and real-time deployment is possible in vessels less than 20 mm in diameter using current 20- and 30-MHz imaging catheters.

References

1. Cavaye DM, Tabbara MR, Kopchok GE *et al.* Three dimensional vascular ultrasound imaging. *Am Surg* 1991; **57**: 751–5.
2. Tabbara MR, White RA, Cavaye DM *et al. In-vivo* human comparison of intravascular ultrasound and angiography. *J Vasc Surg* 1991; **14**: 496–504.
3. White RA, Verbin C, Kopchok G *et al.* Role of cinefluoroscopy and intravascular ultrasound in evaluating the deployment of experimental endovascular prostheses. *J Vasc Surg* 1995; **21**: 365–74.
4. White RA, Donayre CE, Kopchok GE *et al.* Vascular imaging prior to, during, and following endovascular repair. Presented at the Western Vascular Surgery Annual Meeting, Laguna Niguel, CA, February 1996. *J Vasc Surg* (in press).
5. Parodi J. Endoluminal repair of abdominal aortic aneurysms. In: Whittemore A, Bandyk DF, Cronenwett JL *et al.*, eds. *Advances in Vascular Surgery.* St Louis, MI: Mosby-Year Book, 1993: 85–106.

5

Adjunctive manoeuvres for endovascular exclusion of abdominal aortic aneurysm

Krasnodar Ivancev and Timothy A.M. Chuter

Department of Radiology, Malmö University Hospital, Malmö, S-21401, Sweden

Department of Surgery, University of California, San Francisco, USA

Introduction

Endovascular aortic aneurysm exclusion is feasible only when the apparatus is capable of traversing the iliac arteries and when implantation is accurate, secure, and haemostatic. The more versatile the device, the less restrictive the anatomic selection criteria, and the larger the number of suitable patients. But this proportion is not just a function of system design. There are a variety of adjunctive manoeuvres that can help to overcome some of the anatomic obstacles to successful endovascular aneurysm exclusion, thereby extending the range of potential canditates and minimizing the risk of failure.

Iliac artery tortuosity

The aorta and iliac arteries may become longer as an aortic aneurysm dilates. Therefore, patients presenting late in this process often have considerable iliac tortuosity. High degrees of iliac tortuosity rarely impede transfemoral insertion, even when the delivery system is large and rigid, because the iliac arteries are often surprisingly mobile. Transfemoral insertion is prevented when the iliac arteries are tortuous and their mobility is limited either by calcification or by the retroperitoneal fibrosis associated with inflammatory aneurysm (Fig. 5.1). Several factors help to make delivery system insertion easier.

First, the delivery system should be as small, smooth, and tapered as possible. Blunt or open-ended delivery systems, such as that used in the

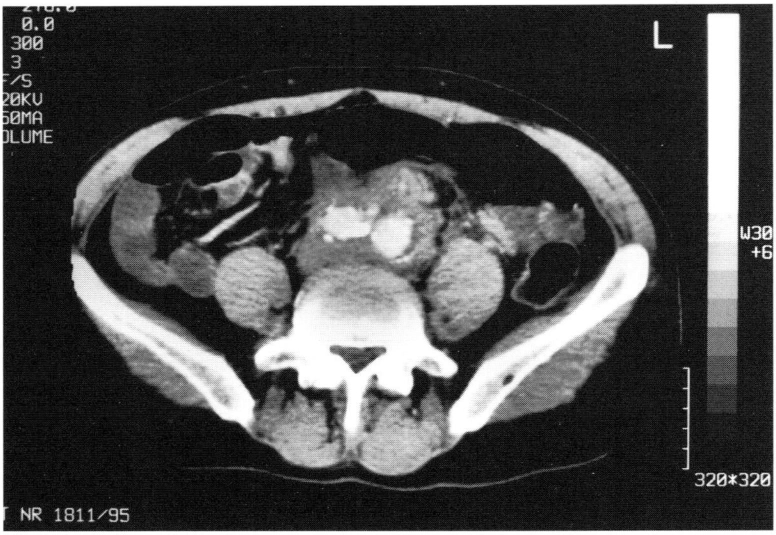

(a)

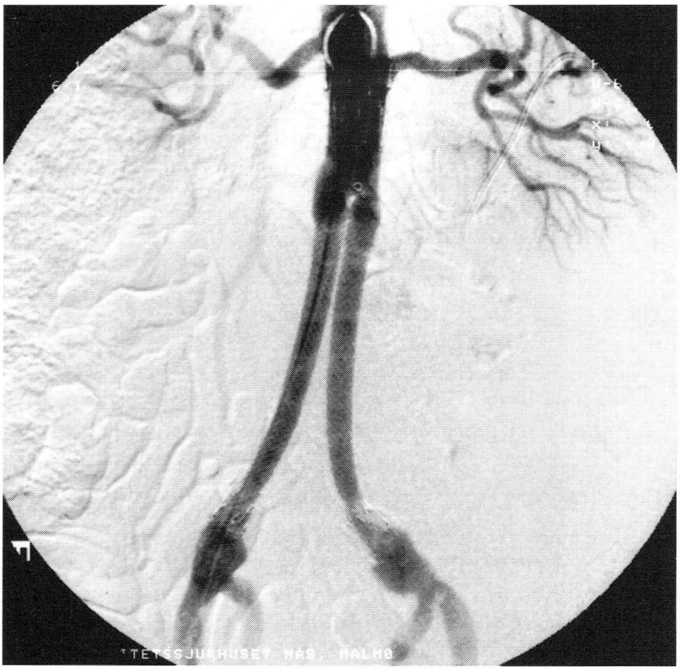

(b)

Fig. 5.1

EGS (Endovascular Grafting System, Endovascular Technologies), often need to be passed through a second sheath. Second, the delivery system should be inserted through the less tortuous iliac system. Third, the delivery system should be inserted over a stiff guidewire; examples include Amplatz Superstiff (Meditech) and Amplatz Extrastiff (Cook). Insertion of a stiff guidewire into tortuous vessels can be facilitated by transcatheter exchange. Angulated radio-opaque catheters (the cobra catheter, for example, has a good all-purpose configuration) and soft-tipped slippery guidewires (e.g. Glidewire (Terumo), Roadrunner (Cook)) may be needed to negotiate very tortuous iliac arteries.

In addition, the femoral artery should be supported, by applying gentle traction, during delivery system insertion. Otherwise, friction at the insertion site will tend to push the femoral artery beneath the inguinal ligament, which increases the redundancy of the external iliac artery and further increases resistance to insertion.

If the common femoral artery is large and diseased, it should be opened longitudinally, following insertion of a guidewire through a needle puncture. This minimizes the risk of creating an arterial dissection. A longitudinal arteriotomy is also preferred when the delivery system is large, because a transverse arteriotomy is more likely to extend circumferentially, especially if the femoral artery is not supported during delivery system insertion.

External iliac artery bends can sometimes be straightened by dividing the inferior epigastric and circumflex iliac branches at the inguinal ligament, and applying traction to the common iliac artery, as described by Parodi.[1]

Common iliac artery bends can sometimes be straightened by pushing the apex of the bend medially and interiorly with a hand on the abdomen, while the aortic bifurcation is being pushed in the opposite direction. The image field should be adjusted carefully to avoid exposure of the operator's hands to radiation.

Finally if the above manoeuvres fail, it may be necessary to expose the iliac artery directly through a retroperitoneal incision. This will allow the iliac artery to be straightened manually. Often a little direct pressure is all that is required. If so, the incision need not be large. On rare occasions it may be necessary to introduce the delivery system

---

Fig. 5.1 (a) Computed tomography showing fibrous encasement of the common iliac arteries in a patient with inflammatory aneurysm. Preoperative angiography showed iliac tortuosity. (b) Angiogram following endoluminal aneurysm repair.

directly into the common iliac artery. This is best done through a short segment of graft, anastomosed to the common iliac artery in a conventional end-to-side manner, as described by May *et al.*[2]

Another consequence of iliac artery tortuosity is kinking of aorto-iliac stent–grafts, whether they are unilateral or bifurcated, particularly with uncrimped woven grafts. To prevent kinking, the length of the distal part of the graft needs to be supported with a stent. If this kind of stent is not an integral part of prosthesis construction, it must be inserted separately. The Wallstent (Schneider) serves this purpose well.

Iliac aneurysm

One of the goals of endovascular aneurysm exclusion is to maintain antegrade flow to the pelvis and buttocks through the internal iliac arteries. To achieve this, the stent–graft has to open distally into the common iliac artery. A uni-iliac approach necessitates contralateral common iliac artery occlusion, so that retrograde flow through the external iliac artery can reach the internal iliac artery, but not the aneurysm. Both distal stent–graft implantation and common iliac artery occlusion can be difficult in the presence of common iliac artery aneurysms, and leakage can occur even when the common iliac artery is only moderately ectatic or irregular.

One option, in the presence of a common iliac artery aneurysm, is to implant the distal end of the graft in the external iliac artery, thereby sacrificing flow to the internal iliac artery. The potential consequences of external iliac artery implantation include colonic ischaemia, buttock claudication, and retrograde perfusion of the aneurysm through the patent internal iliac artery. Although colonic ischaemia seems to be rare, and buttock claudication is often tolerable, the potential consequences of continuing aneurysm perfusion have not been assessed. We take the view that if the internal iliac artery is to be excluded in this way it should be occluded before operation. This can be done percutaneously from the contralateral femoral artery, using detachable occlusion balloons (Interventional Therapeutics) or coils (William Cook Europe), at the time of initial angiography.

Other options, as described by May *et al.*[2] and Marin *et al.*[3], involve direct common iliac artery exposure and ligation of internal iliac artery. These techniques extend the range of suitable patients greatly, but they do require that the patient be able to tolerate the necessary

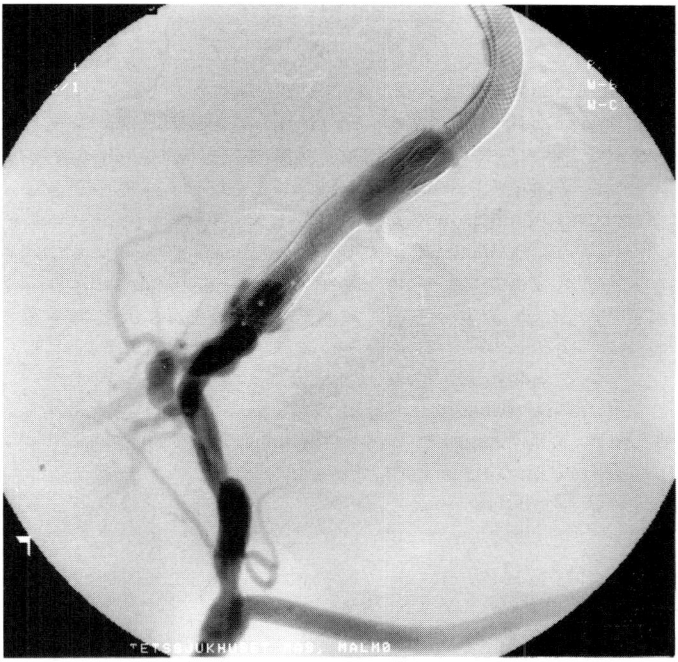

Fig. 5.2 Angiogram following emergency aneurysm exclusion, in which an additional stent–graft was inserted to achieve haemostatic distal implantation. Also shown is the Wallstent which was used to bridge the gap between the implantation site and the distal end of the original graft.

abdominal operation, even though only a small incision with retroperitoneal exposure is required.

Leakage around the end of an *in situ* stent–graft can be treated in a number of ways. Probably the best endovascular option is the addition of a second stent–graft, as a distal extension to the first (Fig. 5.2). This resembles the multicomponent approach used in several of the commercially available devices, such as the Stentor (Mintec). We have found that insertion of the second stent–graft delivery system is easier, and safer, if an additional stent (Wallstent) has been inserted across the junction between the first stent–graft and the distal artery. This stent provides a smooth, straight, stent-lined channel through the distal orifice of the first stent–graft (Fig. 5.2), which minimizes the chance of inadvertent displacement.

Leakage around a common iliac artery occluder can also lead to persistent aneurysm perfusion (endoleak). If there is room in the distal

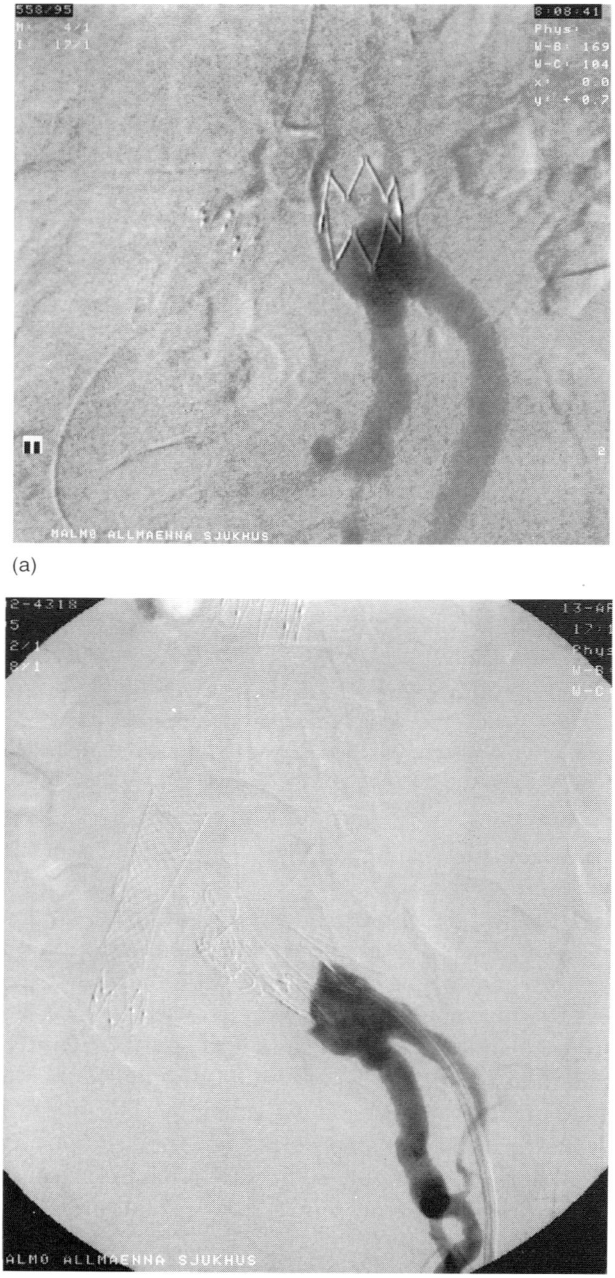

(a)

(b)

Fig. 5.3

common iliac artery, a second occluder can be inserted. If not, the space around the first occluder can be filled with Gianturco coils (Cook Europe), conical pieces of 'chopped up' Wallstents, or pieces of Gelfoam (Ferrosan Denmark), passed through a percutaneously inserted catheter (Fig. 5.3). The most certain cure for a leaky occlusion is ligation of the common iliac artery via a small iliac fossa incision and extraperitoneal exposure.

Aortic tortuosity

High degrees of aortic tortuosity are often associated with large aortic aneurysms. This takes the form of angulation of the neck relative to the suprarenal aorta proximally and to the aneurysm distally. The possible consequences include difficulty in introducing the delivery system, proximal perigraft leak, and kinking of the graft.

Indirect transabdominal pressure is sometimes able to straighten the aorta sufficiently to allow the delivery system to pass from the aneurysm into the neck. A stiff guidewire also helps, particularly if the wire exits the body at two points, so that it can be placed under tension. The use of an axillofemoral guidewire for endovascular stent–graft insertion was first described by Volodos *et al.*[4] An axillofemoral guidewire is inserted through an axillary artery puncture, and directed, using angled catheters, into the descending thoracic aorta, through the aneurysm, and down the femoral artery. This can be difficult if the femoral artery has already been opened, because the catheter will not pass until haemostatic loops are released, which is accompanied by brisk haemorrhage. When the femoral artery has already been incised, the axillary catheter can be retrieved from the iliac artery with a gooseneck snare (Microvena) and pulled out of the femoral artery, through either the haemostatic loops or the valve on a sheath. The transaxillary catheter is left in place to provide some protection to the posterolateral margin of left subclavian artery orifice, around which the axillofemoral catheter and wire turns acutely. This point is subjected to considerable force when the guidewire is placed under tension. The angle between the innominate artery and the aorta is also at risk of damage. Moreover, the right axillary artery is not usually used for this

Fig. 5.3 Angiograms showing (a) leakage around a common iliac artery occlusion device and (b) cessation of leakage after percutaneous insertion of additional closed Wallstents and Gianturco coils.

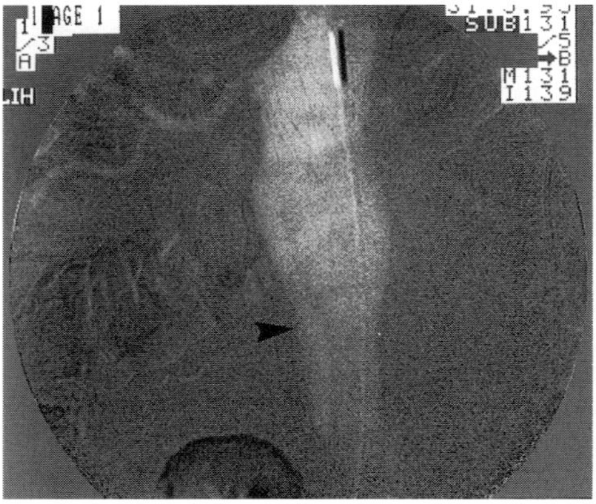

(a)

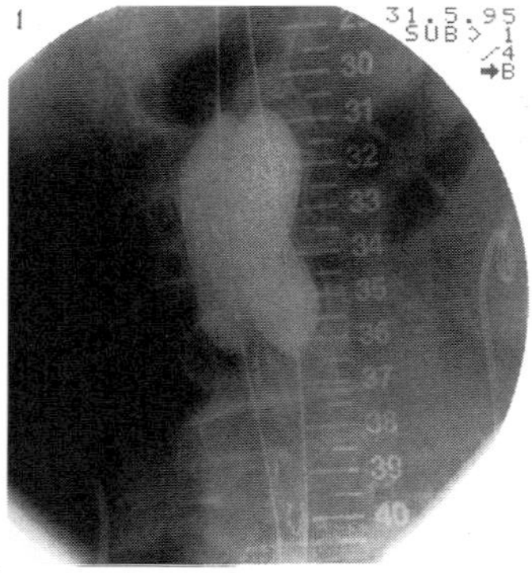

(b)

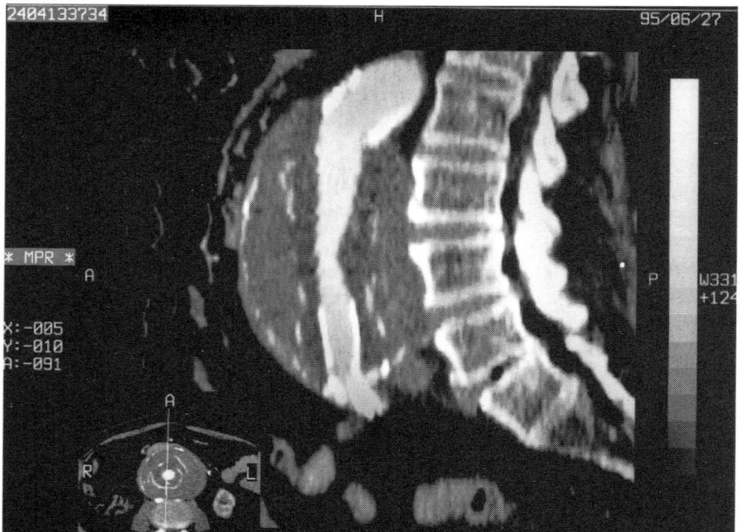

(c)

Fig. 5.4 (a) Intraoperative angiogram showing perigraft leak (arrow). (b) Intraoperative angiogram showing balloon inflation within the proximal stent. (c) Follow-up CT scan showing exclusion of the aneurysm from the circulation.

manoeuvre, for fear of embolism up the right common carotid artery. It is also important to remember to minimize instrumentation of the aneurysm. Although we have not seen arterial emboli originating from the mural thrombus of the aneurysm, this problem has been reported by others,[2,5] and its effects can be devastating. We have seen a case of occipital lobe infarction following use of a left brachiofemoral wire, presumed to be due to embolism into the left vertebral artery.

Another possible effect of aortic tortuosity is proximal perigraft leak ('endoleak'). This results from a disparity between the axial orientation of the proximal stent and of the neck, and occurs most often when the neck is short and angulated. The problem can be corrected by gently inflating a large balloon (such as the Omega balloon (William Cook Europe)) inside the proximal stent (Fig. 5.4). The stent and the neck are forced, by the balloon, to occupy the same longitudinal axis. This orientation is usually retained following balloon deflation, thereby eliminating the cause of the perigraft leak.

Kinking of the wide proximal graft segment is rarely sufficient to compromise luminal diameter significantly. If it does, the remedy is insertion of an additional stent.

Compromised neck

Given the variety of adjunctive manoeuvres, both open surgical and endovascular, that are available for dealing with iliac artery disease, the only absolute prerequisite for endovascular aneurysm repair is a suitable proximal implantation site. Of course, the definition of suitability depends on the characteristics of the prosthesis and its delivery system. Using a Gianturco Z stent-based system, we have found that proximal stent implantation is compromised if the neck is short, angulated, thrombus-lined, irregular, or conical. Together, these can lead to proximal implantation being unstable or leaky. The consequences of neck angulation have been discussed above. The other features of neck anatomy tend to produce malposition of the proximal stent.

If the proximal (modified Gianturco Z) stent is too high, it can be pulled down approximately 5 mm before the barbs fully penetrate the aorta and arrest its movement (Fig. 5.5). If this is noticed when the prosthesis is still attached to the delivery system, traction on the latter will be transmitted to the stent. But if the delivery system has already

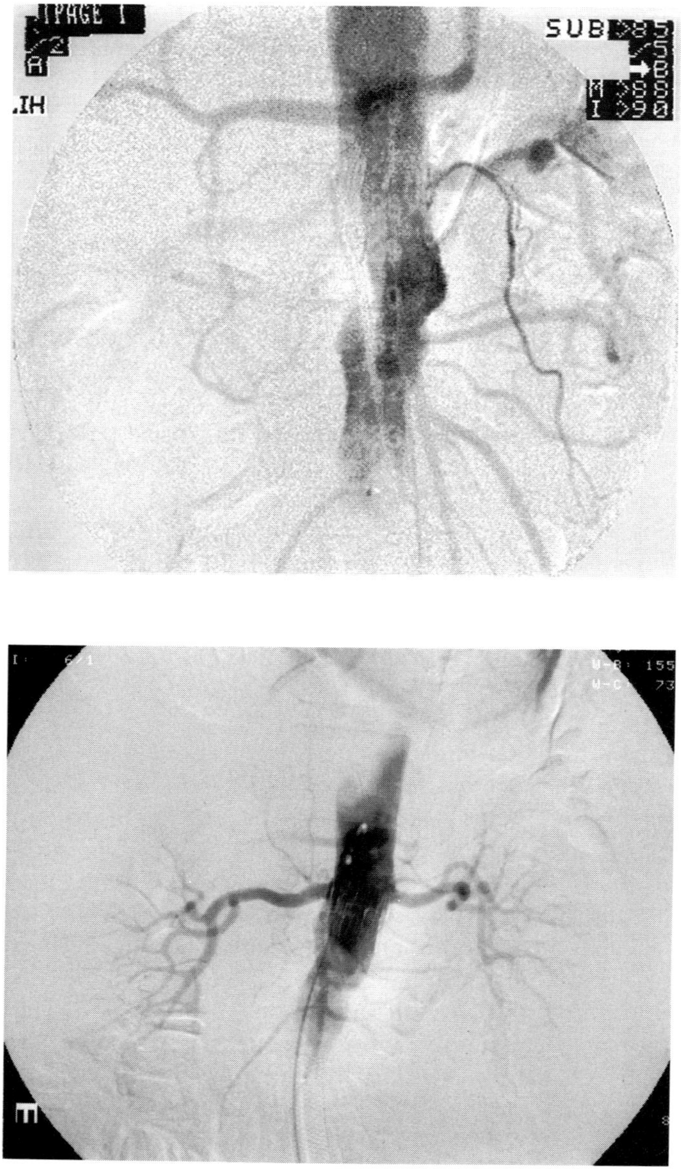

(a)

(b)

Fig. 5.5 (a) Intraoperative angiogram showing partial occlusion of the right renal artery by a malpositioned stent–graft. (b) Follow-up angiogram 6 months later showing flow to both renal arteries. The proximal stent was repositioned during operation so that the right renal artery was covered only by the limbs of the stent and not by the graft fabric.

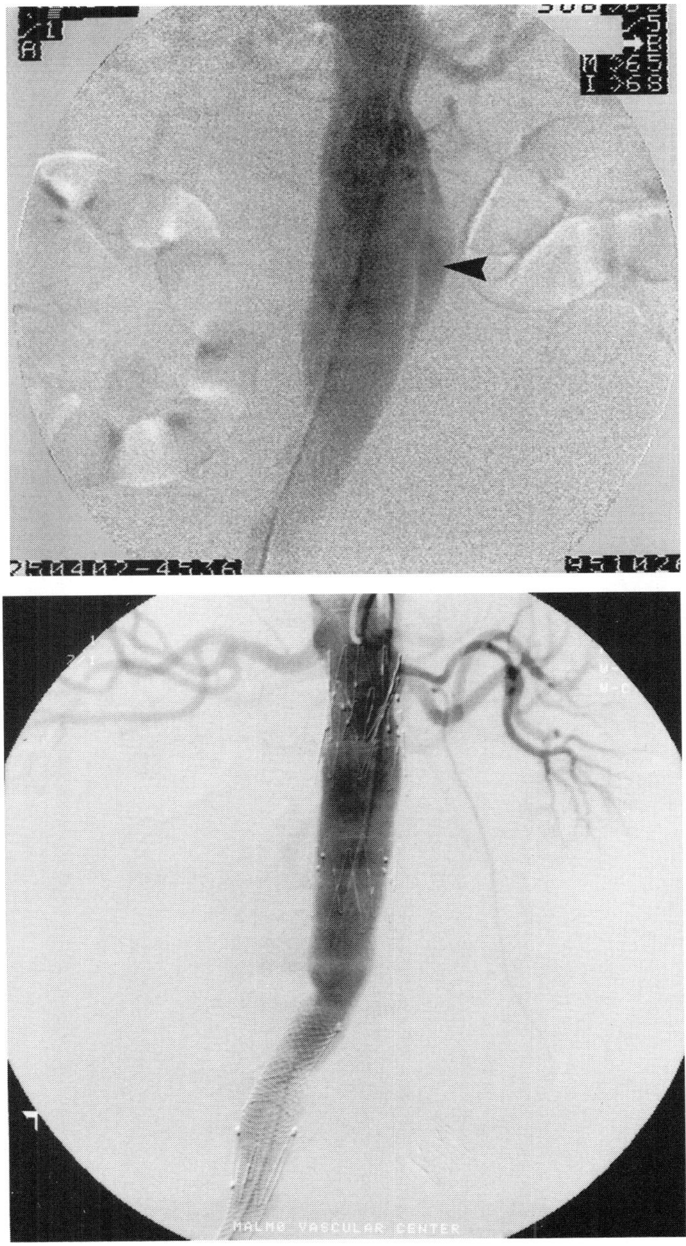

(a)

(b)

Fig. 5.6 (a) Intraoperative angiogram showing perigraft leakage due to malposition of the stent–graft. (b) Follow-up angiogram following insertion of a second stent–graft as a proximal extension.

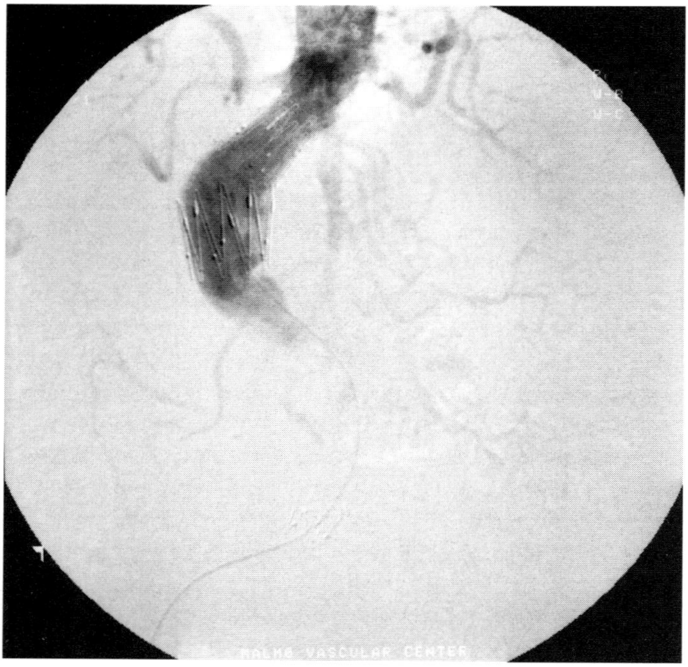

(a)

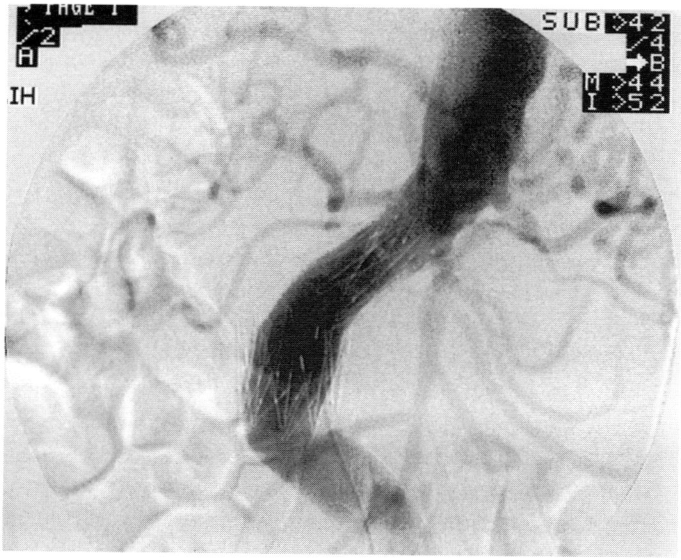

(b)

Fig. 5.7 (a) Angiogram showing separation of the first and second stent–grafts. (b) Angiogram following insertion of additional Wallstents to correct kinking and of an additional stent–graft to bridge the gap.

been removed, a large balloon can be inflated within the stent–graft. This is particularly effective if the stent–graft is tapered or bifurcated, because the balloon wedges into the graft at the transition point.

If the proximal stent is too low, a second stent–graft can be inserted inside the first, as a proximal extension (Fig. 5.6). The second stent–graft should carry barbs distally, because the first stent–graft may not be anchored securely to the aorta, and will migrate unless the second stent–graft provides some means of support (Fig. 5.7). Perigraft leak in the neck of the aneurysm can also be sealed by two or three sequential periaortic ligatures applied at a brief laparotomy. It is relatively easy to apply without clamping the aorta.

Patent collaterals

Patent lumbar and inferior mesenteric arteries provide a potential route for collateral flow into the aneurysm. This is more likely to occur when preoperative evaluation shows little mural thrombus and a large aneurysm, particularly if the patient is coagulopathic or has received anticoagulant therapy.

We have seen only one case in which perigraft perfusion of the aneurysm through collaterals continued after cessation of anticoagulants. The affected lumbar artery was fed through an ascending branch of the internal iliac artery. Percutaneous coil embolization of the feeding vessel resulted in thrombosis of the lumbar artery and perigraft space (Fig. 5.8). A similar case has been reported by Becker *et al.*[6] in which coil embolization was not effective.

Conclusion

Most of the currently available devices (commercial and made in the laboratory) can be relied on to achieve satisfactory endovascular aneurysm exclusion in the presence of straight healthy iliac arteries and long, straight, implantation sites, even if the operator is relatively inexperienced. Unfortunately, such patients comprise a small minority of those with aneurysms greater than 5 cm in diameter. To treat the rest, one needs to be armed with a variety of additional skills and equipment. Given current patterns of training and practice, success depends on teamwork between the surgeon and interventional radiologist.

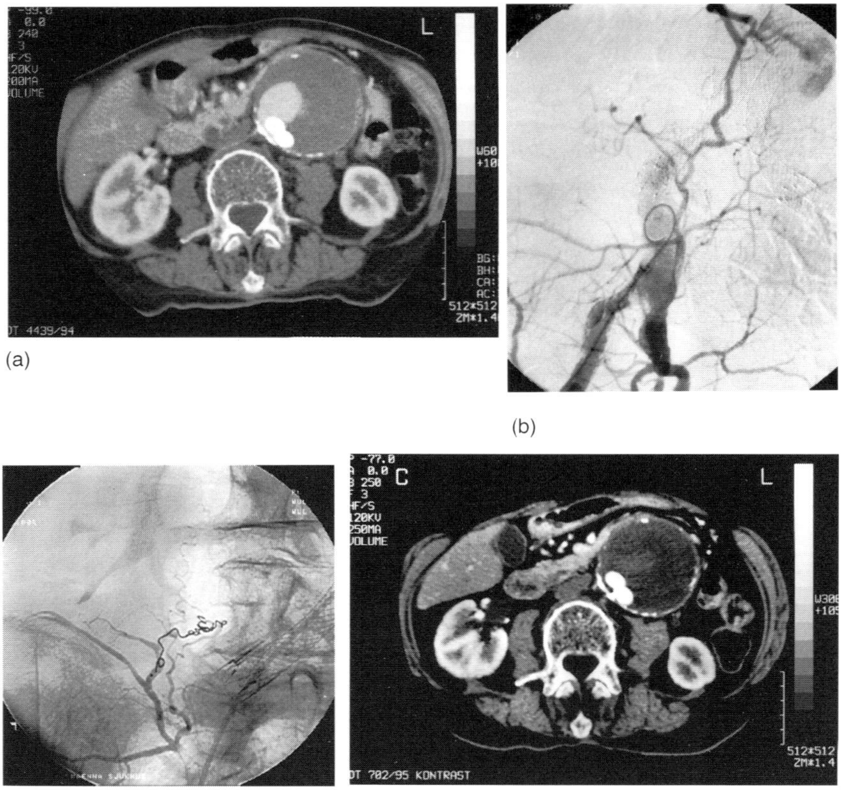

(a) (b) (c) (d)

Fig. 5.8 (a) Computed tomogram showing perigraft perfusion through a patent lumbar artery. (b) Angiogram showing perigraft perfusion through a patent lumbar artery. (c) Angiogram during percutaneous coil embolization of a lumbar tributary arising from the internal iliac artery. (d) Computed tomogram showing no perigraft perfusion.

References

1. Parodi JC. Transfemoral intraluminal graft implantation for abdominal aortic aneurysms. In: Greenhalgh RM, ed. *Vascular and Endovascular Surgical Techniques.* London: WB Saunders, 1994.
2. May J, White G, Waugh R, Yu W, Harris J. Treatment of complex abdominal aortic aneurysms by a combination of endoluminal and extraluminal aortofemoral grafts. *J Vasc Surg* 1994; **19**: 924–33.
3. Marin ML, Veith FL, Cynamon J *et al.* Initial experience with transluminally placed endovascular grafts for the treatment of complex vascular lesions. *Ann Surg* 1995; **222**: 449–69.

4. Volodos NL, Karpovich IP, Troyan VI *et al.* Clinical experience of the use of a self-fixing synthetic prosthesis for remote endoprosthesis of the thoracic and the abdominal aorta and iliac arteries through the femoral artery and as intraoperative endoprosthesis for aorta reconstruction. *Vasa* 1991; **33**: 93–5.
5. Parodi JC. Endovascular repair of abdominal aortic aneurysms and other arterial lesions. *J Vasc Surg* 1995; **21**: 549–57.
6. Becker GJ, Katzen BT, Benenati JF *et al.* Endografts in the treatment of abdominal and thoracic aortic aneurysms and non-aortic lesions: MVI experience. *Eighth Annual International Symposium on Vascular Diagnosis and Intervention*, Miami, FL, 31 January 1996.

6

The MinTec system

Ulrich Blum

Department of Diagnostic Radiology, University Hospital Freiburg, Germany

Components of the endoprosthesis and design of the delivery system

The stent–graft is a self-expanding endoprosthesis constructed of nitinol monofilament (nickel–titanium shape memory alloy) annealed into a tubular zig-zag configuration[1] which incorporates a 0.1-mm woven polyester fabric cover over the nitinol wire stent frame (Fig. 6.1). Each opposing zig-zag is fastened together with a 7–0 polypropylene ligature. This basic stent frame is covered with a polyester fabric of medium permeability. The Stentor (MinTec, Freeport, The Bahamas) has two basic designs addressing varying anatomic requirements for abdominal aortic aneurysms (AAAs), straight (Fig. 6.1a) and bifurcated (Mialhe Stentor) (Fig. 6.1b). The leading and trailing ends of the stent frame are tagged by a platinum marker which allows for proper positioning of the implant. Fixation hooks placed outside the fabric-covered section of the device allow the leading part of the stent to anchor into the proximal aortic neck.

The straight tube is made from a basic nitinol frame (diameter 22–26 mm) covered with a thin Dacron fabric. The bifurcated device has two components which are introduced separately and mated *in loco* (Fig. 6.1b): (1) the aortic part with single limb and (2) the second limb. At the trailing portion of the aortic section, there is a short branch of 10 mm in diameter into which the second contralateral limb is inserted. The juncture into which the two sections are connected is tagged by platinum markers to aid into their mating. The diameter of the aortic section ranges from 22 to 26 mm, and that of the iliac limbs from 10 to 12 mm. The devices are commercially available in standard sizes (diameter 22, 24 or 26 mm, total length 153 or 165 mm; diameter of the iliac limb 10 or 12 mm) or can be custom made.

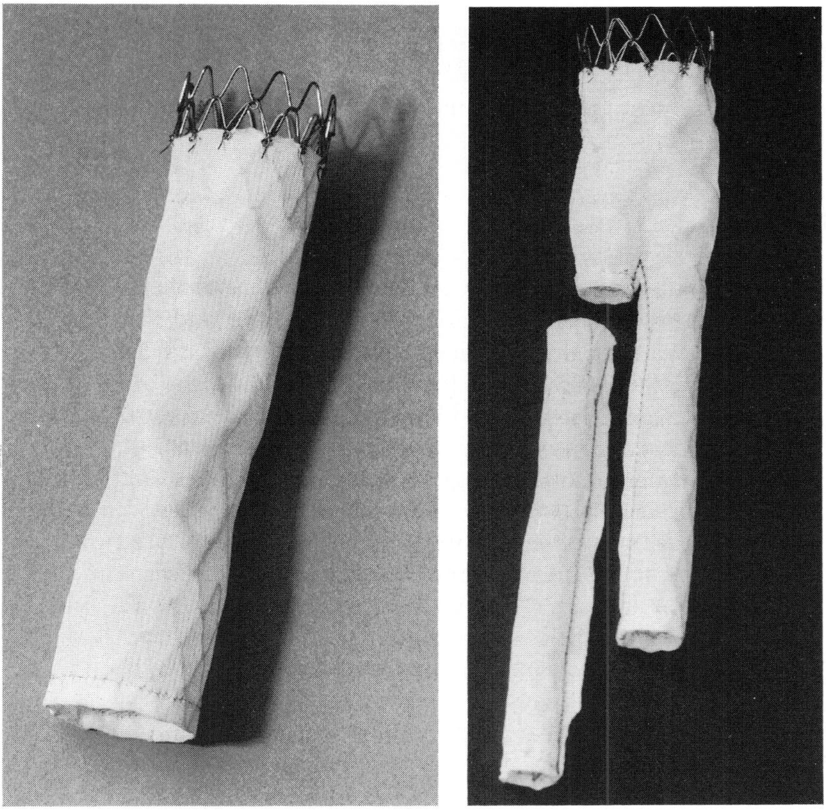

(a) (b)

Fig. 6.1 Basic designs of nitinol stents covered with woven Dacron graft material for infrarenal AAA (Stentor device). (a) Straight tube: the stent frame is covered with a thin woven polyester fabric of medium permeability. The most leading part is uncovered and has a row of barbs for anchoring into the proximal neck of the aneurysm. (b) The bifurcated graft has two components which are inserted separately and mated in place: the aortic section has a single limb and the second limb is inserted contralaterally and implanted in the trailing end of the aortic section.

Insertion of the stent device is achieved by means of a three-stage delivery system with an inner diameter of 18-F comprising three components: an introducer sheath, an aortic pusher and an iliac pusher. The introducer sheath is withdrawn over the aortic and iliac pusher (telescopic system), respectively, to expose the nitinol framework which self-expands below blood temperature. A latex balloon with a maximum diameter of 30 mm and a volume of 15 ml, which is part of the delivery system, permits subsequent modelling of the leading section of the stent frame to facilitate proper fixation of the device against the artery wall.

Patient selection criteria

To select patients properly for eventual endoluminal repair of infrarenal AAA, precise determination of the diameter and length of the abdominal aorta, the iliac arteries, the orifices of the renal arteries, and the anatomy of the aneurysm is fundamental. Multiplane angiography with use of a graduated catheter and spiral computed tomography (CT) were performed at least 1 week before the procedure in all patients considered for stent–graft implantation. Measurements included the distance between the renal arteries to the aneurysm and the aortic bifurcation, the length and the diameter of the proximal and distal neck of the aneurysm, and the diameter of the proximal and distal common iliac artery (CIA). Angiography and spiral CT (including three-dimensional image reconstructions in selected cases) gave accurate representation of luminal shape, aneurysmal wall, size, and direction of infrarenal AAAs.

Patients were selected according to the following criteria:

Inclusion criteria:

- patients eligible or ineligible for surgical treatment with infrarenal aortic aneurysm, with or without iliac involvement (AAA types A–C) (Fig. 6.2).

Exclusion criteria:

- patients whose proximal aortic neck is less than 10 mm in length or more than 25 mm in diameter (AAA type E).
- patients whose distal iliac neck is greater than 12 mm in diameter (bifurcated graft) (AAA type D).
- patients whose distal aortic neck is less than 10 mm in length or more than 25 mm in diameter (straight graft).
- patients with both internal iliac arteries involved in the aneurysm.
- patients with stenosis or occlusion of the superior mesenteric artery.
- patients for whom follow-up is uncertain.

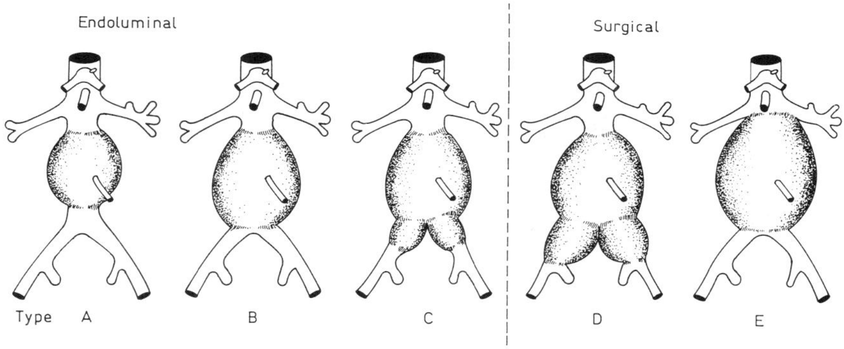

Fig. 6.2 Classification of infrarenal abdominal aortic aneurysm.

Between August 1994 and February 1996 a total of 71 patients (69 men, two women) with a mean age of 70 (range 47–90) years were treated by transfemoral placement of straight tubes (n = 7) or bifurcated grafts (n = 64) for infrarenal AAA with a maximum diameter ranging from 4.4 to 9.8 (mean 5.6) cm. All but eight patients were eligible for surgery and were graded according to the American Society of Anesthesiologists (ASA) physical status as class I (n = 1), class II (n = 29) class III (n = 33) and class IV (n = 8).

Patients considered for endoluminal treatment of AAA were divided into two groups according to the type of AAA:

Group A (AAA type A)

In group A (n = 7) only the abdominal aorta was involved, and implantation of a straight stent–graft was considered suitable (proximal aortic neck length at least 10 mm, diameter 25 mm or less, distal aortic neck length at least 10 mm, diameter 25 mm or less).

Group B (AAA types B and C)

In group B (n = 64) both the aortic bifurcation and the CIA were involved, and the aneurysm was considered suitable for implantation of a bifurcated stent–graft (proximal neck length at least 10 mm, diameter 25 mm or less, no distal neck, ectasia of the CIA, diameter 12 mm or less).

Procedure

Implantation sequence (Fig. 6.3)

All procedures were performed in the angiographic suite as a teamwork approach between vascular surgeons and interventional radiologists under general anaesthesia with the patient prepared for surgical aneurysm repair in case of failed endoluminal technique.

The stent–graft was inserted by its 18-F introduction catheter via a femoral surgical cutdown, a left or right approach. The catheter containing the compressed graft was prechilled with ice-cold saline, advanced over a stiff 0.035-inch guidewire (Amplatz; Medi-tech, Watertown, MA, USA) and positioned at the level of the renal arteries. Under fluoroscopy, the introducer catheter was rotated, so that the platinum marker on the compressed stent–graft came in a lateral position, and to the same side as the femoral cutdown approach indicating the correct rotational axis of the implant for deployment, whereby the most leading marker appeared just below the renal arteries. With the catheter now in the correct rotational and longitudinal axis, and the platinum marker still in the lateral position, the outer sheath was slowly withdrawn by approximately 3 cm. The latex balloon was now positioned in the most leading lumen of the stent graft and inflated, so as to anchor fully the barbs on the neck of the stent graft into the nonaneurysmal wall of the aorta. Deployment of the stent–graft was performed without hypotension.

In the case of straight tubes (Fig. 6.3a), the outer sheath was then withdrawn completely, to deploy the implant fully. Immediately thereafter, balloon modelling with use of the latex balloon in the middle and trailing part of the straight tube was performed. Finally, the introducer system was removed and a 9-F sheath placed while clamping the vessel surgically. After control arteriography had been performed to ensure no leaks were present, the arteriotomy was closed by standard surgical technique. For straight tubes, this was the end of the procedure.

In the case of bifurcated stent–grafts (Fig. 6.3b), with the leading part of the graft deployed, the outer sheath was withdrawn until the radiopaque marker of the iliac stump (connection point of the second iliac limb section) expanded. After balloon modelling of the middle and trailing part of the aortic section, the outer sheath was withdrawn to deploy the fixed ipsilateral iliac limb. Thereafter, the introducer system was removed, leaving the guidewire in position. To complete the bifurcated graft, the second contralateral limb section of the

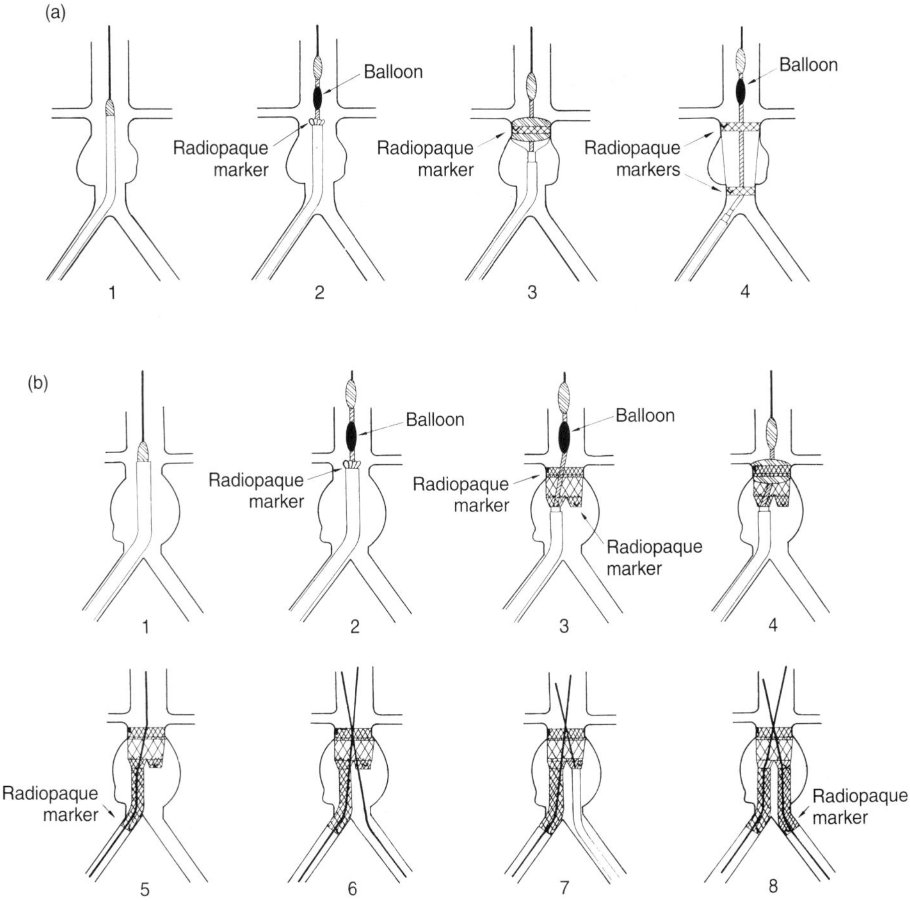

Fig. 6.3 Stent–graft implantation. (a) Straight graft: (1) delivery system containing the graft is advanced to the level of the renal arteries; (2) outer sheath is withdrawn, setting the leading part of the graft with barbs free; (3) balloon dilatation to anchor the leading part of the straight tube; (4) further withdrawal of the outer sheath to complete deployment of the graft. (b) Bifurcated graft: (1–3) (see above); (4, 5) freeing of the ipsilateral iliac limb; (6) insertion of a stiff guidewire into the trailing part of the aortic section; (7) insertion of the delivery system, containing the contralateral iliac limb, into the aortic section; (8) withdrawal of the sheath, thereby deploying the second iliac limb.

implant was then inserted percutaneously on the contralateral side and mated into the primary aortoiliac section previously implanted. Using a standard percutaneous approach a 7-F selective catheter was inserted into the stump of the aortic section. Finally, a 10-F introducer system containing the second iliac limb section was advanced over a stiff 0.035-inch Amplatz guidewire. Once the introducer system had been positioned correctly, it was slowly retracted by about 1 cm so that the leading portion of the second limb began to expand, thereby exposing its radiopaque marker. With the second limb in the correct position, the sheath was then withdrawn completely, to expand the second limb section fully. Thereafter, the whole length of the second limb was dilated with a balloon catheter (Medi-tech, Watertown, MA, USA), applying pressure up to 2 atmospheres.

Depending on the degree of iliac disease, additional extensions (EndoPro system I; MinTec, Freeport, The Bahamas) were necessary ($n = 18$). Completion angiography was performed to determine that the aneurysm has been excluded and that no major leaks existed. Once no residual perfusion of the aneurysm was demonstrated, the introducer and guidewires were removed and the arteriotomy was closed by standard surgical technique.

During the procedure 5000–10 000 IU heparin and a single dose of 2 g cefotiam were given intravenously. After the procedure 20 000–30 000 IU heparin daily were administered intravenously for 2 days to achieve prolongation of the partial thromboplastin time to 50–60 s, followed by a long-term antiplatelet medication (acetylsalicylic-acid 100 mg per day or ticlopidine 250 mg daily).

Introduction of the delivery system

The 18-Fr introducer system could be advanced over a stiff Amplatz guidewire in 69 (97%) of 71 patients despite marked iliac artery tortuosity in 37. In two patients, the introduction was not successful: in one the insertion of the introducer delivery system was impeded owing to a kinked CIA requiring elective surgical repair of the aneurysm. In the other, rupture of the coiled external iliac artery occurred during introduction of the delivery system. Bleeding was controlled via an iliac incision followed by conversion into surgical repair of the AAA.

After stent–graft implantation, there was no evidence of stenosis or occlusion of the iliac limbs even in case of a marked iliac kinking with an angulation up to 90°. In 17 of 71 patients the proximal neck of the AAA showed pronounced anterior ($n = 7$) or lateral ($n = 10$) angulation between the neck and the aneurysm up to about 80°. Even in these subjects the delivery system could be inserted and the endoprosthesis implanted accurately.

Marked calcification at the level of the proximal neck of the aneurysm ($n = 6$) did not influence the anchoring and implantation of the leading part of the aortic section.

Initial technical results

Endoluminal treatment of AAA was technically successful, defined as complete exclusion of the AAA from the circulation, in 60 (85%) of 71 patients.

Group A

All seven patients were successfully treated with a straight tube (diameter 24 or 26 mm, length 9 or 10 cm). After the procedure there was no visible minor or major leak. The procedure time was 30–150 min. In the first patient the intervention took 2.5 hours, decreasing (according to accumulated experience) to 30 min in the last patient. The hospital stay was 4–12 (mean 6) days.

Group B

The initial technical success rate with use of a bifurcated stent–graft was 83%. Apart from the two patients in whom there was difficulty in advancing the introducer delivery system across the iliac arteries, accurate placement of the leading part of the aortic section below the renal arteries was achieved in the remaining 62 patients (97%). The AAA could be excluded completely from blood circulation in 53 of 64 patients (Fig. 6.4a,b). Technical failure with a minor ($n = 6$) or major ($n = 1$) leak originating from the iliac limb was probably because of a Dacron tear in seven patients. A persistent distal leak emerging from the trailing end of the iliac limbs resulting from an inappropriate diameter of the CIA was observed in two patients.

In 16 of 64 patients we had to extend one iliac limb with an additional covered stent to the external iliac artery in order to block retrograde perfusion of the aneurysmal sac. In one patient, we had to extend both iliac limbs with covered nitinol stents, resulting in the

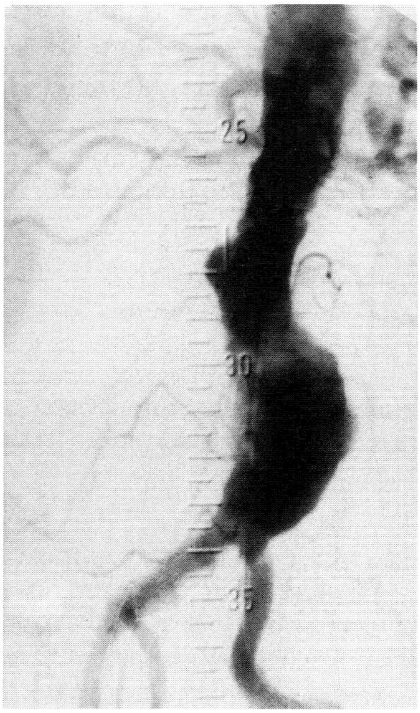

(a)

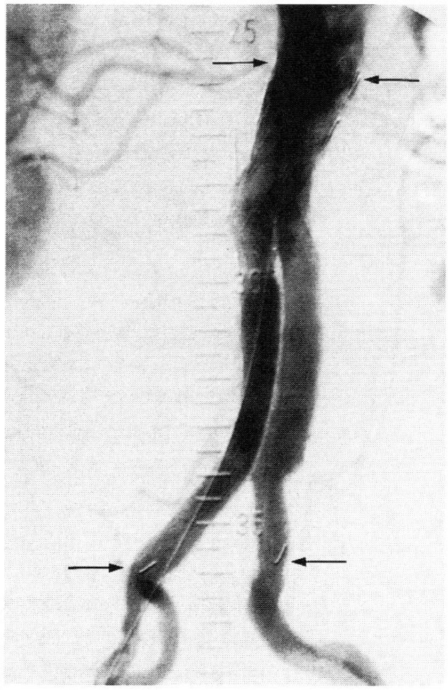

(b)

Fig. 6.4 Implantation of a bifurcated graft in a 72-year-old patient for infrarenal AAA type B. (a) Preprocedural arteriogram demonstrates an infrarenal AAA without involvement of the bifurcation. (b) Completion angiography showing the restored aortic lumen with complete exclusion of the aneurysmal sac. There is no leak at the leading or trailing end (arrows) of the bifurcated endoprosthesis.

obstruction of both internal iliac arteries. However, no problem was created for pelvic or intestinal blood supply.

The duration of the intervention in this group ranged from 50 to 180 min, with an average procedure time of 85 min in the last 30 patients. The average hospital stay was 11.5 (range 4–83) days.

Complications and management

Apart from the rupture of the external iliac artery during introduction of the delivery system via the iliac arteries, minor or major local or

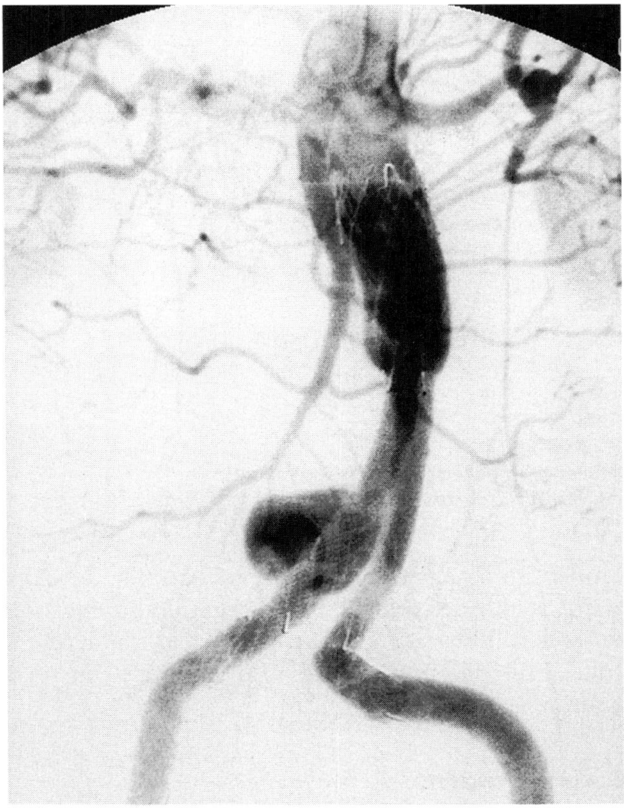

Fig. 6.5 Angiography after 6 months' follow-up in a patient with initially incomplete exclusion of the AAA demonstrating a persistent leak of the right iliac limb.

systemic complications related to the procedure were observed in 13 of 71 patients (Table 6.1).

Local complications

Clinically and angiographically evident peripheral macroembolization in three patients was treated by local thrombolysis ($n = 1$), aspiration thrombectomy ($n = 1$) or Fogarty manoeuvre ($n = 1$). Peripheral microembolization to one toe occurred in one patient and was successfully treated by intra-arterial application of prostaglandin. In another

Table 6.1 Complications following stent–graft implantation for infrarenal AAA.

Complication	*No. of patients (n = 67)*
Local	
Rupture of external iliac artery	1
Peripheral macroembolization	3
Peripheral microembolization	1
Local haematomoa requiring surgery	1
Arteriovenous fistula	1
Lymph fistula	2
Iliac limb occlusion	1
Systemic	
Acute hepatic failure	1
Embolic graft occlusion	1
Renal insufficiency (induced by contrast medium)	2

patient under anticoagulation local haematoma developed at the puncture site, requiring surgical intervention. Lymph fistulas occurred in two patients following the surgical transfemoral access. Arteriovenous fistula developed in one patient at the site of the percutaneous puncture and was corrected surgically.

Systemic complications

One patient with liver cirrhosis (Child–Pugh grade C) died from acute hepatic failure 4 days after the procedure as a result of massive bleeding from a gastric ulcer and hepatorenal syndrome. In another patient with atrial thrombi and fibrillation, embolic occlusion of the left graft limb occurred 4 days after the procedure, and was managed by local thrombolysis. Two days later, however, complete occlusion of the aortic section of the stent–graft was observed. Again, local fibrinolysis was performed for 3 days, leading to complete resolution of the thrombotic material. Finally, the patient had to be treated surgically by fasciotomy because he developed a compartment syndrome. After cardioconversion the patient is now doing well.

Renal insufficiency developed in two patients with renal impairment before the procedure (serum creatinine level 1.5 and 1.6 mg/dl). Serum creatinine concentration rose over a period of 4 days to 3.0 and 3.8 mg/dl, requiring transient haemodialysis.

Postimplantation syndrome

In 42 (59%) of 71 patients fever ranging from 38.0 to 39.7°C developed after the procedure, lasting for 4–14 days without evidence of bacteraemia or graft infection. In all patients laboratory tests showed inflammation with a mild or marked increase in the level of C-reactive protein (CRP) (range 4.0–19.6 ng/dl) and leukocytosis (range 9800–28 500 per mm^3).

Follow-up

The follow-up protocol included intra-arterial digital subtraction angiography (DSA) and spiral CT. The first control study was performed in all patients before discharge, within 7 days after the initial procedure. Thereafter, all follow-up examinations were performed on an outpatient basis with a second control examination after 3 months (CT) and a third after 6 months (intra-arterial DSA with use of a transbrachial approach and CT), followed by a CT control examination after 12 months. Further controls are to be performed every year.

Follow-up ranged from 8 days to 18 months (mean 10.5 months). Fourteen of 71 patients were followed for 12 months and 31 for 6 months. Graft limb thrombosis occurred 4 weeks after stent–graft implantation in one patient with marked angulation of the aneurysmal sac. This patient was treated successfully by local low-dose thrombolysis followed by implantation of an additional covered stent, extending into the orifice of the iliac limb.

Seven of nine patients with an incomplete seal between graft and aorta due to a Dacron tear (Fig. 6.5) or a distal leak at the trailing part of the iliac limb were treated successfully by introduction of a second stent–graft, resulting in complete thrombosis of the AAA. The two remaining patients with minor persistent reperfusion of the aneurysmal sac did not agree to a second intervention.

Once successful exclusion of AAA from circulation had been achieved, accurate CT evaluation of the original aortic lumen and the aneurysmal sac did not reveal any reperfusion after stent–graft placement according to determination of density values at defined levels during follow-up (Fig. 6.6). There was no evidence of retrograde blood flow via the lumbar arteries or the inferior mesenteric artery. In addition, apart from one patient with successful endoluminal treatment for an inflammatory AAA, careful measurement of the infrarenal

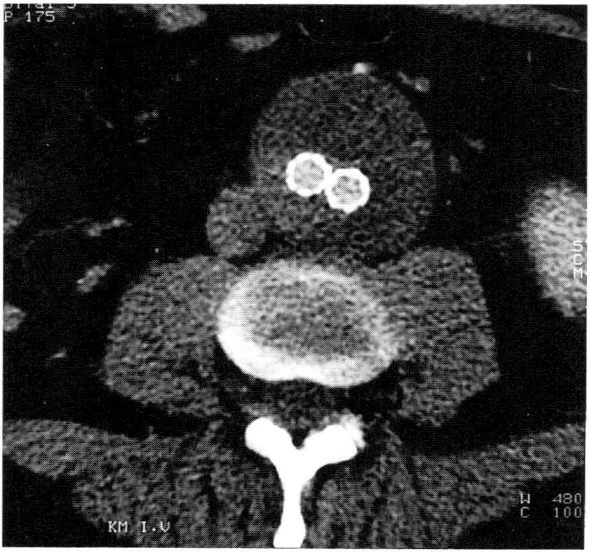

Fig. 6.6 Control CT examination after 12 months confirms complete exclusion of the AAA with absence of contrast enhancement within the aneurysmal sac.

aorta at 6 and 12 months did not reveal substantial reduction in the diameter of the aneurysmal sac.

Summary

Since 1951 elective surgical repair with use of a synthetic graft has proved to be the method of choice for the treatment of AAA to prevent rupture, associated with an acceptable perioperative mortality rate of 1.4–6.5%.[2] In the past 20 years different stent concepts have been developed to decrease complications and risks associated with the current surgical treatment.

In 1991 Parodi *et al.*[3] reported on the first five patients treated for AAA with a nonbifurcated, knitted, crimped Dacron graft sutured to a balloon-expandable stent at both ends. All five interventions were technically successful and the grafts were patent during a short follow-up. The initial concept of this group, however, was limited to AAA not involving the bifurcation or iliac arteries. Recently, Parodi[4] published the results of a series of 50 patients with AAA treated with an 80% primary success rate.

The clinical use of different stented or nonstented graft combinations has been reported in a limited number of patients.[5–10] Scott and Chuter[5] and Yusuf *et al.*,[6] using the stent–graft designed by Chuter *et al.*,[7] successfully treated six patients with a bifurcated graft. White *et al.*[8] and May *et al.*,[9] using a new nonstented balloon-expandable graft consisting of a conventional Dacron graft incorporating metallic implants (Sydney endograft), successfully treated patients with AAA without involvement of the bifurcation or iliac arteries by straight tubes and a limited number of patients with bifurcated grafts ($n = 5$), with an initial success rate of 81%.

We implanted a new nonbifurcated or bifurcated stent–graft type for the endoluminal repair of AAA in 26 patients based on a self-expandable nitinol framework covered with a thin polyester fabric[10] and have now treated a total of 64 patients with use of a bifurcated stent–graft. Careful and detailed preinterventional assessment of the anatomy of each AAA allowed appropriate selection of our patients. Apart from the two patients in whom introduction of the delivery system was not successful, the 18-F delivery system could be advanced even in patients with pronounced tortuosity of the iliac arteries followed by accurate placement of the graft below the renal arteries. The high flexibility of the nitinol frame permitted the proximal part of the graft to be anchored safely into the proximal neck and the iliac limbs to be implanted even in marked angulation between the proximal neck and aneurysm. The primary technical success rate in patients treated with straight tubes was 100% and with bifurcated grafts 83%. During follow-up, a persistent leak at the level of the iliac limb could be treated successfully with implantation of an additional stent–graft followed by complete exclusion of the AAA and restoration of normal blood flow. Intervention-related major or minor complications occurred in 14 (20%) of 71 patients. Local complications were rupture of the external iliac artery ($n = 1$), peripheral embolization ($n = 4$), local haematoma at the puncture site ($n = 1$) and arteriovenous or lymph fistulas ($n = 3$). One patient with liver cirrhosis (Child–Pugh grade C) developed acute hepatic failure and died 8 days after the procedure. One other patient with atrial thrombi and fibrillation developed an occlusion of the stent–graft. Renal insufficiency induced by contrast medium (in two patients with impaired renal function before the procedure) required transient haemodialysis.

Laboratory findings indicating inflammation with a mild or marked increase in the level of CRP and leukocytosis was observed in all patients, fever in more then half. However, there was no evidence of bacteraemia or graft infection. The mechanism of this self-limiting inflammatory process, which we call postimplantation syndrome, is still unclear. While no stent–graft infection was demonstrated, we are at present performing experimental studies to understand this phenomenon. Preliminary results of laboratory studies suggest a non-specific inflammatory reaction with release of proinflammatory substances, such as cytokines, resulting in the increase in CRP levels and leukocytosis.

With increasing experience, the time required for the procedure was acceptable and decreased to a mean total procedure time of approximately 85 min in the last 30 patients receiving bifurcated stent–grafts, which is comparable to the surgical procedure.

Until now, our experience has been limited and the follow-up period too short to draw definite conclusions. In addition to technical concerns, several basic aspects have to be addressed. (1) Once stent–grafts are in place, can retrograde blood flow via patent lumbar arteries result in a subsequent increase in intra-aneurysmal pressure with eventual rupture? (2) Are stent–grafts and fixation systems durable (material fatigue)?

Refinements of the stent framework and its fabric as a result from our initial experience are in progress. Enlargement of the diameter of the aortic section and iliac limbs will increase the number of patients suitable for endoluminal management.

In conclusion, on the basis of our results and the short-term follow-up, endoluminal repair of infrarenal AAA with use of straight or bifurcated grafts is safe and clinically effective. The stent concept, therefore, may be a therapeutic option, especially in patients with high surgical risks.

References

1. Cragg AH, De Jong SC, Barnhart WH, Landas SK, Smith TP. Nitinol intravascular stent: results of preclinical evaluation. *Radiology* 1993; **189**: 450–8.
2. Ernst CB. Abdominal aortic aneurysm. *N Engl J Med* 1993; **328**: 1167–72.
3. Parodi JC, Palmaz JC, Barone HD. Transfemoral intraluminal graft implantation for abdominal aortic aneurysms. *Ann Vasc Surg* 1991; **5**: 491–9.
4. Parodi JC. Endovascular repair of abdominal aortic aneurysms and other arterial lesions. *J Vasc Surg* 1995; **21**: 549–57.
5. Scott RAP, Chuter TAM. Clinical endovascular placement of bifurcated graft in abdominal aortic aneurysms without laparotomy. *Lancet* 1994; **343**: 413.
6. Yusuf SW, Baker DM, Chuter TAM, Whitaker SC, Wenham PW, Hopkinson BR. Transfemoral endoluminal repair of abdominal aortic aneurysm with bifurcated graft. *Lancet* 1994; **344**: 650–1.

7. Chuter TAM, Green RM, Ouriel K, Fiore WM, DeWeese JA. Transfemoral endovascular aortic graft placement. *J Vasc Surg* 1993; **18**: 185–97.
8. White GH, Yu W, May J, Stephen MS, Waugh RC. A new nonstented balloon-expandable graft for straight and bifurcated endoluminal bypass. *J Endovasc Surg* 1994; **1**: 16–24.
9. May J, White GH, Yu W *et al.* Surgical management of complications following endoluminal grafting of abdominal aortic aneurysms. *Eur J Vasc Endovasc Surg* 1995; **10**: 51–9.
10. Blum U, Langer M, Spillner G *et al.* Abdominal aortic aneurysms: preliminary technical and clinical results with transfemoral placement of endovascular self-expanding stent–grafts. *Radiology* 1996; **198**: 25–31.

7

Chuter–Gianturco bifurcated stent–grafts for abdominal aortic aneurysm exclusion

Timothy A.M. Chuter

Department of Surgery, University of California, San Francisco, USA

Design of the delivery system and endoprosthesis

Several basic features of the bifurcated system dictate the rest of system design.

1. The prosthesis is prefabricated in bifurcated form, with a large aortic orifice proximally and two small iliac orifices distally.
2. There are self-expanding Gianturco Z stents at all three graft orifices.
3. The prosthesis is attached, proximally and distally, to a catheter-based central carrier.
4. The delivery system has a single primary sheath, which is inserted with the prosthesis already loaded.

To permit insertion of the loaded delivery system (sheath, central carrier, and prosthesis), a tapered obturator is present at the upstream end of the central carrier, because the single sheath could not be inserted with an open proximal orifice and the presence of the prosthesis precludes use of a full dilator. The central carrier is also responsible for controlling the position of the prosthesis during deployment by means of reversible attachment to the proximal and distal stents.

Because the contralateral limb (usually the left) is delivered in the same sheath as the rest of the prosthesis, it must initially lie somewhere along the line of delivery system insertion. Therefore, the delivery system has to incorporate some means of pulling the left limb from the aorta or ipsilateral iliac artery into the contralateral common iliac artery, and some means of preventing premature distal stent deployment, which would prevent translocation of the left limb. The means of left limb transposition is a catheter attached to its distal end. The distal stents are prevented from deploying prematurely by small sheaths of their own. These basic design considerations are embodied in the following mechanisms.

The stent–graft is attached to the central carrier by two pairs of suture loops, one pair proximally and another pair distally. These loops pass around the inner catheter of the carrier, and cannot be released while the inner catheter remains in the carrier. The tension in the suture loops moors the stent–graft in a fixed position and orientation, relative to the carrier.

The inner diameter of the introducer sheath (18 Fr) matches the outer diameter of the central carrier at its tip. The resulting smooth transition from one to the other gives the delivery system the external profile necessary for insertion.

The sheath on the left limb stent is attached to a 2.5-Fr catheter (the left limb catheter), which is used during deployment to tow the left limb of the graft out of the aorta into the left common iliac artery. A suture loop runs the length of this catheter and holds the stent within the sheath. The compressed right limb distal stent also has a sheath, which runs along the central carrier to the outside.

Components used in the endoprosthesis

The graft component of the bifurcated prosthesis has been changed recently. The version used in most of the early experience ($n = 46$) is hand-sewn from tubular segments of Cooley Verisoft fabric (Meadox Medicals, Oakland, NJ, USA). Recently, we have begun a multicentre study in Europe with a commercial version of this device ($n = 8$), which uses a thin-walled fabric. This is woven in bifurcated form, not sewn. The two versions also have a slightly different configuration. The hand-sewn version has 16-mm wide 'bell-bottoms' on the ends of its 8-mm limbs. The thin-walled version has limbs of uniform diameter, which correspond to half the diameter of the proximal segment.

The proximal Gianturco Z stent has eight points at each end, connected by the 16 limbs in between. Coils soldered to eight of the limbs provide points of attachment for the graft. Small pairs of barbs are also mounted on four of the proximal stent limbs. One barb of each pair extends proximally to the level of the stent angles, where it bends caudally to form a hook. The other barb extends distally, parallel to the long axis of the stent. The terminal portion of this barb is curved outward, away from the long axis of the stent.

The distal stents are smaller than the proximal stent, measuring 15 mm in length and 17 mm in diameter. They have six bends at each end, and no barbs.

The proximal stent is attached to the graft so that an 8-mm segment has no fabric covering, whereas the distal stent protrudes only 2 mm beyond the distal end of the graft.

Patient selection criteria

Patient selection depends on anatomic and physiologic criteria. The anatomic criteria relate to assessment of the feasibility of endovascular aneurysm exclusion, and the physiologic criteria to assessment of the patient's cardiopulmonary reserve or the 'anaesthetic risk'. Both sets of criteria have changed as the study has progressed. We started with patients who could clearly tolerate conversion to an open repair, should that be necessary, and who clearly had suitable anatomy for endovascular exclusion. By gradually broadening the inclusion criteria (Table 7.1) we have treated patients with anatomic features that are associated with a higher chance of failed endovascular exclusion.

Patients recruited to the industry-sponsored study (Cook–Meadox trial) meet different criteria. They must be fit for operation and have favourable anatomy. However, they represent a small part of the total experience. We apply more liberal criteria to all other patients. We are prepared to treat patients with difficult anatomy, as long as they are reasonably fit, and those at high risk, as long as their anatomy is favourable.

Table 7.1 Features of arterial anatomy in the first 20 patients compared with those in the second 20

	First 20	*Second 20*
Neck angulation $>60°$	1	6
Neck length ≤ 15 mm	1	7
Iliac angulation $>90°$	2	8
Aneurysm diameter >6 cm	4	11

Table 7.2 Relative contraindications to endovascular aneurysm exclusion

Proximal
Short neck (less than 10 mm)
Angulated neck (more than 75° to the long axis of the aneurysm)
Conical neck (widening by more than 4 mm from proximal to distal)
Thrombus-lined neck
Distal
Severe iliac artery tortuosity (angulation of more than 90° at any point)
Severe iliac artery calcification
Iliac artery dilatation (wider than 16 mm) at, or distal to, the implantation site
Bilateral iliac disease

The overall assessment is multifactorial. Even the anatomic criteria are not clear-cut. The additive effect of two sets of contraindications are weighed. The first set determines the feasibility of proximal stent implantation, and includes characteristics of the neck (Table 7.2). The second set determines the feasibility of device insertion and distal stent implantation, and includes the characteristics of the iliac arteries, the common iliac artery in particular (Table 7.2). However, none of these exclusion criteria is absolute. Isolated features, such as short neck, angulated neck, or tortuous iliac arteries (Fig. 7.1), are not considered absolute grounds for exclusion.

The assessment of feasibility and subsequent prosthesis sizing both depend on the findings of preoperative imaging. The method has varied from centre to centre, depending on the technology available. In Malmö the preoperative investigation includes contrast-enhanced computed tomography (CT) with transaxial images at 3-mm intervals, and angiography with intra-arterial contrast and marked calibrating catheters. The CT data are the primary basis for graft sizing. Angiography is used mainly to assess the iliac arteries.

Procedure

The steps in bifurcated graft insertion are:

1. Bilateral access through the surgically exposed femoral arteries.
2. Heparin 10 000 units intravenously 5 min before the application of vascular clamps.
3. Placement of a cross-femoral catheter. The specific method is not

(a)

(b)

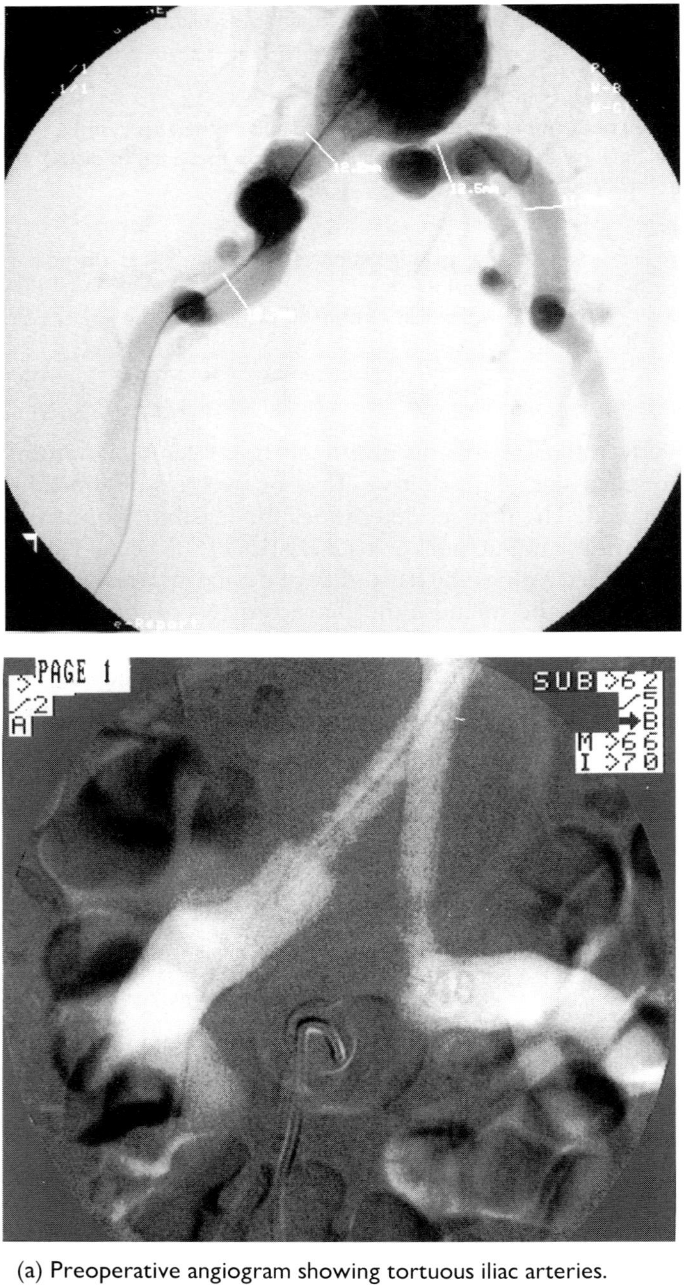

Fig. 7.1 (a) Preoperative angiogram showing tortuous iliac arteries. (b) Completion angiogram in the same patient.

important. The catheter can be passed over a guidewire, which has itself been passed through the iliac arteries from one femoral artery to the other, using angulated catheters and standard radiologic techniques. Alternatively, the catheter can be retrieved from the aneurysm with a snare or basket. Whatever the method, it is important to minimize intra-aortic manipulation. We attribute the lack of any detectable embolism to this policy.

4. Insertion of a stiff guidewire through the right femoral artery. A double-lumen dilator is used to ensure that the guidewire and cross-femoral catheter do not wind around each other in the right iliac artery.
5. Insertion of an angiographic catheter, from the left femoral artery to the level of the renal arteries.
6. Insertion of the delivery system through the right femoral artery (Fig. 7.2a).
7. Deployment of the proximal stent by withdrawal of the sheath (Fig. 7.2b). The proximal stent is usually deployed immediately beneath the renal arteries.
8. Creation of a connection between a small catheter, attached to the left limb of the graft (the left limb catheter), and the cross-femoral catheter (Fig. 7.2c). In the past this connection was made with sutures, but a screw connection has been developed for use in future systems.
9. Translocation of the left limb catheter from the right femoral artery to the left, by applying traction to the cross-femoral catheter.
10. Traction on the left limb catheter at the left groin to pull the left limb of the graft into the left common iliac artery (Fig. 7.2d).
11. Deployment of the right limb stent (Fig. 7.2e).
12. Release of the prosthesis from the delivery system by withdrawing the innermost catheter.
13. Removal of the delivery system (Fig. 7.2f).
14. Deployment of the left limb stent (Fig. 7.2g,h).

Complications: management and prevention

The first bifurcated graft insertion was in October 1993.[1] By January 1995 the series included 40 patients.[2] To show the effects of increasing experience, the results in these first 40 patients will be examined in two groups of 20 patients each. Table 7.3 compares the complication rates

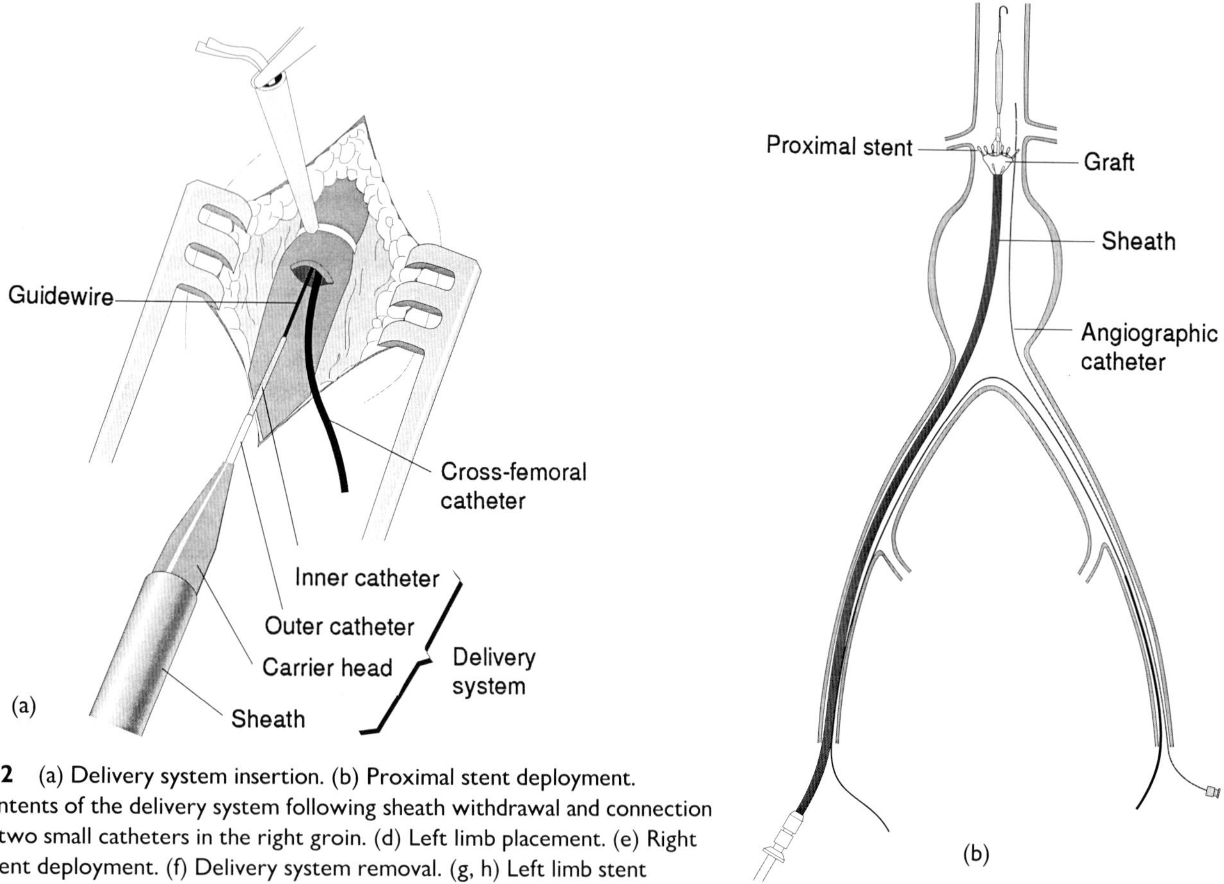

Fig. 7.2 (a) Delivery system insertion. (b) Proximal stent deployment. (c) Contents of the delivery system following sheath withdrawal and connection of the two small catheters in the right groin. (d) Left limb placement. (e) Right limb stent deployment. (f) Delivery system removal. (g, h) Left limb stent deployment.

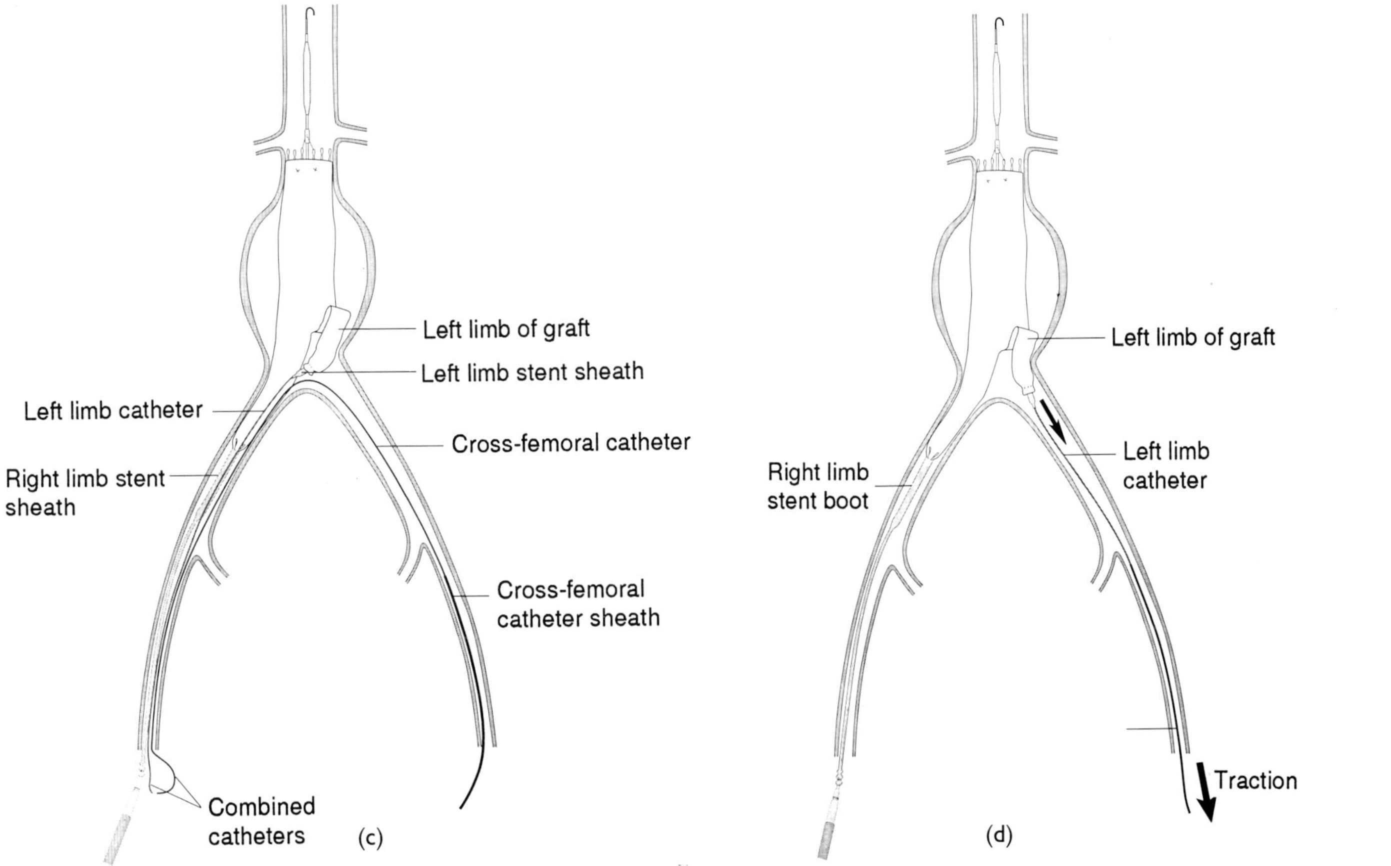

Fig. 7.2 *continued overleaf*

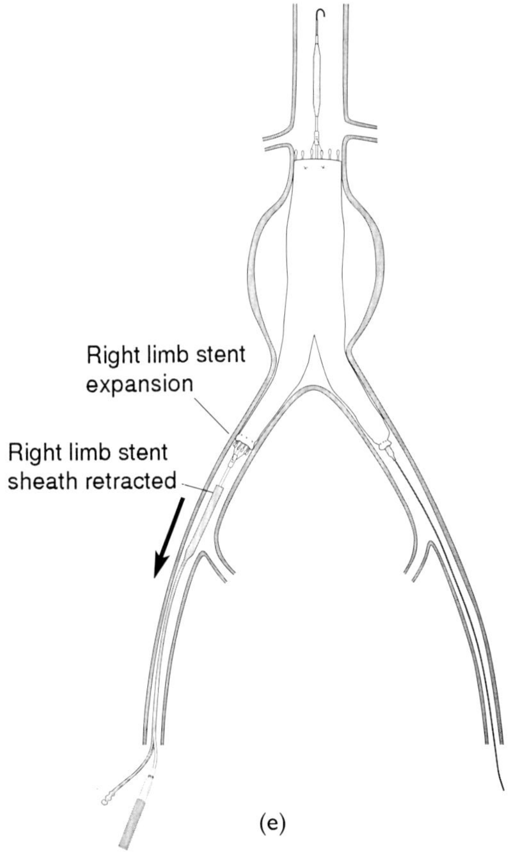
Right limb stent
expansion
Right limb stent
sheath retracted

(e)

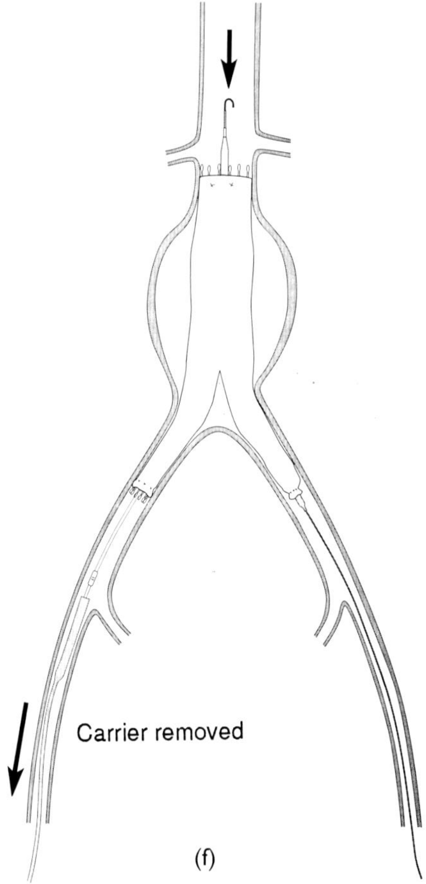
Carrier removed

(f)

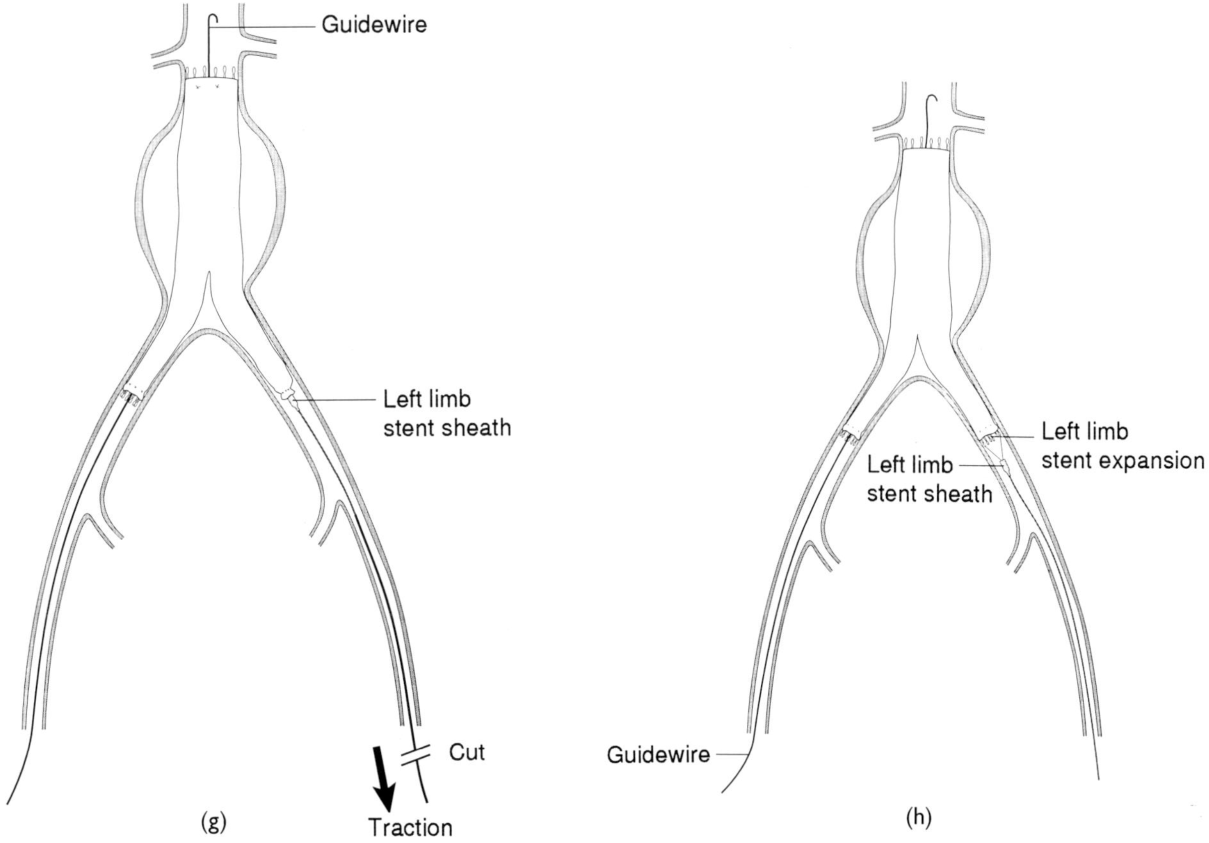

Fig. 7.2 *continued*

Table 7.3 Incidence of complications in groups 1, 2 and 3

	Group 1 ($n = 20$)	*Group 2* ($n = 20$)	*Group 3* ($n = 15$)
Failed deployment	2	1	0
Early perigraft leak	4	3	0
Twisted graft limbs	0	1	0
Graft thrombosis	5	0	0
Graft infection	1	0	0
Migration	1	0	0

in the first 40 patients (groups 1 and 2), with the subsequent experience comprising a further 14 cases.

There are striking differences between the three groups in the rates of failed deployment, perigraft leak, and graft thrombosis. These are reflected in the morbidity, mortality, and success rates shown in Table 7.4.

The most important cause of morbidity and conversion among the first 20 patients was graft thrombosis. This resulted from a high incidence of uncorrected kinking, due to the rigidity of the uncrimped, woven fabric. The routine insertion of adjunctive stents (Wallstents) eliminated the kinks and prevented graft thrombosis in all cases except one. In this case, the left limb of the graft thrombosed 3 months after

Table 7.4 Morbidity, mortality, and outcome in groups 1, 2 and 3

	Group 1 ($n = 20$)	*Group 2* ($n = 20$)	*Group 3* ($n = 15$)
Combined morbidity and mortality			
30-day	6 (30)	3 (15)	0 (0)
Overall	9 (45)	3 (15)	0 (0)
Mortality	1 (5)	2 (10)	0 (0)
Immediate conversion	2 (10)	1 (5)	0 (0)
Early conversion or death	1 (5)	2 (10)	0 (0)
Late conversion	5 (25)	0 (0)	0 (0)
Persistent perigraft leak	0 (0)	0 (0)	0 (0)
Total converted or leaking	8 (40)	3 (15)	0 (0)
Success	12 (60)	17 (85)	15 (100)

Values in parentheses are percentages.

the procedure. The cause of thrombosis was probably a combination of damage to the iliac artery and unsatisfactory deployment of the Wallstent. In the most recent eight cases the Cooley Verisoft fabric has been replaced with a crimped thin-walled woven fabric, which is less prone to kinking. However, it is doubtful whether this will eliminate the need for adjunctive stenting. The new graft is less likely to kink, but its straight-limbed configuration makes it prone to longitudinal folding, as we have discovered by means of intravascular ultrasonography. These longitudinal folds responded just as well to the insertion of Wallstents as the earlier kinks. Although Wallstent insertion is effective, it is also expensive and time consuming. For this reason, a version of the system is currently being tested in which additional stents (not Wallstents) are incorporated into the initial stent–graft delivery.

The most important cause of death was aneurysm rupture in the early postoperative period due to perigraft leak. We now take an aggressive approach to the treatment of perigraft leak. Any patient with contrast enhancement of the perigraft space on CT is investigated angiographically to identify the source, and treated.[3] None of these patients has required conversion to conventional operative repair, and none has been left with perigraft leak.

At the time of writing, 20 grafts have been in place for more than 2 years, and 20 others for more than 1 year. There have been only two significant late complications.

The first was a case of presumed graft infection, based on persistently high leukocyte count and C-reactive protein concentration, and CT findings suggestive of inflammation. This graft was removed at the time of open aneurysm repair. At operation, no purulence was seen and no organisms have grown from any of the intraoperative cultures.

The second was a case of proximal stent migration. The proximal stent migrated approximately 1 cm distally, based on serial abdominal radiography. The patient was converted to open repair. It is possible that the thrombus seen within the neck of this aneurysm impaired attachment of the proximal stent. Careful review of radiographs and CT scans has demonstrated proximal stent migration of 3–5 mm in several other patients (Fig. 7.3). This degree of migration is understandable in the light of our experience with the deliberate relocation of malpositioned stents. There have been two cases in which the proximal stent of a similar system was inadvertently placed above the level of the renal arteries. In these cases, it was possible to pull the proximal stents down approximately 5 mm before their progress was arrested by barb penetration.

(a)

(b)

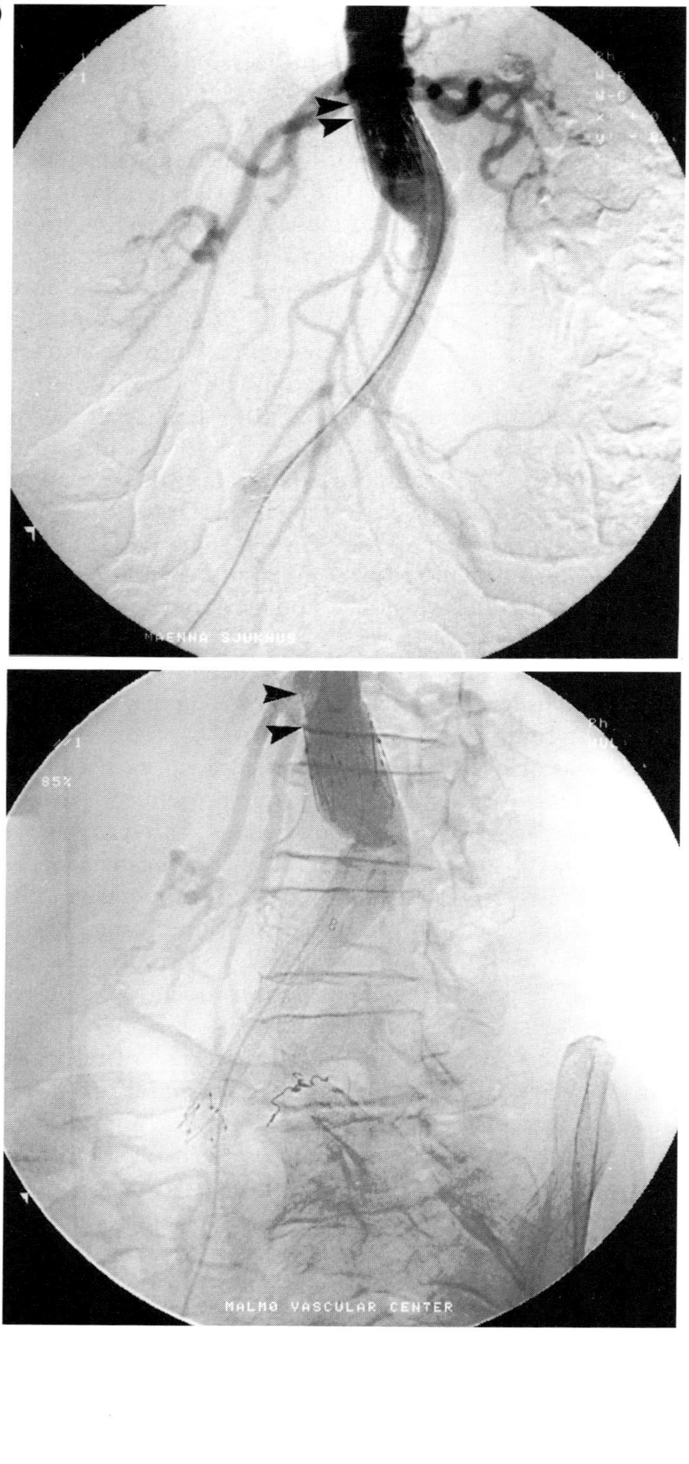

Comparison

It is clear that the distal end of a stent–graft needs to be implanted at the iliac level. Implantation in the distal aorta is neither haemostatic nor secure.[4,5] There are two alternative configurations for aortoiliac stent–grafts: the straight aortouni-iliac and the bifurcated aortobi-iliac.

A straight aortouni-iliac stent–graft is easy to implant, but it excludes flow to the contralateral limb and leaves the contralateral common iliac artery open as a potential route for flow into the aneurysm.[4–7] When a graft of this type is used to exclude an abdominal aortic aneurysm, these problems must be corrected by femorofemoral bypass and common iliac artery occlusion.

In contrast, bifurcated aortobi-iliac stent–graft insertion requires neither extra-anatomic bypass nor common iliac artery occlusion, because antegrade flow to both iliac arteries is maintained through separate graft limbs. However, the initial stent–graft deployment is more complicated, because one limb has to be placed in the contralateral common iliac artery, which lies outside the line of delivery system insertion.

All bifurcated stent–grafts currently under investigation fall into one of two categories, unitary or modular, depending on the way they solve the problem of contralateral graft limb placement. Bifurcated stent–grafts with a unitary construction are inserted as a single component. The contralateral limb of the graft is then pulled into place and stents are deployed to fix it in position.[2] Bifurcated stent–grafts with a modular construction are assembled inside the aorta from tubular components.[8] The relative advantages and disadvantages of the two methods are listed in Table 7.5.

The most common short-term problem with a modular approach has been leakage through the junction between the component stent–grafts. To create a haemostatic seal at this point the recipient site on the main stent–graft and the added limb need to be coaxial. This can be difficult to achieve when the iliac arteries enter the aorta at wide angles, or the axial orientation of the main stent–graft is slightly off, because

---

Fig. 7.3 (a) Angiogram 1 month after endovascular aneurysm repair with a bifurcated graft, showing the position of the proximal stent (arrowed) relative to the right renal artery (arrowed). (b) Angiogram in the same patient 17 months after endovascular aneurysm repair with a bifurcated graft, showing distal migration of the proximal stent (arrowed) relative to the renal artery (arrowed).

Table 7.5 Differences between modular and unitary approaches to bifurcated stent–graft reconstruction of the aorta

Modular	*Unitary*
Requires catheterization of the recipient site on the main graft	Requires insertion of a cross-femoral catheter
Simple stent–graft components and delivery systems	More complex graft construction and delivery system
Nonidentical limbs easy to customize from stock components	Customization must be performed at the time of graft manufacture
Graft–graft junction created within the aneurysm; potential site for leakage and breakage	Bifurcation sewn, knitted, or woven into the graft; predictable durability
Easy to deliver in a fully stented form	Difficult to deliver fully stented; additional stents must be added as needed.

or the axial orientation of the main stent–graft is slightly off, because the fully stented components lack flexibility. This accounts for the high rates of leakage seen initially with devices of this kind. Another problem has been disassembly.[8] In approximately 10% of cases the component stent–grafts have separated, resulting in leakage through the gap.

In our experience, the main drawback of the unitary approach has been the lack of stent support in the graft limbs. The bifurcated stent–graft could not be delivered in a fully stented form using the current delivery system. Additional stents had to be added once the graft was in place. Systems are now being tested which address this problem by incorporating the additional stents along with delivery of the primary stent–graft.

References

1. Chuter TAM, Donayre C, Wendt G. Bifurcated stent–grafts for endovascular repair of abdominal aortic aneurysm: preliminary case reports. *Surg Endosc* 1994; 8: 800–2.
2. Chuter TAM, Risberg B, Hopkinson BR *et al.* Clinical experience with a bifurcated endovascular graft for abdominal aortic aneurysm repair. *J Vasc Surg* (in press).
3. Ivancev K, Chuter TAM, Lindblad B, Lindh M, Brunkwall J, Risberg B. Endovascular treatment of perigraft perfusion following transfemoral aneurysm repair. *World J Surg* 1996; 20: 673–8.

4. Parodi JC. Endovascular repair of abdominal aortic aneurysms and other arterial lesions. *J Vasc Surg* 1995; **21**: 549–57.
5. White G. Endoluminal grafting of AAA: review of more than 100 cases. Presented to the International Symposium on Vascular Diagnosis and Intervention, Miami, FL, 31 January 1996.
6. Yusuf SW, Baker DM, Hind RE *et al.* Endoluminal transfemoral abdominal aortic aneurysm repair with aorto-uni-iliac graft and femorofemoral bypass. *Br J Surg* 1995; **82**: 916.
7. Marin ML, Veith FL, Cynamon J *et al.* Initial experience with transluminally placed endovascular grafts for the treatment of complex vascular lesions. *Ann Surg* 1995; **222**: 449–69.
8. Stelter W. Transluminal repair of AAA with the Stentor system. Presented to the International Endovascular Symposium, Sydney, 12 December 1995.

8

The EndoVascular Technologies system

Ivo A.M.J. Broeders, Jan D. Blankensteijn and Bert C. Eikelboom

Department of Vascular Surgery, Academic Hospital Utrecht, Heidelberglaan 100, 3584 CX Utrecht, The Netherlands

Introduction

The medical device development company EndoVascular Technologies (EVT), located in Menlo Park, California, was founded in July 1989. EVT focuses on transfemoral endovascular repair of abdominal aortic aneurysm. The company has further developed and patented the concept of endovascular aneurysm treatment from Lazarus.[1] The principle of this concept is fixation of an endoluminal graft to the arterial wall. This is achieved by producing a prosthesis that contains self-expanding attachment systems with fixation pins. These pins are driven into the wall of nondilated segments of the infrarenal aorta above and below the aneurysm by means of balloon inflation.

After completion of *in vitro* and animal testing, the first *in vivo* implantation of a Tube Endograft occurred in February 1993. The first Bifurcated Endograft procedure followed in September 1994. At present the EVT Endograft is the only device for endovascular aneurysm repair that has received Food and Drug Administration (FDA) approval for clinical investigation in the USA. In December 1995 implantations were started with third-generation Endograft prosthesis and delivery systems. This chapter discusses the design of the Endograft, the implantation procedure, patient selection and clinical trials, and the results of implantation of the first- and second-generation Endograft endoprosthesis.

Design of the Endograft and implantation utilities

The latest generation of EVT Endograft systems for the treatment of AAA include the implants and catheter delivery system as well as the devices that have been developed to assist the implantation procedures. These devices are the EVT marker board, AngioScale angiography catheter and expandable sheath. The contralateral torque catheter and iliac balloon catheter are additional devices required for the bifurcated version of the Endograft.

The Tube and Bifurcated Endograft

The Endograft consists of a vascular graft and proximal and distal attachment systems. The attachment systems are constructed to meet the objective of providing a self-expanding endoluminal vascular graft that is independent of the inward radial forces of the vascular wall to maintain its optimal position. The superior attachment system of the Tube and Bifurcated Endograft (Fig. 8.1) and the inferior attachment system of the Tube Endograft are identical. The metal frame is fashioned in a zig-zag configuration and is self-expanding. When this frame is released from a compressed state it increases its diameter by increasing the angles between the straight segments.

Because the diameter of the metal frame in resting position exceeds that of the vascular segment at the implantation side, the attachment system will maintain an outward radial force on the arterial wall. In

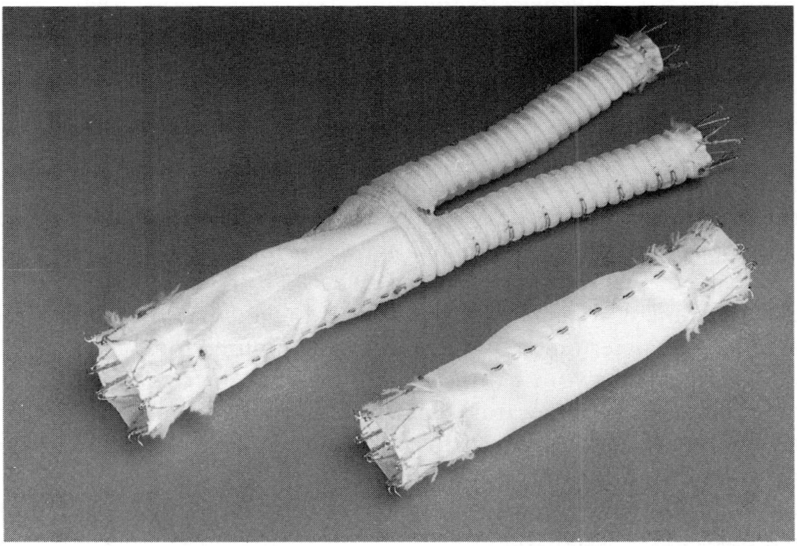

Fig. 8.1 Tube and Bifurcated Endograft.

this the attachment system differs from vascular stents which are balloon expanded to a static diameter during implantation and depend on inward forces of the arterial wall to maintain position. The EVT Endograft attachment systems contain eight angled hooks which project outward in a radial direction. They penetrate the aortic wall with the aid of balloon distension to fix the graft permanently in its deployed position and prevent migration.

The iliac attachment systems of the Bifurcated Endograft are different from its aortic attachment system. Although they have an identically designed zig-zag self-expanding frame, they have only three hooks to keep the graft in position.

The attachment systems are hand-sewn to the vascular graft. The vascular graft of the tube endoprosthesis and the 'trunk' section of the bifurcated endoprosthesis are composed of noncrimped woven polyester. The 'limbs' of the bifurcated endoprosthesis are crimped. Animal studies have demonstrated that crimping of the limb segments offers the vascular graft more resistance to the kinking or angulation caused by tortuosity of the common iliacs.[2] Thin clusters of polyester 'fuzz' are sewn to the outside of the vascular graft at the proximal and distal ends to promote tissue attachment and sealing. Platinum radiopaque markers are sewn along the length of the tube graft 180° apart, and extend along the lateral sides of the limbs of the bifurcated prosthesis. The markers on the limbs have a rectangular design and are sewn on the graft perpendicular to the limb axis. This allows detection of rotation without markers on the medial side of the limbs.

The marker board

The EVT markerboard is a radiolucent plastic casing that contains two radiopaque bars. The bars can be moved up and down by remote control. The angle of the bars relative to the long axis of the casing can be changed. The radiopaque bars serve as a tool in the positioning of the attachment systems. The position of the aneurysm relative to the spine can be determined by preoperative computed tomography (CT), especially when two- or three-dimensional reconstructions are available. This helps the operating team to position the fluoroscopy unit and to move the radiopaque bars to the area of deployment without using contrast. Fine adjustments of the radiopaque bars require peroperative angiography but repositioning of the fluoroscopy unit with resulting parallax can be avoided in this way.

The AngioScale angiography catheter

The length of the selected endoprosthesis has to be determined from measurements on the preoperative CT scan and angiography. At the beginning of the procedure angiography with the EVT AngioScale angiography catheter is used to verify the correct size of the implant '*in vivo*'. This 6-Fr multihole pigtail catheter contains 15 to 25 platinum marker bands at intervals of 10 mm. When introducing the angiography catheter in the area of implantation, the radiopaque bands will allow measurements that are not disturbed by the effects of magnification, tortuosity, or parallax.

The expandable sheath

The EVT expandable sheath serves two purposes. First, it facilitates the introduction of the delivery system by straightening out the common and external iliac, thus dilating minor areas of narrowing and minimizing vessel tortuosity along the route of introduction. Second, the valve system will help to reduce blood loss during the implantation procedure.

The valve system is composed of spring and thumbwheel diaphragm valves which are a few centimetres apart. Haemostasis is maintained by introducing instruments into the chamber between the valves by opening the spring valve. Access into the sheath is then obtained by opening the thumbwheel valve. The expandable sheath has a 27-Fr outer diameter which contains a tapered dilator to fully expand the sheath. After removing the dilator the delivery system can be introduced.

The delivery system

The EVT delivery system is a 23-Fr coaxial catheter that enables introduction and implantation of a compressed Endograft. The delivery system is a co-axial system composed of a single-lumen main catheter, an inner triple-lumen balloon catheter and an outer jacket. The Endograft is folded around the balloon catheter. Its attachment systems are housed in a compressed state by superior and inferior metal capsules. The capsule of the superior attachment system is fixed to the balloon catheter. The capsule of the inferior or ipsilateral attachment system is fixed to the main catheter. The system contains two handles. The distal handle is connected to the balloon catheter and controls movement of the superior capsule and thereby the release of the superior attachment system. The proximal handle is connected to the main catheter. It enables retraction of the inferior capsule. The capsule of the contralateral attachment system of the Bifurcated Endograft is connected to a pull-wire assembly which is guided in the opposite direction to the contralateral limb and runs along the prosthesis beyond the tip of the delivery system. The jacket covers the capsules, the endoprosthesis with pull-wire assembly (bifurcated graft), and the distal part of the main catheter. It can be retracted over the main catheter.

The contralateral torque catheter (Bifurcated Endograft)

The EVT contralateral torque catheter is a single-lumen flexible tube that can be inserted over the pull-wire assembly through a 12-Fr introducer sheath. It has a locking system at the distal end to hook on to the contralateral capsule. A luer lock mechanism at the proximal end helps to maintain haemostasis. The contralateral torque catheter serves to correct for twist in the contralateral limb and is subsequently used to retract the contralateral capsule to release the contralateral limb attachment system.

The iliac balloon catheter (Bifurcated Endograft)

The hooks of the distal attachment systems of the bifurcated prosthesis have to be implanted into the arterial wall with a separate balloon catheter. The EVT iliac balloon catheter is introduced over the wire through the 12-Fr introducer sheath on the contralateral side and the through main sheath on the ipsilateral side. The balloon diameter ranges from 9 to 13 mm. Because balloon size can be adjusted to the diameter of the distal attachment systems, optimal control of distal attachment system implantation can be achieved.

The implantation procedure

Patient preparation

Implantation is performed under regional or general anaesthesia in a fully equipped operating room or in an angiography suite that has been appropriately designed to serve as a fully functional surgical operating theatre. The marker board is positioned under the patient on a radiolucent operating table. Operating field preparation and draping is configured to permit immediate conversion to standard abdominal aneurysm surgery should this become necessary. Either a mobile or a ceiling-mounted fluoroscopy unit with dual-screen road-mapping capability and video recording is required. Under fluoroscopy control the radiopaque bars of the marker board are moved to the estimated area of implantation.

The Tube Endograft

In most cases a preferable access side can be selected on the basis of anatomic details of the iliac and common femoral arteries. Factors that interfere with smooth introduction of the expandable sheet and delivery system are occlusive arterial disease and pronounced tortuosity or angulation of these arteries. If both sides are suitable for access, a right-handed surgeon will select the right common femoral artery (Fig. 8.2).

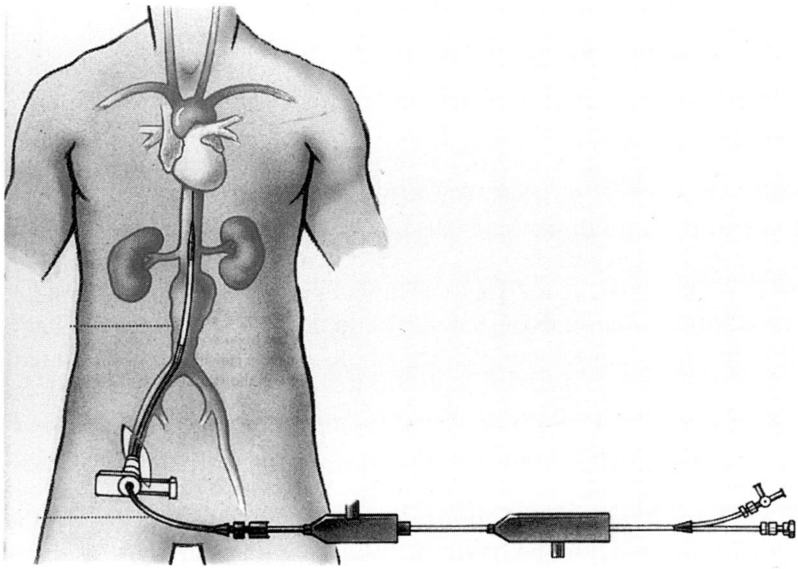

Fig. 8.2 Introduction of the Endovascular Grafting System®.

All movements of guidewires and implantation devices are performed under fluoroscopy control.

The common femoral artery is exposed to provide device access. When preoperative imaging has revealed tortuosity of the iliac artery, ligation of the circumflex iliac and deep epigastric arteries together with partial incision of the inguinal ligament will be helpful in mobilization. A guidewire is introduced to allow positioning of the AngioScale catheter. An angiogram and road-map are obtained and the radiopaque bars are positioned at the exact levels of deployment. Length measurements are performed to confirm selection of the correct graft size. The AngioScale catheter is replaced by a 0.035-inch superstiff EX guidewire and the patient is heparinized with 5000 units heparin intravenously. The expandable sheath is introduced over the superstiff guidewire through a transverse arteriotomy in the common femoral artery and positioned in the upper common iliac artery. The dilator is advanced and left in place for 1 min to expand the sheath fully. The mean arterial pressure is reduced to 60–70 mmHg. After removal of the dilator, the delivery system is introduced and advanced into the aorta until the hooks of the superior attachment system are positioned at the upper radiopaque bar, which has been placed just below the most caudal renal artery ostium. The outer jacket is retracted until its tip marker projects over the central part of the tube graft. Using the control knob on the distal handle, the superior capsule is advanced upward to deploy the proximal attachment system. The balloon is positioned centrally in the attachment system and inflated with 20% dilute contrast up to 2 atmospheres. The jacket is now fully retracted (Fig. 8.3). Two more inflations of 1 min are performed. During inflation, correction for twist can be made by rotating the main shaft relative to the balloon catheter. If necessary the position of the distal attachment system can also be corrected. An endolocking mechanism prevents sliding of the inferior attachment system out of its capsule.

After balloon deflation the balloon catheter is advanced to stabilize a pusher button platform beneath the hooks of the inferior attachment system. The inferior capsule is retracted by turning the control knob on the proximal handle and the inferior attachment system is released. The balloon is repositioned within the deployed inferior attachment system and repeatedly inflated to drive the hooks into the aortic wall. If the aorta bifurcation configuration prevents full expansion of the balloon catheter, a 'kissing balloon' technique can be used by inserting a second balloon catheter through the contralateral limb. The delivery system is retracted into the jacket and removed. A postimplantation

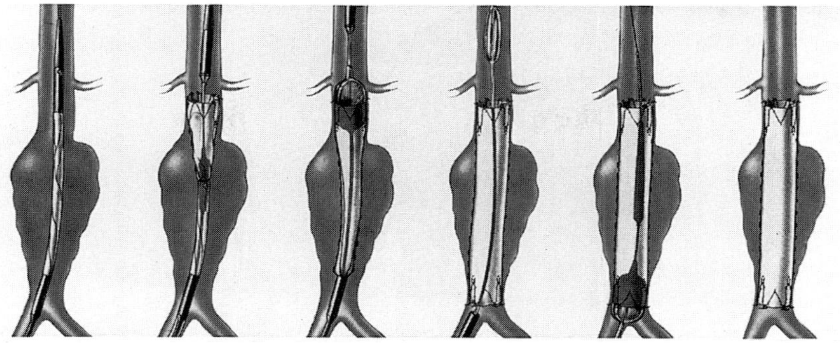

Fig. 8.3 Implantation of a Tube Endograft.

angiography is performed in anteroposterior and lateral direction to exclude perigraft flow. The expandable sheath is then removed and the arteriotomy and wound are closed.

The Bifurcated Endograft

The common femoral artery is exposed on both sides. The procedures of length measurements and positioning of the proximal radiopaque bar are similar to those of tube graft implantation. Markers are placed on the monitor screen to mark the position for deployment of the iliac attachment systems. The patient is heparinized. The expandable sheath is introduced on the preferable access side and a 12-Fr sheath is inserted into the contralateral femoral artery. A snare loop is introduced through the 12-Fr sheath and the loop is positioned just proximal to the aortic bifurcation. The J tip of the pull-wire assembly is introduced at the ipsilateral side and passed through the loop (Fig. 8.4). The snare loop with the captured pull-wire assembly is pulled out through the sheath. While maintaining tension on the distal end of the pull-wire assembly on the contralateral side, the proximal end of the pull-wire assembly followed by the delivery system is introduced through the expandable sheath at the ipsilateral side. The delivery system is advanced into the aorta until the bifurcated prosthesis has passed the aortic bifurcation.

The outer jacket is retracted completely. The iliac limbs are then placed distally into the respective iliac arteries by retracting the main catheter and the pull-wire assembly.

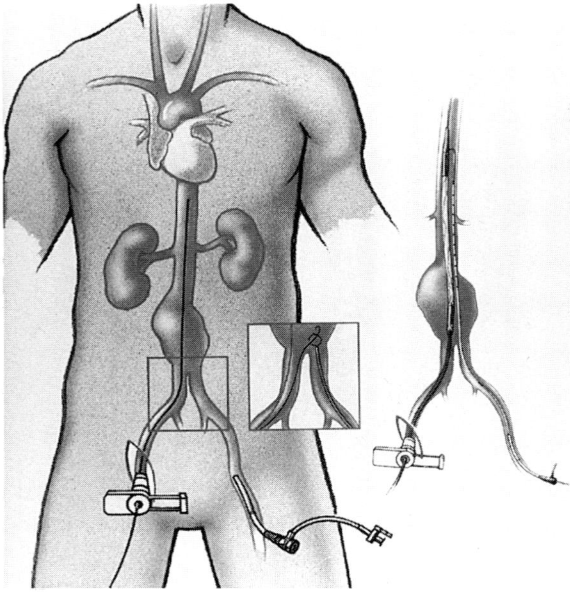

Fig. 8.4 The snare loop captures the pull-wire assembly.

A crucial part of the implantation procedure (Fig. 8.5) is correction for torsion of the superior part of the trunk at this point. Once the tension is lowered to a mean of 60–70 mmHg, the aortic attachment system is positioned, released, and fixed in position by balloon inflation. During inflation any remaining twist in the trunk of the prosthesis is corrected. The torque catheter is introduced through the 12-Fr

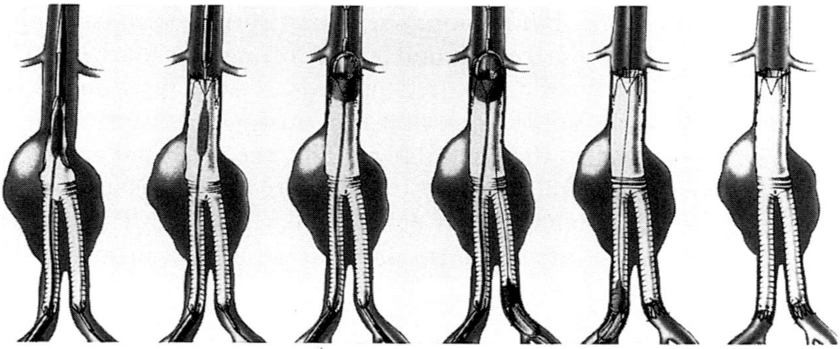

Fig. 8.5 Implantation of a Bifurcated Endograft.

sheath and hooked on to the contralateral capsule. A locking mechanism connected to the pull-wire assembly prevents premature deployment of the contralateral iliac attachment system. The contralateral limb is corrected for twist by manipulating the torque catheter, and the attachment system is positioned. The torque catheter and the outer part of the pull-wire assembly are retracted to strip the capsule off the attachment system, leaving a guidewire in place within the graft limb. After removal of the torque catheter the iliac balloon catheter is positioned over the guidewire into the attachment system and repeatedly inflated at 2 atmospheres.

The iliac balloon catheter is removed and the position of the outer jacket and expandable sheath on the ipsilateral side is checked to be certain that they are below the iliac bifurcation and will not interfere with implantation of the ipsilateral iliac attachment system. The implantation procedure of this attachment system is similar to that of the inferior attachment system of the Tube Endograft, except for the balloon inflation. Full inflation of the aortic balloon may damage the common iliac artery. For this reason the delivery system is removed and balloon inflation is performed with the iliac balloon catheter. The sheaths are removed after performing control angiography and the arteriotomies and wounds are closed.

Patient selection and clinical trials

Patient selection

Treatment of the abdominal aortic aneurysm by endoprosthesis implantation is confined to the infrarenal aorta. The physical condition of the patient should allow abdominal aneurysm repair in case of conversion to standard surgery. The main criteria for patient selection apply to anatomic details of the vascular tree between the renal arteries and the iliac bifurcation. A nondilated segment of at least 15 mm is needed between the most caudal renal artery ostium and the beginning of aneurysmal dilatation to position the superior attachment system safely. Implantation the inferior attachment system of the Tube Endograft requires an inferior 'cuff' of 12 mm between the distal end of the aneurysm and the aortic bifurcation. The diameter of the superior and inferior neck may vary between 18.5 and 26.4 mm. The available graft lengths are 9.0–16.0 cm, with 5-mm increments. At least one femoral and iliac artery system must be accessible by a 23-F delivery system. If only the iliac artery can accommodate the 23-Fr delivery system, a vascular graft is temporarily anastomosed upon the external iliac artery to allow entry into the vascular lumen.

Only a minority of patients with an abdominal aneurysm appear to meet these criteria. Data reported from two centres demonstrated that 13–15% of the candidates were suitable for Tube Endograft implantation, even after preselection by referring surgeons.[2,3] In most cases patients were rejected because of absence of an adequate inferior neck. The introduction of the Bifurcated Endograft has overcome this problem and will allow a much larger percentage of abdominal aneurysms to be treated with an endoprosthesis.

Implantation of the iliac attachment systems of the Bifurcated Endograft requires at least 15 mm of nonaneurysmal common iliac arteries at corresponding levels. Common iliac artery diameters may range from 9.5–13.4 mm. The bifurcated graft can be produced in lengths from 11.0–19.5 cm.

Table 8.1 Inclusion and exclusion criteria.

Inclusion criteria	*Exclusion criteria*
Age 21 years or more	Ruptured aneurysm
Male or infertile female	Active infection
Superior neck at least 15 mm long	Weight over 159 kg
Inferior neck at least 12 mm long (tube graft) or common iliac necks at least 15 mm long (bifurcated graft)	Currently being treated with another investigational drug or device
Anaesthesia clearance (class 1–4)	Significant femoral or iliac artery occlusive disease or ectasia requiring aortofemoral/ aortoiliac bypass
Life expectancy more than 2 years	
One femoral or iliac artery permitting access by a 23-Fr (7.7-mm) device	Requires additional vascular or nonvascular surgical procedure at time of operation
Contralateral femoral or iliac artery permitting access by a 12-Fr (4.0-mm) device (bifurcated graft only)	Evidence of thromboatheromatous projections in the flow channel
	Transplant subjects or subjects requiring organ transplant
	Noniatrogenic bleeding diathesis
	Aneurysm etiology other than degenerative or arteriosclerosis

CT and arterial angiography with a calibrated catheter are required to obtain the preoperative length and diameter measurements. Two-dimensional multiplanar reconstructions of spiral CT images are of great help to size the graft.[4] A complete overview of inclusion and exclusion criteria for the clinical trials sanctioned by the FDA is presented in Table 8.1.

Clinical studies

Patients selected for Endograft implantation are enrolled in one of the three clinical studies that are being supervised by EVT.

Patients who require a bifurcated graft are included in a phase 1 clinical study in the USA. The object of this study is to evaluate the short-term safety and efficacy of the Bifurcated Endograft. The safety will be evaluated based on rates of occurrence of procedure- or device-related complications. These are complications that may ensue with endovascular as well as conventional aneurysm repair. Efficacy is evaluated by observing device-specific complications. These include implantation failure, arterial trauma, perigraft and branch flow with aneurysm enlargement, prosthesis twist, dilatation or migration, and attachment system dysfunction. The study is being performed in five selected centres. As soon as sufficient data have been gathered, EVT will submit a phase 2 study protocol to the FDA to investigate long-term safety and efficacy in comparison with conventional aneurysm repair.

Candidates for a Tube Endograft who are treated in the USA are enrolled in the phase 2 clinical study EnACT–T (Endovascular Aneurysm Clinical Trial – Tube). This study will evaluate the safety and efficacy of endovascular repair with the Tube Endograft compared with standard surgical repair. A comparison will be made based on complications common to both types of operation in the first year. Patients are observed in concurrent control groups. Candidates suitable for standard tube graft repair with infrarenal clamping but who do not meet the criteria for endovascular tube graft repair form the control group. Some 120 patients will be enrolled in each group. Efficacy of the device will be evaluated based on rates of device-specific complications and will be fulfilled separately from the concurrent control study.

Patients treated with a Tube or Bifurcated Endograft outside the USA are enrolled in an international clinical study that is designed to

Table 8.2 Clinical study protocol.

	Preoperative	*Discharge*	*6 weeks*	*3 months*	*6 months*	*12 months*	*18 months*	*2 years or annually*
Physical examination	Yes	Yes	Yes	In case of PGF	Yes	Yes	In case of PGF	Yes
Ankle: brachial index	Yes	Yes	Yes		Yes	Yes		Yes
Laboratory investigation	Yes	Yes	Yes					
Arterial angiography	Yes	*						
Ultrasonography		Yes		In case of PGF	Yes	Yes	In case of PGF	Yes
Contrast-enhanced CT	Yes	Yes		In case of PGF	Yes	Yes	In case of PGF	Yes
Abdominal radiography		Yes		Yes	Yes	Yes		Yes

*Only if indicated; PGF, perigraft flow.

establish the long-term safety and efficacy of the device and the procedure. Some 200 candidates for tube and 200 for bifurcated endoprostheses will enter this study.

A protocol for evaluation before, during and after operation has been designed to apply to all candidates for endovascular repair in all three studies (Table 8.2).

Contrast-enhanced CT and ultrasonography give information on aneurysm and prosthesis dimensions and may reveal the origin of perigraft flow. Abdominal radiography is used to evaluate the integrity of the attachment systems and to exclude migration of the prosthesis. All radiological and ultrasonographic studies are reviewed by a core laboratory to ensure unbiased analysis of imaging data and evaluation of the status of the endografts in all subjects.

Results of previous studies

In the 2-year period before the commencement of the current studies discussed above, a total of 102 tube and 12 bifurcated grafts were implanted worldwide. Based on clinical experience, significant changes have been made to the design of the prosthesis and delivery system. Following FDA approval, clinical studies were restarted in December 1995 with a third-generation device. Results have been published from a total of 77 first- and second-generation Tube Endografts. Forty-six of these grafts were implanted in 13 centres in the USA, as part of a phase 1 clinical study.[5] Thirty-one patients were incorporated in the international clinical study in centres in Australia, England, The Netherlands, and Sweden.[6]

Implantation was successful in 69 patients (90%). Two additional patients were converted during follow-up (3%). There was one procedure-related death (1%). In this patient puncture of the contralateral femoral artery led to intimal damage and arterial insufficiency of the lower limb. Local exploration, limb revascularization, and fasciotomy had to be performed. Renal failure developed and the patient died on the 11th postoperative day from multiorgan failure. The average duration of the procedure, from incision to skin closure, was 194 min for the US patients. The mean hospital stay was 3.8 days; 72% of patients with a successful procedure were discharged within 3 days. The median duration of the procedure at the international centres was 125 min; the median hospital stay was 7 days.

Device-related complications included implantation failure, vascular damage, and thromboembolic complications, perigraft flow, and attachment system fractures.

Implantation failure

In eight patients (10%) implantation was unsuccessful. Five failures occurred with the first-generation Tube Endograft. Using the second-generation Tube Endograft, 94% of procedures were completed successfully. Failures were caused by a short distal neck, an endoprosthesis too short leading to perigraft flow, proximal displacement, subintimal deployment, and iliac stenosis (four cases).

Vascular damage and thromboembolic complications

Damage to the femoral or iliac arteries was reported in 12 cases (16%). Local repair at the level of the arteriotomy could be accomplished in eight instances. A femorofemoral (one) or iliofemoral (two) bypass was performed in three patients. One procedure was converted to standard aortobifemoral repair. Thromboembolic events were noted in five patients. In four this was manifested by petechiae in the skin of the lower limbs. In one case a toe amputation was performed after several weeks.

Perigraft flow

Leakage of blood into the aneurysm sac was found by postimplantation peroperative angiography, postoperative ultrasonography, and contrast-enhanced CT in 24 (34%) of 70 cases. The source of perigraft flow could be identified at the proximal attachment side in nine patients and at the distal attachment side in 13. In the remaining two patients perigraft flow may have been caused by side branches remaining patent. Eleven (46%) of the 24 leaks resolved spontaneously. One patient was converted on the second postoperative day. Five patients were treated with balloon angioplasty; this was successful in one case and in another the procedure was converted to standard surgery. Seven patients still had perigraft flow at the last control evaluation without signs of prosthesis malfunction or aneurysm enlargement.

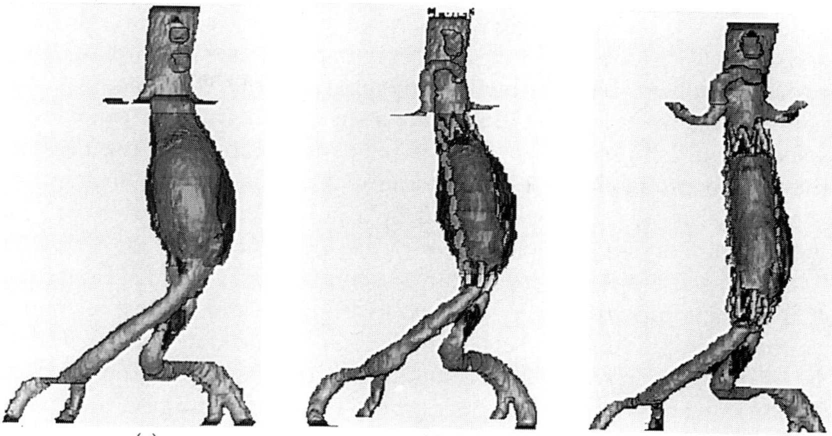

(a) (b) (c)

Fig. 8.6 Three-dimensional scan (a) before the procedure, (b) after operation, and (c) at 1-year follow-up.

Attachment system fractures

An attachment system fracture was discovered after graft explant and conversion to standard aneurysm repair in one patient who demonstrated a 1-cm distal migration of the superior attachment system. Immediate review of all follow-up abdominal radiographs that had previously been reported as normal revealed additional fractures in some of the patients, all of whom were doing well. Clinical studies were suspended immediately. The design of the attachment system has been improved and intensive fatigue laboratory testing has given confidence that the problem has been solved. After approval by the FDA, clinical studies were restarted in December 1995 with a third-generation device.

In a total of 11 patients (16%) with a first- or second-generation tube graft, attachment system breaks were discovered. As noted, one conversion was performed because of persistent perigraft flow. In the remaining patients no adverse clinical consequences have been noted yet (Fig. 8.6).

Discussion

Phase 1 clinical studies have demonstrated that abdominal aneurysms suitable for endovascular repair can be treated safely and efficiently with the EVT Tube Endograft. Several factors have contributed to the satisfactory results. All investigators involved in the implantation procedures have been trained by members of the EVT medical and engineering team. This training consisted of instruction on patient selection and clinical study design, device function, table-top deployment, flow model deployment, and animal training. In the near future the animal model will be replaced by a pulsatile flow model with an artificial aneurysm mimicking *in vivo* circumstances.

All implantation procedures have been attended by an EVT support team. Their growing experience contributed to the success of many endograft implantations. Selection of suitable candidates has proven to be of vital importance. All investigating centres have selected patients by the same criteria, and preoperative CT scans and angiograms were reviewed by the EVT medical team before approval on implantation.

The development of the Bifurcated Endograft will increase the proportion of patients with an abdominal aneurysm suitable for endovascular repair with an EVT Endograft. Preliminary experience is promising but has also demonstrated that implantation of a bifurcated graft is quite a challenge compared with the tube graft, because tortuosity of the iliac vessels may induce torsion on the individual segments of the endoprosthesis. Advanced imaging techniques such as CT and magnetic resonance imaging with three-dimensional reconstruction will contribute to selection of the correct candidates for this device.

Several important questions on endovascular aneurysm repair remain unanswered. Volume scans have demonstrated that the thrombus mass and the total aneurysm volume actually shrink after successful implantation of a Tube Endograft.[7] This suggests that the primary goal of the procedure – eradication of risk of rupture – can be achieved. On the other hand, vascular disease may proceed and lead to increase in the diameter of the aorta in the region of the attachment sites. Also the long-term effects of persisting perigraft or branch flow require further study. Delayed rupture has already been reported after endovascular aneurysm repair with a different type of device.[8]

Treating patients with a technology of which the long-term safety and efficacy have not yet been established can be justified only when supported by a prospective multicentre clinical study that is controlled in an efficient and reliable manner. The EVT studies, under control of the FDA and supported by a radiology laboratory, meet these requirements and have the potential to answer the above questions.

References

1. Lazarus HM. Intraluminal graft device: system and method. *US Patent No. 4,787,799*. 1988.
2. Quiñones-Baldrich WJ, Deaton DH, Mitchell RS *et al.* Preliminary experience with the Endovascular Technologies bifurcated endovascular aortic prosthesis in a calf model. *J Vasc Surg* 1995; **22**: 370–81.
3. Balm R, Eikelboom BC, De Smet AMGA, Mali WPThM. Treatment of an infrarenal aortic aneurysm with an endoprosthesis introduced via the femoral artery; first experience in nine patients in the Netherlands. *Ned Tijdschr Geneeskd* 1995; **139**: 717–22.
4. Balm R, Eikelboom BC, van Leeuwen MS, Noordzij J. Spiral CT–angiography of the aorta. *Eur J Vasc Surg* 1994; **8**: 544–51.
5. Moore WS, Rutherford RB. Transfemoral endovascular repair of abdominal aortic aneurysm. Results of the North American EVT phase 1 trial. *J Vasc Surg* 1996; **23**: 543–53.
6. Balm R, Eikelboom BC, May J, Bell PRF, Swedenborg J, Collin J. Early experience with transfemoral endovascular aneurysm management (TEAM) in the treatment of aortic aneurysms. *Eur J Vasc Endovasc Surg* 1996; **11**: 214–20.
7. Balm R, Kaatee R, Blankensteijn JD, Mali WPTM, Eikelboom BC. CT–angiography of aortic abdominal aneurysms after transfemoral endovascular aneurysm management: diameter and volume management. *Eur J Vasc Endovasc Surg* 1996 (in press).
8. Lumsden AB, Allen RC, Chaikof EL *et al.* Delayed rupture of aortic aneurysms following endovascular stent grafting. *Am J Surg* 1995; **170**: 174–8.

9

The Corvita system

Jean Pierre E. Dereume and Jose Ferreira

Department of Vascular Pathology, Erasmus University Hospital (ULB), Route de Lennik 808, 1070 Brussels, Belgium

Design of the endoprosthesis and delivery system

The Corvita endovascular graft

The Corvita endoluminal graft (CEG) is composed of a metallic, self-expanding, braided wire stent and an inner liner comprised of polycarbonate–urethane microfibres.[1] The inner liner is bound to the stent by means of a polycarbonate–urethane adhesive.

The metallic stent

The metallic stent design was first described by Didcott[2] for oesophageal applications in 1967. The braid is made from cobalt–chromium–nickel alloy wires with diameters ranging from 0.10 to 0.23 mm. Some 24 to 96 wires are braided simultaneously with specially adjusted braiding machines in a diamond patterned, double-helical spring structure (Fig. 9.1). The spring properties of the metallic wire are enhanced by precipitation hardening in an inert environment. Following heat treatment, a special surface treatment is applied to ensure a surgical, implant grade, surface quality with low surface contamination.

To achieve secure placement of the device at the predetermined site, as well as to provide a blood-tight seal against the native artery, the metallic stent is designed to exert a radial pressure against the vessel wall. The radial pressure depends on several physical parameters including the ratio of oversizing the CEG in relation to the vessel diameter, the diameter of the wires, the number of wires, the angle at which the stent is braided, the type of braiding (one over and one under

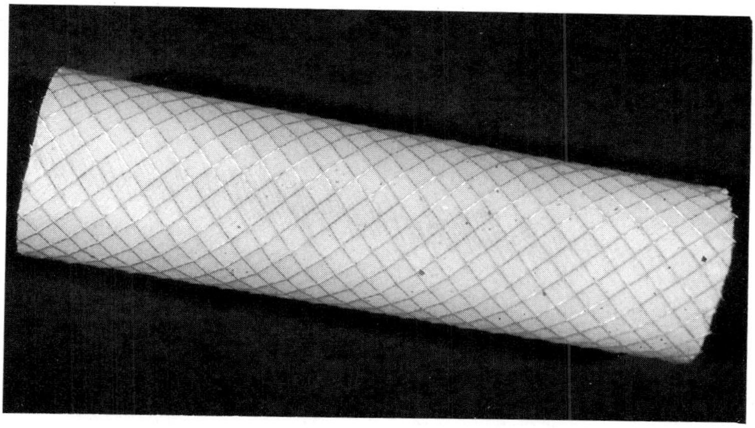

Fig. 9.1 Early version of a tubular 30-mm diameter endoluminal graft with 36 wires.

versus two over and two under), the thickness of the liner, the type of alloy, and the heat treatment process.

To enhance the anchoring of the CEG further, the ends are flared slightly outward, thereby causing the wires to embed in the vessel wall and preventing the CEG from migrating upstream or downstream. The flare is designed into the device by controlling wire tensions during braiding, by means of artificial mechanical deformation and by other proprietary procedures (Fig. 9.2). More recent designs of the CEG utilize paired wires instead of single wires to enhance radial pressure further (Fig. 9.2).[3]

Another design also under investigation makes use of hyperbolic geometry (Fig. 9.3): both ends of the stent increase continuously in diameter from a central locus, thereby enabling the user to cut the device to the appropriate length and diameter at the operating table.[4] The hyperbolic design allows a high degree of outward pressure to be focused at the ends of the CEG, which is important when placing the device across an aneurysm where the anchoring site is limited to short healthy necks on either side of the aneurysm. Often the aneurysmal disease extends to the distal abdominal aorta and the iliac vessels, where the aortoiliac bifurcation is frequently cone shaped and oversized. It is under these difficult conditions that the hyperbolic shape ensures close contact of the CEG against the wall of the enlarged aortoiliac bifurcation.

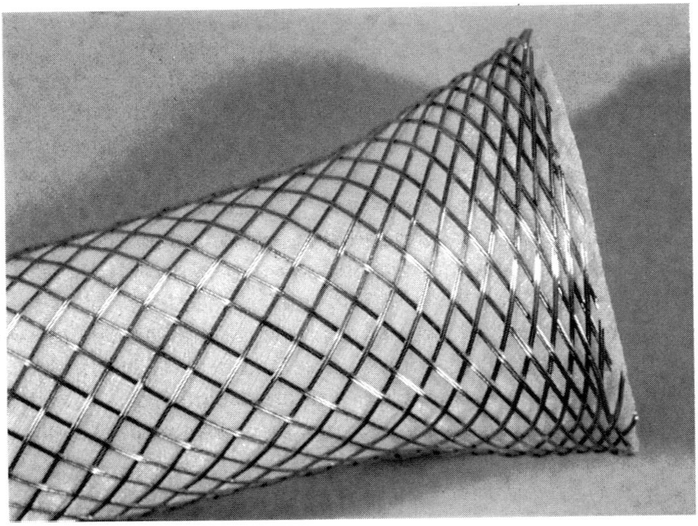

Fig. 9.2 End portion of a Corvita endoluminal graft with double-wire configuration and outside flaring wire ends.

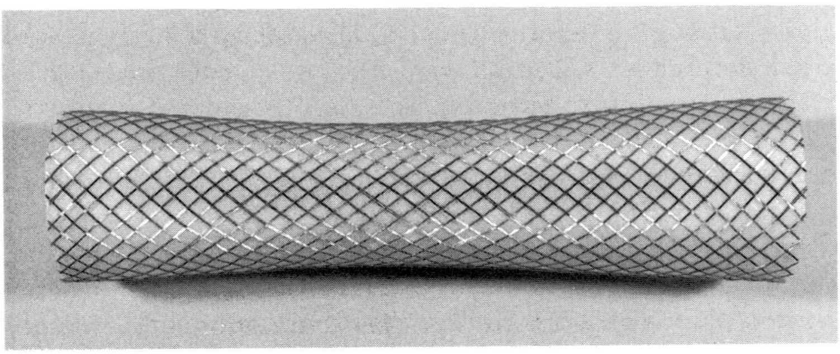

Fig. 9.3 Corvita endoluminal graft with hyperbolic shape.

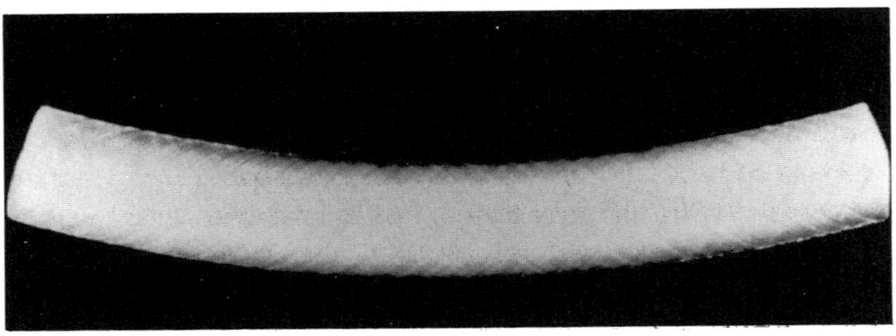

Fig. 9.4 The polycarbonate–urethane fibre liner.

The liner

The polycarbonate–urethane fibre liner (Fig. 9.4) is manufactured by extruding polycarbonate–urethane solution (Corethane; Corvita Corporation, Miami, FL, USA)[5] from a spinerette on to a rotating mandrel. The spinerette system is reciprocated along the axis of the mandrel to produce a controlled pitch angle. Each fibre layer is bound to underlying fibre layers to produce an integral non-woven structure (Fig. 9.5).[6] Control of the pitch angle allows for precise matching of the pull-down characteristics of the nonwoven Corethane component to that of the Didcott metallic stent, thereby preventing wrinkling of the liner and minimizing the profile of the delivery system. The diameter of the fibres comprising the liner range from 10 to 20 μm and the interfibre distance measures 20–50 μm. The high porosity of this fibrous structure permits ingrowth of living tissue into the liner.[7–9] The porous elastomeric liner is integrally bound to the inner surface of the metallic stent by means of an adhesive layer comprised of a slightly modified polycarbonate–urethane polymer.

Corethane is an elastomeric material that differs from other commercially available polyurethanes used in the medical device industry (e.g. pacemaker lead insulators) by the use of a carbonate linkage in the

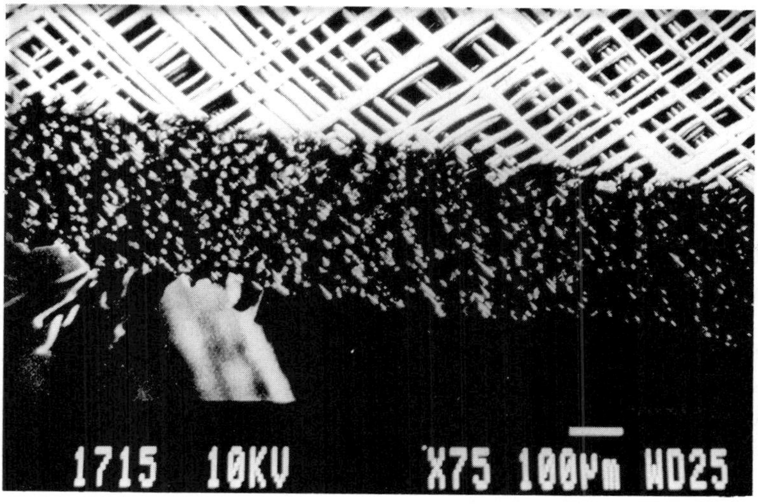

Fig. 9.5 Scanning electron micrograph of the liner (original magnification × 75) showing the multilayer porous fibre structure with fibres crossing each other at a defined pitch angle.

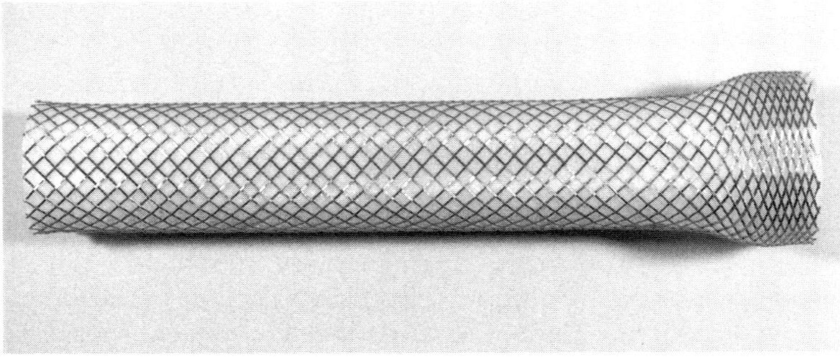

Fig. 9.6 The bifurcated Corvita endoluminal graft as seen from the outside with a strong proximal flare for improved anchoring and sealing.

backbone of the polymer rather than the more conventional ether or ester linkages. It has been found that the carbonate linkage is significantly more stable than both ether and ester linkages with regard to oxidative and hydrolytic degradation.[10] Although Corethane has been proven to be more stable than conventional polyurethanes,[11] the long-term biostability as a load-bearing member remains to be proven. For this reason, the Corethane liner is placed inside the stent with the stent wires being the load-bearing members.

Some 400 layers of Corethane fibres are typically used to ensure mechanical resistance of the device to blood pressure for bridging abdominal aortic aneurysms. CEGs ranging in diameter from 20 to 40 mm are used to accommodate the various geometric requirements of aneurysm morphology.

The exact required length of the CEG is determined either by on-table angiography using an external radiopaque tape measure or, more precisely, with an invasive endoluminal sizing device. The CEG can then be simply cut to the desired length with scissors in the operating room just before insertion.

A bifurcated configuration of the CEG has recently been developed (Fig. 9.6) to accommodate patients presenting with aortic aneurysmal disease who demonstrate an extension of the disease into the iliac arteries with an absence of a distal aortic neck.[12] The bifurcated design comprises an aortic tubular trunk where the inner middle third portion of the anterior and posterior walls of the Corethane tube are sewn along the longitudinal axis of the device into a 'double-barrel' configuration (Fig. 9.7). After placement of the aortic portion of the

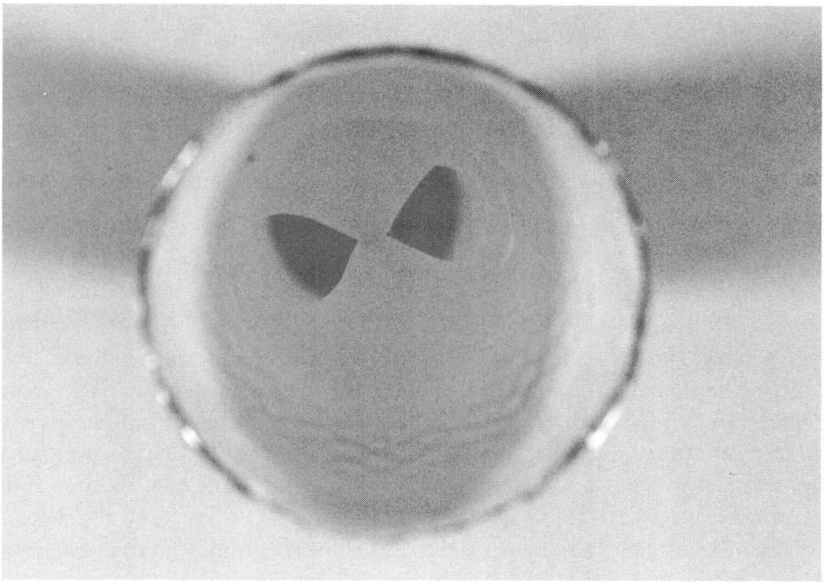

Fig. 9.7 Interior of the Corvita bifurcated endoluminal graft with a portion of the inner liner sewn together to form a 'double-barrel' configuration.

endoluminal graft into the abdominal aorta, two smaller CEG limbs of 14–16 mm in diameter, previously cut to the appropriate length, are deployed into the 'barrels' of the aortic trunk and extended distally into a healthy segment of each iliac artery (see Fig. 9.9c).

The advantages of this fully stented elastomeric endoluminal graft are:

1. It can be reliably anchored in proximal and distal necks by the radial pressure of the metallic structure and the outside flare of the wire ends.
2. The application of the liner against the arterial wall ensures a blood-tight seal.
3. It can be inserted into a sheath of very small diameter (compression ratio 6 : 1).
4. The blood contact surface is polycarbonate–urethane whose healing properties and secondary endothelialization have been demonstrated during a multicentre trial of the Corvita peripheral graft.[8]
5. The device can be cut to length at the operating table.

The delivery system

The delivery system for implantation of large-diameter (20–40 mm in the fully expanded state) abdominal aortic CEGs consists of three components:

1. An external sheath of 15- or 18-Fr internal diameter (BALT, Montmorency, France).
2. An internal 'holding catheter'.
3. A dilator tip.

The holding catheter is basically a plunger used to hold the trailing portion of the CEG stationary while the external sheath is retracted during deployment. The CEG is cut to the desired length with scissors in the operating room and manually compressed and introduced over a stiff guidewire into the external sheath. Once the CEG has been fully inserted into the delivery sheath, the leading part of the sheath is capped with a soft, flexible, conically shaped tip (Fig. 9.8). By tying a surgical knot near the leading extremity of the guidewire, the dilator tip is retrieved at the end of the procedure when the guidewire and sheath are removed. An alternative to tying a knot around the guidewire is to use a super-stiff guidewire with a metal olive tip permanently fixed to the distal extremity (BALT). In the bifurcated CEG version, the iliac limb CEGs (up to 16 mm in diameter) are delivered to the aortic trunk in a similar manner using a 12-Fr diameter delivery system (BALT).

In case a precise measurement of the CEG length required to bridge the aneurysmal defect is difficult to obtain owing to tortuosity of the vessel or parallax deformation, the CEG length can be oversized by up to 20% to seat the device safely. In this case, after normal release of the

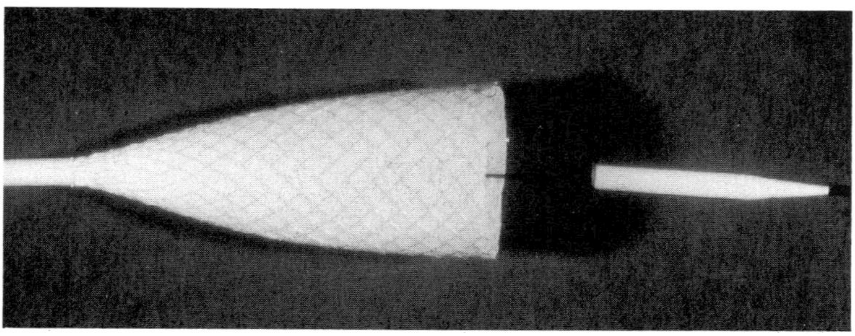

Fig. 9.8 CEG partially introduced into the delivery sheath and with the closing soft tip over the guidewire.

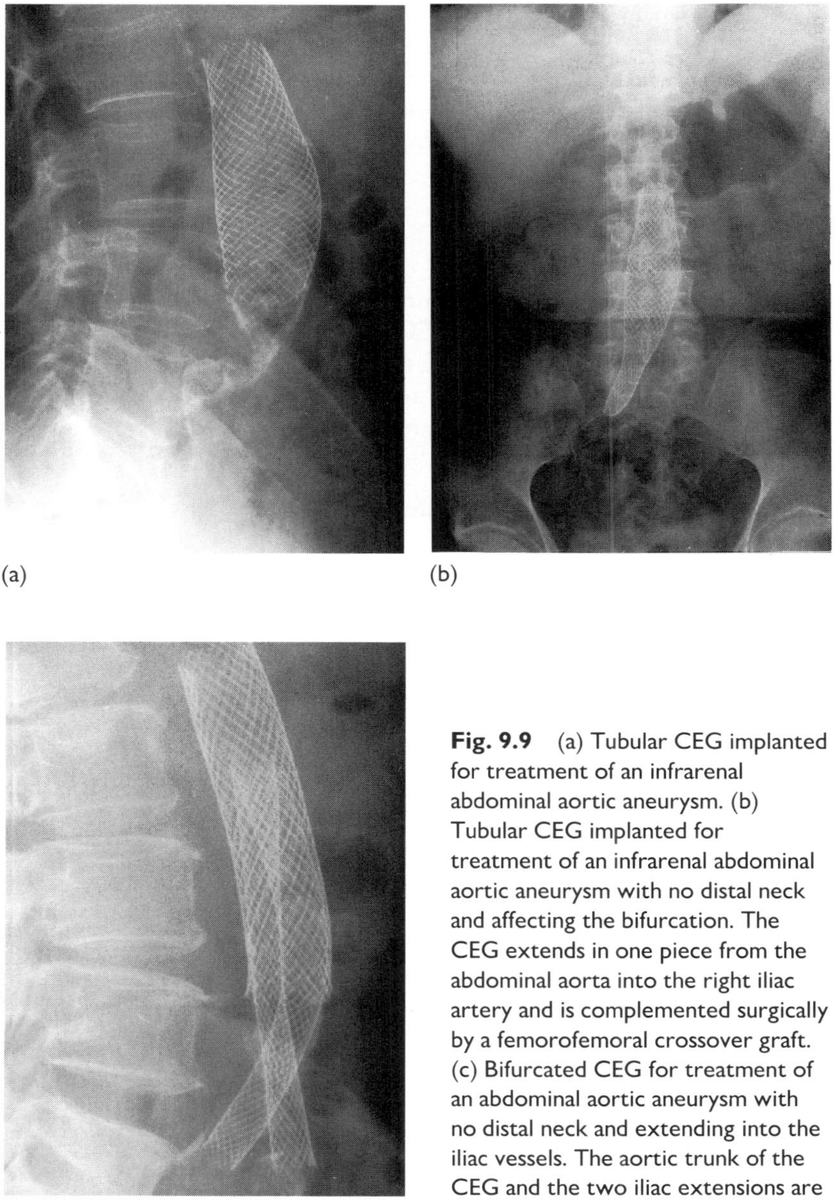

(a) (b) (c)

Fig. 9.9 (a) Tubular CEG implanted for treatment of an infrarenal abdominal aortic aneurysm. (b) Tubular CEG implanted for treatment of an infrarenal abdominal aortic aneurysm with no distal neck and affecting the bifurcation. The CEG extends in one piece from the abdominal aorta into the right iliac artery and is complemented surgically by a femorofemoral crossover graft. (c) Bifurcated CEG for treatment of an abdominal aortic aneurysm with no distal neck and extending into the iliac vessels. The aortic trunk of the CEG and the two iliac extensions are visible.

proximal portion of the CEG, the final (trailing) portion is compressed longitudinally by an upward push at the end of the release procedure. The body of the CEG then takes a balloon shape in the aneurysmal pouch; this does not, however, impair the functionality and structural stability of the device (see Fig. 9.9a).

Patient selection criteria

Eighty-six CEG implant procedures were performed between July 1993 and February 1996. The CEG was successfully delivered to the intended site in 78 patients. The device was unsuccessfully delivered in eight patients because of severe tortuosity of access vessels in five patients and misplacement in three. The success rate was directly related to:

1. The experience gained by the surgical team: while six failures occurred in 23 implantations (26%) during the period from July 1993 to November 1994, only two occurred in 63 implantations (3%) in the period from November 1994 to February 1996.
2. An improvement of the CEG and its delivery system, made subsequent to November 1994 with the incorporation of a paired-wire configuration of the metallic stent, flared extremities of the stent, and the introduction of the bifurcated design.

The CEG was implanted in various arterial locations (Table 9.1) to repair different arterial lesions – mostly for bridging abdominal aortic aneurysms in high-risk patients falling into the American Society of Anesthesiologists (ASA) grade III classification.

From November 1994 to December 1995 the authors conducted a prospective trial (feasibility study) using CEGs in 37 successive high-risk patients for treatment of abdominal aortic aneurysms. Inclusion criteria for entry into the trial were: (1) presence of an abdominal aortic aneurysm with a diameter greater than 50 mm requiring active treatment; (2) severe concomitant disease which classifies the candidate as ASA grade III or IV; (3) presence of a healthy proximal neck of the abdominal aortic aneurysm with a minimum length of 15 mm below the level of the renal arteries; and (4) informed consent of the patient.

Exclusion criteria were (1) sepsis; (2) reduced life expectancy of less than 2 years; and (3) occluded or severely diseased access vessels (iliac arteries) which prohibit passage of the CEG delivery system.

Table 9.1 Arterial site of CEG placement and indications.

Implant location	*Successful CEG placements*	*Unsuccessful CEG placements*
Thoracic aorta	6 Descending thoracic aortic aneurysms 1 Aortic arch aneurysm 1 Acute rupture of ulcerated plaque	1 Descending thoracic aortic aneurysm
Abdominal aorta	51 Abdominal aortic aneurysms 2 Perforated ulcers 1 Aortoureteral fistula 1 Stenosis	3 Abdominal aortic aneurysms
Iliac arteries	10 Stenoses, dissections, arteriovenous fistulas, false aneurysms	3 Aneurysms
Subclavian and axillary arteries	5 Stenosis, arteriovenous fistulas, false aneurysm	1 Stenosis
Total ($n = 86$)	78	8

Procedure

Severity of concomitant disease is extensively evaluated during the preoperative period. Cardiac, pulmonary, and renal function are measured in order to define the operative risk of a conventional, standard, surgical procedure. The anatomy of the abdominal aortic aneurysm is defined with conventional digital subtraction aortography and by spiral computed tomography (CT) with longitudinal reconstruction, to obtain a precise measurement of the length of the proximal neck.

The implant procedure is performed in an operating room in the presence of an anaesthesiologist who can adapt the specific type of anaesthesia to the individual clinical case. Also helpful is an interventional radiologist in the event that difficulties occur in gaining access to the abdominal aorta through severely diseased access vessels. The operating room should have a good-quality C-arm fluoroscope with vascular imaging capabilities (road-mapping). A high-flow injection pump for performing accurate angiography when controls are required is a useful accessory.

After induction of general anaesthesia, endotracheal intubation, and mechanical ventilatory assistance, a radiopaque tape measure is placed under the patient, parallel to the left border of the lumbar spine. The patient is draped as for a conventional surgical procedure to enable conversion to a surgical procedure in the event of bleeding, CEG misplacement, or unsuccessful access to the abdominal aorta. The right or left common femoral artery is exposed and punctured with a needle. A soft hydrophilic coated, 0.035-inch guidewire is passed through the needle and placed in the suprarenal aorta. An 11-Fr angiography catheter of 61.5 cm length (BALT) with a dilator is threaded over the guidewire and advanced to the aorta at the level of the renal arteries. After removing the dilator, a bolus of contrast medium is injected under fluoroscopy through the 11-Fr sheath to establish the precise location of the ostia of the renal arteries. A contrast angiogram is taken of the proximal neck and stored on the left monitor of the C-arm apparatus (GE Medical Systems, Loncin, Belgium). The precise diameter and length of the proximal neck can be measured with the aid of the radiopaque tape measure. The sheath is then pulled down to the bifurcation and angiography of the aortoiliac bifurcation is performed and stored in the computer memory.

The soft guidewire is retrieved from the sheath and replaced with a super-stiff guidewire (Schneider, Bülach, Switzerland) around which a surgical knot is tied at the distal extremity to allow retrieval of the soft tip of the delivery device at the end of the procedure. More recently we have used a stiff guidewire with an olive at its extremity (BALT). Depending on the anatomy of the aneurysmal disease, one of three different implant situations can occur, each requiring a different CEG configuration or surgical strategy:

1. If the aneurysm has a good proximal and distal neck above the bifurcation, a simple straight-tube CEG that has been cut to the desired length, as measured previously on the angiogram, is delivered (Fig. 9.9a).
2. If the aneurysm extends to the iliac vessels with no distal neck, a straight-tube CEG can be deployed from the aorta, just below the renal arteries, to a distal healthy segment of one iliac artery. Because the CEG can adapt to different diameters, ranging from 30 mm to less than 10 mm, a single length of CEG can be placed from the level that is just distal to the renal arteries to either the

common iliac artery or the external iliac artery (Fig. 9.9b). With this configuration, revascularization of the contralateral limb is mandatory and assured by a crossover femorofemoral bypass graft (polytetrafluoroethylene ring-supported, 8-mm diameter graft (IMPRA, Tempe, AZ, USA)) at the end of the procedure. Perfect closure of the contralateral common iliac artery is obtained simply by delivering within this artery a short additional iliac CEG whose distal end is closed with a surgical ligature, thereby acting as an occluding device.

3. If the aneurysmal disease extends to huge bilateral iliac aneurysms, the use of the bifurcated-type CEG becomes mandatory. As described previously, the bifurcated aortic trunk ('double-barrel' design) is first placed in the aorta below the renal arteries. Thereafter, two additional extension iliac CEGs are simultaneously delivered from each 'barrel' to the healthy portion of the iliac arteries (Fig. 9.9c).

At the end of these procedures, a control angiography is obtained to confirm the position of the CEG below the renal arteries and to verify the absence of paraprosthetic leaks. After reversal of heparin (a bolus of 10 000 units heparin was administered intra-arterially at the beginning of the procedure) by protamine, the wound is closed and the patient is monitored in the recovery room. All patients receive prophylactic antibiotic coverage with intravenous administration of 1 g cefazolin. This prophylactic treatment is continued for 24 hours. Postoperative anticoagulants or antiplatelet drugs are not administered.

Results, complications and management

This section describes a series of successive CEG implants for correction of abdominal aortic aneurysms in 37 patients over a time period of 1 year (November 1994 to December 1995). All these patients presented unacceptable operative risks (ASA grades III and IV). During the same period, a further 35 patients received standard surgical procedures, and three were operated on for ruptured abdominal aortic aneurysms.

Among the 37 patients with CEGs, two were unsuccessfully placed: one because of dislodgement of the device inside the aneurysmal sac during the placement procedure; the other because of iatrogenic rupture of the iliac vessel which required conversion to standard surgery. The implant procedure was successful in the remaining 35 cases (95%). Thirty-four patients were male, three female and the mean age was 73 years. Amongst the successful cases, the aneurysm type was fusiform in 30 patients, ectatic in three and two cases consisted of false aneurysms. The mean maximum transverse diameter of the aneurysms in this study was 58 mm. General anaesthesia was used for all patients except three with severe respiratory disease, who received epidural anaesthesia.

The access vessel used to introduce the CEG was the femoral artery in 30 patients. Five patients with severely diseased femoral arteries required a retroperitoneal access with direct approach to the iliac arteries. Depending on the anatomic configuration, an aortic tubular CEG was used in 17 patients and an aortoiliac tubular CEG, in conjunction with a femorofemoral crossover bypass graft, was used in 15. The bifurcated CEG was used in only three of the more recent cases owing to the unavailability of this device in the early part of the study. The extension of vascular disease in 11 patients necessitated telescopic placement of two or more CEG elements to cover long segments of damaged artery. In these cases the caudal CEG element was deployed in overlap with the more proximal CEG element to ensure a blood-tight seal between successive elements.

Local complications associated with abdominal aorta aneurysm implant procedures were:

- Two iatrogenic dissections of access vessels (iliac arteries) were induced by the size of the delivery system and treated by intraoperative semiclosed endarterectomy.
- Two distal macroembolizations were treated by embolectomy and venous bypass reconstruction.
- Two retroperitoneal haematomas were observed; one necessitated surgical drainage.
- One perioperative crossover occlusion was treated with a repeat crossover operation 3 days later.
- Four ischaemic complications due to the occlusion of internal iliac vessels by the CEG were observed: one was a temporary gluteal ischaemia; three were reversible ischaemic colitis of the sigmoido-rectal junction and were detected by colorectal endoscopy 2 days after operation. These low-grade colonic ischaemic events reversed spontaneously.

General complications principally related to severe concomitant disease included:

- Four coronary ischaemic attacks necessitating monitoring in the intensive care unit.
- Two reversible deteriorations of previous chronic renal failure.
- One case of gastroduodenal bleeding from an acute gastric ulcer, which was medically treated.
- One case of pancreatitis.
- One case of prolonged ileus.
- Two patients with pulmonary infection.
- Three major hypotensive episodes of unknown origin requiring fluid replacement.
- Nine patients demonstrated inflammatory reactions with a raised sedimentation rate, fever and increased C-reactive protein values associated with a lowered platelet count. The inflammatory reactions began on the second postoperative day and subsided spontaneously 1 week later. There was no evidence of bacteraemia or infection of the CEG. The mechanism of this postimplantation syndrome is unclear. Accumulation and activation of platelets trapped on the luminal surface of the CEG might induce release of proinflammatory substances like cytokines and thus induce the observed inflammatory reaction.

Perioperative mortality:

- One patient died during the first postoperative week from acute myocardial infarction (perioperative mortality rate of 3%).

Late mortality:

- One patient developed a perforated diverticulitis and died 2 months after surgery from sepsis.

To evaluate the efficacy of the CEG treatment in excluding aneurysms with the absence of residual leaks that could maintain pressure on the aneurysmal sac, a control CT reconstruction with contrast medium was systematically performed during the first postoperative week. The precise location of any residual leaks detected on the CT scan was then further elucidated by contrast angiography. The findings were as follows:

1. Twenty-two (63%) of 35 patients had immediate blood-tight CEGs.

2. Thirteen (37%) of 35 patients demonstrated some residual leaks, which were further defined according to the anatomic site of entry of the leak, the nature of outflow vessels from the leak, and the blood velocity through the leak:
   (i) Five patients demonstrated low-flow leaks that occluded spontaneously during the first 4 postoperative months.
   (ii) Two patients with high-flow leaks underwent successful interventional radiologic treatments with coils and GEL-FOAM® (The UPJOHN Co, Kalamazoo, MI) embolizations of outflow vessels.
   (iii) Two patients with high-flow leaks underwent repeat operations: one required the placement of an adjunctive proximal CEG tube segment to close the proximal leak; the other required an outflow tract ligature of one hypogastric artery, inducing thrombosis of the leak.
   (iv) Of the remaining four patients with residual leaks (11%), two are scheduled for additional interventional radiologic treatment and two refused further treatment.

To evaluate further the efficacy of this endovascular treatment to prevent growth of the aneurysmal sac and the associated risk of rupture, CT scans of 19 patients with a follow-up of more than 6 months were examined. In 16 patients with blood-tight CEGs, the mean reduction of the maximum transverse diameter of the aneurysmal sac was 1 mm after 6 months. Calcification of the wall of the aneurysmal sac and presence of mural fibrin deposits might have slowed the reduction in aneurysm size after thrombosis. Of three patients with residual leaks, an increase in diameter of 3.7 mm was observed after 8 months, indicating that residual leaks maintain pressure on the arterial wall and do not suppress the risk of late rupture. The main cause of leaks is the presence of underlying atherosclerotic disease causing a 'cobblestone' surface at the arterial necks and provoking an incomplete friction seal between the CEG and the arterial wall. Immediate postoperative blind leaks with no outflow vessels seem to have a good prognosis for future thrombosis. However, high-flow leaks with patent outflow vessels have to be treated aggressively by adjunctive radiologic embolization of outflow vessels. Alternatively, the leak can be suppressed by occluding the leak entry site(s) in a CEG repeat intervention.

Conclusions

Advantages

High success rate In this prospective trial from November 1994 to December 1995, all successive high-risk cases with a proximal neck length of 1.5 cm were offered CEG treatment; all patients voluntarily accepted. The endoluminal graft was successfully implanted in 35 of the 37 patients (success rate 95%).

High versatility With the exception of aneurysms extending to the renal arteries with short or no proximal neck, the straight-tube device and the bifurcated configuration permitted application of the technique in nearly all cases.

Low level of complications Because of the shape of the device and its structural stability, no migration of the device was observed during the follow-up period. The small profile of the delivery system and the immediate release of the aortic portion of the CEG, which immobilizes the fibrin clots in the aneurysmal sac, could explain the low occurrence of only minor embolic events (2 of 35) (6%).

Sealing Good healing properties of the Corethane coating, already observed in the Corvita peripheral vascular graft[8] and demonstrated in two CEG specimens harvested during necropsy, demonstrate rapid invasion of fibrous tissue in the pores and formation of a neointima on the luminal surface covered with neoendothelial cells. The initial mechanical sealing by the CEG in the neck of the aneurysm is eventually replaced by a physiologic seal of healthy tissue.

Blood flow Because of the porosity of the liner, blood flow is only minimally disturbed during the CEG release procedure. No haemodynamic clamping effect was observed in the series.

Disadvantages

Biodegradation Virtually all synthetic polymers, including Dacron, degrade over time.[13] The polycarbonate type of urethane demonstrates a stronger resistance to biodegradation compared with conventional implant-grade polyurethane elastomers.[10] Experience gained over

5 years with microfibrous Corethane in a similar embodiment in the peripheral graft shows structural integrity of the graft despite some signs of degradation of the polycarbonate fibres. This degradative phenomenon could weaken the liner of the CEG during long-term implantation. Although the metallic stent itself is the load-bearing member of the device, and not the Corethane liner, this treatment should be reserved for older patients until more data on the long-term performance of the device have been obtained.

Leaks Residual leaks were observed in 11% of patients despite additional attempts to close the entry or outflow tracts of the leaks. Leaks localized at the proximal neck are the result of poor apposition of the CEG against the arterial wall, mostly secondary to irregular surfaces induced by atherosclerotic plaques. Increasing the radial force by oversizing the CEG, the use of paired wires, and the increase of mechanical flaring of the proximal extremity could reduce the frequency of proximal leaks. Distal leaks are most often due to poor apposition of the distal part of the CEG against a conical distal neck. Distal leaks can be treated successfully by interventional radiologists, who may chose to embolize the run-off vessels of the leak with coils and/or GELFOAM® (The UPJOHN Co, Kalamazoo, MI) particles. Availability of the bifurcated CEG should also dramatically reduce the number of distal leaks as a result of better sizing of the device as well as better sealing of the device on a healthy segment of iliac artery.

The appearance of late new leaks, which has been described by Parodi,[14] may be attributed to enlarging necks. This phenomenon may be avoided with the CEG as a result of the enhanced healing observed with microporous Corethane, as could be demonstrated in one thoracic CEG. Complete healing of the CEG has been observed in some explanted cases as early as 1 month after surgery.

Acknowledgements

The authors thank A. Cohen, N. Frid, H. Köntges and L. Pinchuk for technical assistance and Mrs N. Huant for the preparation of the manuscript.

References

1. Dereume JP. Endoprothèse luminale et son procédé de préparation. European patent no. 93203572.8.

2. Didcott CC. Oesophageal strictures: treatment by slow continuous dilatation. *Ann R Coll Surg* 1973; **53**: 112–26.
3. Frid N. Tuteur auto-expansible pour dispositif médical à introduire dans une cavité d'un corps, et son procédé de preparation. Belgian patent application no. 09500334.
4. Frid N. Tuteur auto-expansible pour dispositif médical à introduire dans une cavité d'un corps, et dispositif médical muni d'un tel tuteur. Belgian patent application no. 09500335.
5. Pinchuk L, Esquivel MC, Martin JB Jr. Corethane: a novel thermoplastic elastomer for biomedical applications. *Proceedings of the Society for Plastic Engineering* 1991; **3**: 1812–14.
6. Leidner J, MacGregor DC, Wilson GJ, Wong E. A novel process for the manufacturing of porous grafts: process description and product evaluation. *J Biomed Mater Res* 1983; **17**: 229–47.
7. Wilson GJ, MacGregor DC, Klement P *et al.* The composite Corethane/Dacron vascular prosthesis: canine *in vivo* evaluation of 4 mm diameter grafts with 1 year follow-up. *Trans Am Soc Artif Organs* 1991; **37**: 475–6.
8. Dereume JP, Van Romphey A, Vincent G, Engelman E. Femoro-popliteal bypass with a compliant, composite polyurethane Dacron graft: short-term results of a multicenter trial. *Cardiovasc Surg* 1993; **1**: 499–503.
9. Dereume JP, Ferreira J, El Douaihy M *et al.* Clinical experience with an integrated self-expandable stented graft (Corvita) for the treatment of various arterial lesions. In: Veith FJ, ed. *Current Critical Problems in Vascular Surgery*; **6**. St Louis, MO: Quality Medical Publishing, 1995.
10. Pinchuk L. A review of the biostability and carcinogenicity of polyurethanes in medicine and the new generation of 'biostable' polyurethanes. *J Biomater Sci Polym Ed* 1994; **6**: 225–67.
11. Zhao Q, Casas-Bejar J, Urbanski P *et al.* Glass wool–$H_2O/CoCl_2$ test system for *in vitro* evaluation of biodegradative stress cracking in polyurethane elastomers. *J Biomed Mater Res* 1995; **29**: 467–75.
12. Moritz JD, Rotermund S, Keating DP, Oestmann JW. Infrarenal abdominal aortic aneurysms: implication of CT evaluation of size and configuration for placement of endovascular aortic grafts. *Radiology* 1996; **198**: 463–66.
13. Vinard E, Eloy R, Descottes J *et al.* Prothèses vasculaires en Dacron chez l'homme. Performances mécaniques, lésions et stabilité moléculaire. *Presse Med* 1990; **19**: 709–14.
14. Parodi JC. Endovascular repair of abdominal aortic aneurysms and other arterial lesions. *J Vasc Surg* 1995; **21**: 549–57.

10

The Sydney experience

James May, Geoffrey H. White and Weiyun Yu

Department of Vascular Surgery, Royal Prince Alfred Hospital and Department of Surgery, University of Sydney, Australia

Introduction

The first endoluminal repair of an abdominal aortic aneurysm (AAA) at the Royal Prince Alfred Hospital was undertaken in May 1992. Between then and January 1996 the endoluminal method has been used to repair AAAs in 103 patients (seven women). The mean age was 70 years and co-morbidity was present in 45 patients (Table 10.1). It was our aim to use new systems and devices as they became available. In this way a comparison of these devices is possible when used by one group of surgeons in one medical centre. As a result of this policy the following methods of endoluminal repair were used: the modified Parodi, the Sydney (White–Yu), the Endovascular Technologies (EVT), the Chuter–Gianturco and the Mintec Stentor (Miahle). Table 10.2 indicates the number of patients receiving the different devices used with these methods, together with the configuration of the prostheses.

Table 10.1 Co-morbidity in 103 patients undergoing endoluminal AAA repair.

	No. of patients
Poor left ventricular function (and renal impairment in three)	25
Renal failure on dialysis	1
Chronic obstructive airway disease	7
Bilateral thoracoplasty	1
Chronic liver disease	4
Hostile abdomen	7
Total	45

Table 10.2 Devices used and graft configurations.

System	Graft configuration			
	Tube	*Aortoiliac or aortofemoral*	*Bifurcated*	*Total*
Modified Parodi	3	6	1	10
Sydney (White–Yu)	38	17	11	66
EVT	11	0	4	15
Chuter–Gianturco	0	0	1	1
Stentor	0	0	11	11
Total	52	23	28	103

Design of the delivery system and endoprostheses

The design of the different delivery systems and endoprostheses used have been reported previously.[1–6] As our largest experience is with the Sydney endograft developed by White and Yu in our own endovascular laboratory, the design of this delivery system and endoprosthesis will be summarized in this chapter.

The Sydney endograft is a balloon-expandable device constructed of commercially available woven Dacron of thickness 0.24 mm (Fig. 10.1). The endoprosthesis is anchored by means of metallic graft attachment devices which are incorporated into the fabric of the graft. The endoprosthesis is mounted on an 8 cm long, non-compliant balloon (William Cook, Eight Mile Plains, Australia). The diameter is sized from preoperative computed tomography (CT) and angiography. The endoprosthesis and balloon are packaged into a Teflon loading sheath matched to the size of a longer introducing sheath. The 24- or 20-Fr introducing sheath with its mandrel is passed into the aortic aneurysm over an extra stiff guidewire via the femoral and iliac arteries. The mandrel is removed and the loading sheath 'docked' over the guidewire to the introducing sheath by means of a Silastic sleeve (Fig. 10.2). A coaxial pusher is used in combination with the balloon catheter shaft to advance the endoprosthesis into the aortic aneurysm. The endoprosthesis is deployed immediately below the renal arteries by withdrawing the introducing sheath and inflating the balloon.

Because the entire length of abdominal aorta between the renal arteries and the aortic bifurcation has the potential to become aneurys-

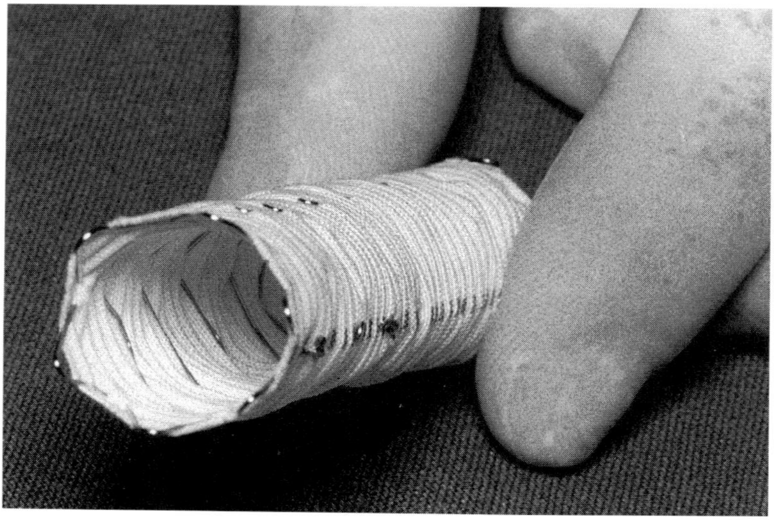

Fig. 10.1 The Sydney endograft, a balloon-expandable Dacron prosthesis developed by White and Yu. (From May *et al. J Endovasc Surg* 1995; **2**: 240–7, with permission.)

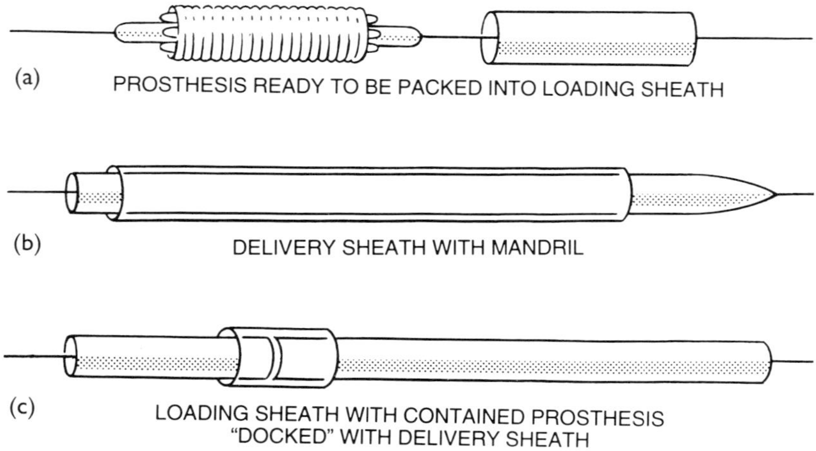

Fig. 10.2 Preparation of the Sydney endograft for delivery. (a) The Sydney prosthesis is mounted on a balloon catheter for packing into the loading sheath. (b) The appearance of the introducing sheath with mandrel. (c) The loading sheath and introducing sheath connected. (From May *et al. J Endovasc Surg* 1995; **2**: 240–7, with permission.)

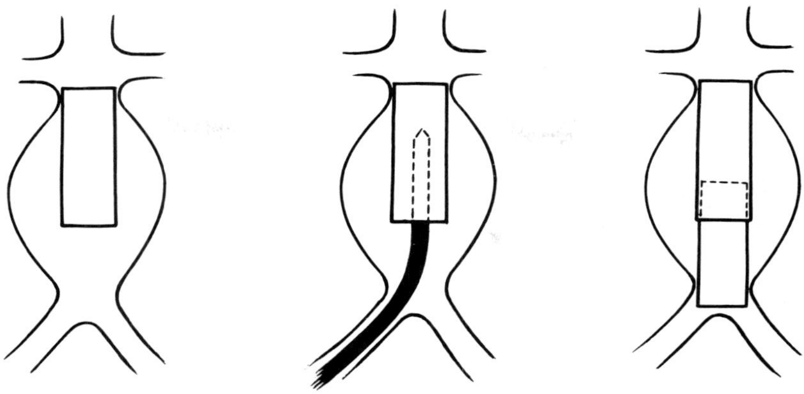

Fig. 10.3 (a) The first endograft is deployed immediately below the renal arteries. (b) The introducing sheath with its mandrel is reintroduced and lies within the first endograft. (c) The mandrel is removed and the second endograft delivered through the introducing sheath to lie within and overlapping the first endograft. (From Yu *et al. Asian J Surg* 1996; **19**: 37–40, with permission.)

mal, it is desirable that any endoprosthesis used covers this segment in its entirety irrespective of the length of the aneurysm. In some cases the 8-cm long Sydney endograft can achieve this aim. In the majority of patients, however, a second endograft has to be introduced using the overlapping double prosthesis or 'trombone technique'[7] (Fig. 10.3). This allows a second endograft to be deployed within and overlapping the first endograft. The procedure is performed under radiographic control and post-procedure angiography is used to confirm exclusion of the aneurysm sac.

Patient selection criteria

The basic criteria for selection was a proximal neck of thrombus-free aorta of 1.5 cm or greater and diameter of 28 mm or less. Patients were further divided into two subgroups. Aneurysms with a proximal neck, as described, and a distal neck of thrombus-free aorta between the aneurysm and the aortic bifurcation of 1.5 cm or more and non-tortuous iliac arteries of diameter 8 mm or greater were suited for endoluminal repair with a tube endoprosthesis and were designated

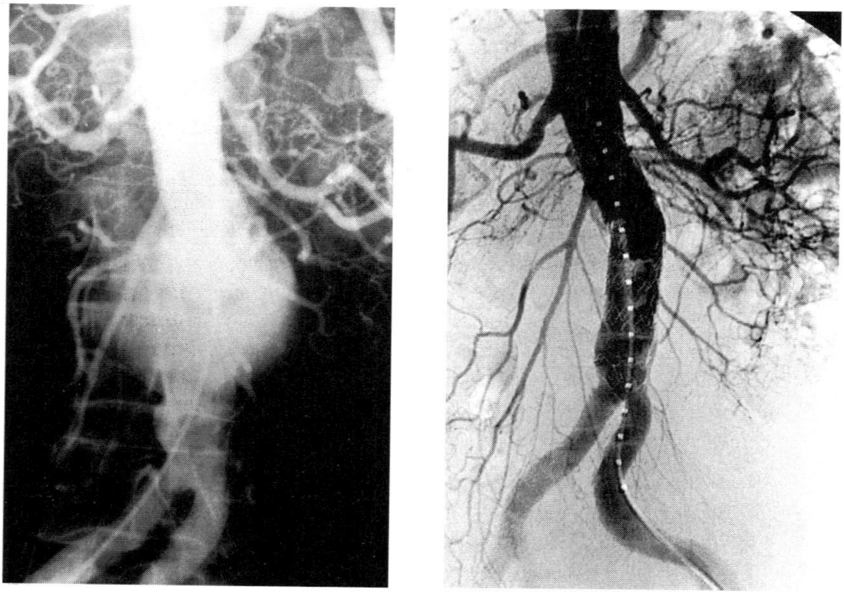

(a) (b)

Fig. 10.4 (a) Preoperative aortogram demonstrating a type I abdominal aortic aneurysm suitable for endoluminal tube graft repair. (b) Postoperative aortogram after endoluminal repair with Sydney endograft, demonstrating normal flow within the prosthesis and exclusion of the aneurysmal sac from the general circulation. (From May *et al. Asian J Surg* 1996; **19**: 37–40, with permission.)

type I[8] (Fig. 10.4). Type II aneurysms were those with a proximal neck as described but lacking one or more of the criteria for inclusion in type I. These aneurysms were suited for endoluminal repair with either a tapered aortoiliac or aortofemoral graft or a bifurcated graft. The requirement of 1.5 cm in length for the distal neck was relaxed in six patients who had an endoluminal tube graft. The co-morbidities mentioned previously led to rejection for open operation in one-third of the patients.

Procedure

The procedure was carried out in the operating room with the patient prepared and draped for open operation in the event of failed endoluminal repair. The procedure was performed entirely by the endoluminal route in 80 patients and by a combination of the endoluminal and extraluminal routes in 23. The techniques for the combined procedures have been described in detail in previous reports.[3,9,10] The aim was to use an endoluminal tube graft wherever possible. Initially this resulted in type I aneurysms being treated by the endoluminal route and type II aneurysms by a combination of the endoluminal and extraluminal routes. With the development of a bifurcated version of the Sydney endograft and the availability of bifurcated EVT and Stentor devices, type II aneurysms are now more commonly managed by the endoluminal route alone.

Complications and management

The outcome of these 103 patients undergoing endoluminal AAA repair is shown in Table 10.3, broken down according to the endoluminal method used. Overall there were 12 primary conversions from endoluminal to open repair at the original operation and six secondary conversions at subsequent operation. All but two of the six endoleaks were corrected by secondary endoluminal repair or had secondary conversion to open repair. One of these two patients had an unrelated cerebrovascular accident and further intervention is not planned, while the endoleak in the second patient sealed spontaneously. There have been six perioperative deaths, all procedure related, and six non-procedure-related late deaths.

Of the 103 patients undergoing endoluminal AAA repair, 72 are currently alive and well with the AAA excluded from the circulation.

Complications have been classified according to the recommendations of the *ad hoc* committee of the Society for Vascular Surgery (SVS) and International Society for Cardiovascular Surgery (ISCVS) on uniform reporting standards for AAA. The local vascular complications are listed in Table 10.4 and the remote general complications in Table 10.5.

Follow-up

The follow-up protocol has included physical examination and contrast-enhanced CT within 10 days of operation, at 6 months, 12 months and annually thereafter. Duplex ultrasonography and

Table 10.3 Outcome.

System	*No. of procedures*	*Conversion*		*Endoleak*	*Death*	
		Primary	*Secondary*		*Perioperative*	*Late*
Modified Parodi	10	5	1	0	1	1
EVT tube	11	0	0	1	0	3
EVT bifurcated	4	2	0	0	1	0
Stentor	11	0	1	0	1	0
Chuter–Gianturco	1	0	0	0	0	0
Sydney tube	38	1	4	5	2	2
Sydney aortoiliac	17	1	0	0	0	0
Sydney bifurcated	11	3	0	0	1	0

Table 10.4 Local vascular complications.

	No. of patients
Femoral artery repair	3
Perforation of iliac artery	2
Graft stenosis	2
Common iliac artery occlusion	3
Paragraft flow (endoleak)	
Spontaneous seal	1
Corrected endoluminally	2
Converted to open repair	2
Untreated	1
Bleeding	2
Wound complication	4
Total	22

Table 10.5 Systemic remote complications.

	No. of patients
Renal insufficiency	
Obstructive	2
Contrast media induced	5
Cardiac	
Congestive failure	2
Myocardial infarction	4
Cardiac arrhythmia	2
Stroke or transient ischaemic attack	3
Total	18

angiography have been used selectively. No patient has been lost to follow-up.

The changes in morphology of AAAs that have been observed by follow-up CT have been reported previously.[11,12] In all but three patients the maximum transverse diameter of the AAA diminished progressively with time. This incremental diminution was 0.4 cm at 6 months, 0.8 cm at 12 months and 1.1 cm at 18 months. Concurrent with this diminution in diameter of the aneurysmal sac was a paradoxical increase of approximately 10% in the mean diameter of the proximal and distal neck of the aneurysm. Unlike the aneurysmal sac measurements, however, the increase in mean diameter of the aneurysmal necks was not progressive. Two of the three patients who demonstrated an increase in maximum transverse diameter of the aneurysmal sac at 6 months showed a subsequent reduction in maximum transverse diameter at the 12-month follow-up. The increase in diameter in the third patient was 2 mm over 12 months.

Summary

In discussing the advantages and disadvantages of the endoluminal systems that we have had the opportunity of using, it should be stated at the outset that it is unreasonable to compare the outcome of one system used early during the learning curve of experience with the more sophisticated systems available more recently. Notwithstanding this, a commentary on the strengths and weaknesses of the various systems as observed by one group may be instructive for others.

The strengths of the Parodi system were twofold. First, this device demonstrated the principles of debulking, delivering and deploying the endoprosthesis, and underlined how clearly and carefully Parodi had considered and understood the endoluminal method of AAA repair. Second, his system was simple enough to allow others to use it and to modify it through their own efforts, independent of commercial manufacturers.

EVT had the advantage of producing a device that could be supplied with a set of instructions rather than a method that obliged users to assemble their own device. The EVT device also combined the advantages of a self-expanding and balloon-expandable device. The balloon served to drive the hooks on the attachment devices through the aortic wall. The authors' experience with only one late endoleak using the EVT tube endoprosthesis is encouraging. The incidence of endoleaks, however, in other reports emphasizes the unforgiving nature of the tube endograft with regard to the sizing of the diameter and length of the device.[4,13] Our experience with the EVT bifurcated device and the Chuter–Gianturco bifurcated device is too small for useful comment to be made.

The Stentor device has the advantage of being comparatively small in size (18 Fr) and flexible. These features enabled the endoluminal method to be used in our limited experience in one woman with small iliac arteries and in three men with tortuous iliac arteries who would not otherwise have been suitable for this method.

The strengths of the Sydney endograft include: (i) technical similarity to conventional angioplasty, permitting easy adaptation to the technique; (ii) precise implantations are possible due to controlled gradual expansion and deployment; and (iii) additional strength of the multiple graft attachment devices compared with a single self-expanding stent at the proximal end of other prostheses. Although rarely encountered, the main risk associated with this technique lies with potential vessel rupture resulting from graft or balloon oversizing.

References

1. Parodi JC, Palmaz JC, Barone HD. Transfemoral intraluminal graft implantation abdominal aortic aneurysms. *Ann Vasc Surg* 1991; **5**: 491–99.
2. White GH, Yu W, May J *et al.* A new non-stented endoluminal graft for straight or bifurcated endoluminal bypass. *J Endovasc Surg* 1994; **1**: 16–24.
3. May J, White G, Yu W, Waugh R, Harris JP. Treatment of complex abdominal aneurysms by a combination of endoluminal and extraluminal aorto-femoral grafts. *J Vasc Surg* 1994; **19**: 924–33.
4. Moore WS, Vescera CL. Repair of abdominal aortic aneurysm by transfemoral endovascular graft replacement. *Ann Surg* 1994; **220**: 331–41.
5. Chuter TA, Green RM, Ouriel K, Fiore WM, DeWeese JA. Transfemoral endovascular aortic graft placement. *J Vasc Surg* 1993; **18**: 185–95.
6. Yusuf SW, Baker DM, Chuter TAM, Whitaker SC, Wenham PW, Hopkinson BR. Transfemoral endoluminal repair of abdominal aortic aneurysm with bifurcated graft. *Lancet* 1994; **344**: 650–1.
7. Yu W, White GH, May J, Stephen MS. Endoluminal repair of abdominal aortic aneurysms using the trombone technique. *Asian J Surg* 1996; **19**: 37–40.
8. May J, White GH, Yu W, Waugh RC, Stephen MS, Harris JP. Results of endoluminal grafting of abdominal aortic aneurysms are dependent on aneurysm morphology: presented at SVS/ISCVS Joint Meeting, Seattle, *Ann Vasc Surg* 1996; **10**: 254.
9. May J, White G, Yu W *et al.* Endoluminal repair of complex abdominal aortic aneurysms. In: Yao JST, Pearce WH, eds. *Arterial Surgery*: Management of Challenging Problems. Norwalk, CT: Appleton & Lange. 1995; 237–46.
10. May J, White GH. Specialised endovascular techniques: combined surgical and endovascular approaches. In: White RA, Fogarty TJ, eds. *Peripheral Endovascular Interventions*. St Louis, MI: Mosby Year Book. 1996; 433–48.
11. May J, White GH, Yu W, Waugh RC, Stephen MS, Harris JP. A prospective study of changes in morphology and dimensions of abdominal aortic aneurysms following endoluminal repair; a preliminary report. *J Endovasc Surg* 1995; **2**: 342–7.
12. May J, White GH, Yu W, Waugh RC, Stephen MS, Harris JP. A prospective study of anatomico-pathological changes in abdominal aortic aneurysms following endoluminal repair: is the aneurysmal process reversed? *Eur J Vasc Endovasc Surg* 1996; **11**.
13. Balm R, Eikelboom BC, May J, Bell PRF, Swedenborg J, Collin J. Early experience with Transfemoral Endovascular Aneurysm Management (TEAM) in the treatment of aortic aneurysms. *Eur J Vasc Endovasc Surg* 1996; **11**: 214–20.

11

The Ivancev–Malmö system of endovascular aneurysm exclusion

Krasnodar Ivancev, Timothy A.M. Chuter and Bo Risberg

Department of Radiology, Malmö University Hospital, Malmö, S-21401, Sweden

Department of Surgery, University of California, San Francisco, USA

Department of Surgery, Malmö University Hospital, Malmö, S-21401, Sweden

Design of the delivery system and endoprosthesis

The Ivancev–Malmö system of endovascular aneurysm repair is a direct descendant of the system used in a series of animal experiments performed at M.D. Anderson Cancer Center, Houston, Texas, USA in the mid-1980s[1,2] and a relative of the system used by Dake *et al.*[3] at Stanford to repair thoracic aortic aneurysms. The Ivancev–Malmö prosthesis is based on a barbed Gianturco Z stent, and employs a similar sheath–dilator combination for access to the aorta. The primary difference between the Ivancev system and the others is the means by which the prosthesis is advanced through the sheath and into the aorta. The Ivancev–Malmö system uses a central cannula and suture loop to pull on the cranial end of the prosthesis, whereas the other systems use a blunt-ended dilator to push on the caudal end of the prosthesis. The Ivancev–Malmö system is also distinguished by the absence of a loading capsule. Instead, the sheath has a conical Teflon fitting at its outer end to assist in compressing the prosthesis during loading.

The Ivancev–Malmö system was adapted, for aortic aneurysm repair, from a system of esophageal stent delivery manufactured by William Cook, Europe. This delivery system comes in two sizes: 24 and 20 Fr. These nominal sizes refer to the inner diameter; the corresponding outer diameters are 28 and 23 Fr respectively. We used the smaller of the two for grafts up to 34 mm in diameter. The larger system was needed only for the 38-mm grafts sometimes used in thoracic aneurysm repair.

The pusher component has a long shaft, which resembles the shaft of the dilator, and a 20-cm long metal cannula with a smooth bulbous tip at its upstream end. A central lumen runs through them all, from the bulbous tip to the end of the shaft.

We have tried a variety of common iliac artery occluders, but all represented some type of closed-ended stent–graft, comprising a fabric bag and an unbarbed Gianturco Z stent. In some cases the graft was closed at both ends, like a pillow, and in others it was closed at only one end, like a pillow case. The diameters have varied according to the diameter of the iliac artery, ranging from 15 to 25 mm. Each of the occluders has its own delivery system. Sometimes the occluder is preloaded into the inner sheath of a double-sheath system. On other occasions, the occluder is loaded into the outer end of a single-sheath system with a loading capsule. The sheaths used to deliver the conventional fabric (Cooley Verisoft, Meadox Medicals) occluders range in outer diameter from 18 to 23 Fr, depending on the diameter of the occluder. The sheaths used to deliver thin-walled graft occluders range in outer diameter from 14 to 16 Fr.

The size and shape of the prosthesis also vary from case to case, depending on the location, dimensions, and pathology of the vessel. The same basic system has been used to treat true aneurysms of the thoracic aorta, abdominal aorta, and iliac arteries, false aneurysms of the thoracic aorta,[4] and abdominal aorta,[5] and a single case of common iliac arteriovenous fistula. But the vast majority of cases (30 in the past 2 years) have involved aneurysms of the abdominal aorta. All but one of these were treated with a tapered aortoiliac prosthesis, in conjunction with femorofemoral bypass and contralateral common iliac artery occlusion, as described by Parodi and others.[6–9] These cases not only comprise the bulk of our experience, they also have the longest follow-up, and form the basis of the most important lessons. For these reasons, abdominal aortic aneurysm repair is the focus of this chapter.

The graft size is individualized for each patient, according to the findings of preoperative imaging. All grafts are tapered to match the diameters of the aorta proximally and the common iliac artery distally. Some of the early grafts were sewn with a longitudinal seam and a smooth taper. This was changed for two reasons. First, there was a concern that the wall tension generated by arterial pressure might eventually disrupt a long hand-sewn suture line. Second, adjunctive stenting requires constant wall diameter in the stented portion. Currently we use a graft made from two cylindrical segments of different diameters, which are spatulated and sutured end-to-end using CV-6 Gortex (W.L. Gore).

Components used in the endoprosthesis

The fabric of the stent graft is a standard woven polyester (Cooley Verisoft, Meadox Medicals, Oakland, NJ, USA). When supplied the graft has crimps, but these are ironed out so that the graft can be compressed into the rather limited space available in the delivery system.

Both proximal and distal graft orifices are supported by modified venous Gianturco Z stents (William Cook, Europe). The proximal stents have nine angles at each end, and 18 limbs, each 25-mm long. The resting diameter of the stent is 45 mm. The limbs of the stent together have nine attachment points for the graft, and eight caudally oriented barbs. The distal stents have no barbs, and a resting diameter of only 20 mm.

Patient selection

One of our original goals was to determine the functional limits of the system. To do this, we initially took an aggressive approach to patient inclusion, and analysed cases where endovascular aneurysm exclusion failed, in order to determine whether the system, or the technique, could be modified to avoid the problem, or whether similar anatomic features would, in future patients, be grounds for exclusion. Under these circumstances, it was not possible to include patients who were unable to withstand conventional open repair. However, as the method and the criteria of patient selection evolved, we were able to predict the results with greater accuracy, which permitted the inclusion of some high-risk patients.

We still have no absolute exclusion criteria, except the absence of a neck, but we recognize several factors that make endovascular repair more difficult and dangerous. These represent relative contraindications to the endovascular approach, and include the following:

1. Short neck (less than 10 mm).
2. Angulated neck (more than 75° to the long axis of the aneurysm).

3. Conical neck (widening at a rate more than 3 mm per 10 mm from proximal to distal).
4. Thrombus-lined neck.
5. Severe iliac artery tortuosity (angulation of more than 90° at any point).
6. Severe iliac artery calcification.
7. Iliac artery dilatation (wider than 20 mm) at, or distal to, the implantation site.
8. Short common iliac artery (<30 mm long).

Using this approach, approximately 70% of the abdominal aortic aneurysms treated in Malmö during the last 9 months have had endovascular stent–graft insertion. This proportion reflects not only the limitations of the technique, but also difficult anatomy and poor cardiopulmonary condition, which are common in this tertiary referral population of patients with large aneurysms. On one hand, difficult anatomy may preclude endovascular treatment. On the other, poor physical condition may preclude conventional repair.

In most cases, the basis for these decisions is spiral computed tomography (CT) with intra-arterial contrast, using a table speed of 5 mm, collimation width of 5 mm and reconstruction in 3 mm thick scans. In addition to the usual transaxial slices, we often represent spiral CT data as a shaded surface display or multiplanar reconstruction to assist in assessment of the aortic shape and dimensions. Angiography is also part of the routine preoperative evaluation, mainly to assess the iliac arteries, which are frequently found to be too calcified and too tortuous to be assessed well by CT alone.

Procedure

All patients are treated in an operating room, using a mobile C-arm fluoroscopy unit (Siremobil 2000; Siemens, Erlangen, Germany), equipped for digital subtraction angiography, road-mapping, and hard copy output. The steps in stent–graft insertion are as follows:

1. The prosthesis is mounted over the metal cannula of the pusher, with the proximal end of the prosthesis next to the bulbous dilatation. A single unknotted length of multifilament thread is passed through opposite angles at the proximal end of the proximal stent. Both ends of this suture are tied to a guidewire and pulled through the central lumen of the pusher, from the

bulbous end to the end of the shaft, where they are clamped under a small amount of tension. Thus the suture loop is used to attach the prosthesis to the pusher, so that when the pusher is advanced through the sheath, the prosthesis is towed along behind it.

2. Both femoral arteries are exposed surgically.
3. Catheters and guidewires are passed into the proximal aorta from femoral arteries. A stiff guidewire (Amplatz Extra Stiff, Cook) is left on the side selected for delivery system insertion, and a 5-Fr straight-tipped, multiple side-hole, angiographic catheter is left in the other femoral artery.
4. Heparin 150 units/kg is administered intravenously before application of arterial occlusive clamps and snares.
5. In most cases, the sheath and dilator of the delivery system are inserted through a longitudinal femoral arteriotomy and passed over the stiff guidewire into the aorta (Fig. 11.1), until the end of

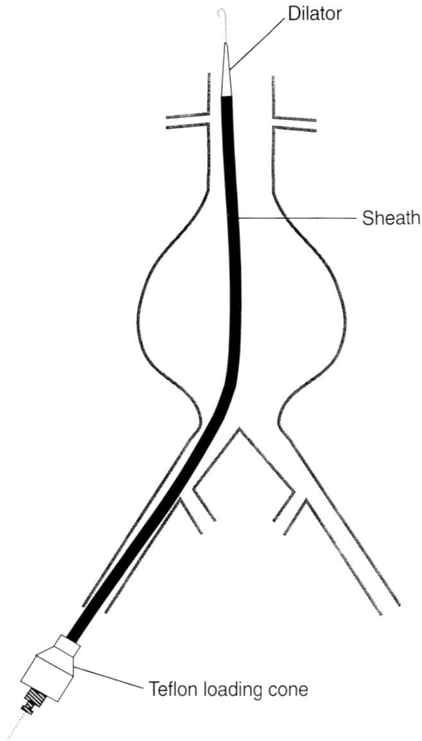

Fig. 11.1 Insertion of the introducer sheath and its dilator over a stiff guidewire.

the sheath is above the level of the renal arteries. Retroperitoneal exposure is sometimes used to straighten tortuous iliac arteries and facilitate introduction of the delivery system, but direct iliac artery access has been required only once.

6. The dilator is removed from the sheath, and Fogarty clamps are applied to the sheath at the femoral level as the dilator is removed, to prevent brisk haemorrhage.
7. The pusher and stent–graft are squeezed into the cone of the sheath. The pusher is then used to advance the stent–graft up the sheath, through its suture attachment to the proximal stent.
8. The Fogarty clamps are removed to allow the pusher and stent–graft to pass up the sheath. Haemostasis, at this point, is provided by the bulk of the stent–graft and the shaft of the dilator, both of which plug the lumen of the sheath.
9. When the proximal stent reaches the level of the aneurysm neck, angiography is repeated to confirm the position of the renal arteries. This has proved to be particularly important when the neck is short or tortuous. If the neck of the aorta is angulated sharply anteriorly, the C arm has to be rotated into a more cranial–caudal axis.
10. The position of the proximal stent is maintained by manipulating the pusher as the sheath is withdrawn slowly.
11. The self-expanding proximal Z stent deploys as soon as it emerges from the upstream end of the sheath. Angiography is often repeated immediately before full deployment to allow last-minute adjustments of stent position (Fig. 11.2). Serial angiography is important in cases of severe aortic tortuosity, because the presence of the rigid pusher alters the configuration of the aneurysm neck, and movement of the pusher would sometimes be associated with movement of the aneurysm neck, none of which can be appreciated and accommodated without angiographic visualization.
12. Further withdrawal of the sheath completes stent–graft deployment. Expansion of the distal stent indicates that the entire stent–graft is outside the sheath.
13. The stent–graft is released from the pusher by removing the suture loop, after first checking to make sure that there are no knots that might snag on the proximal stent and cause it to be dislodged.

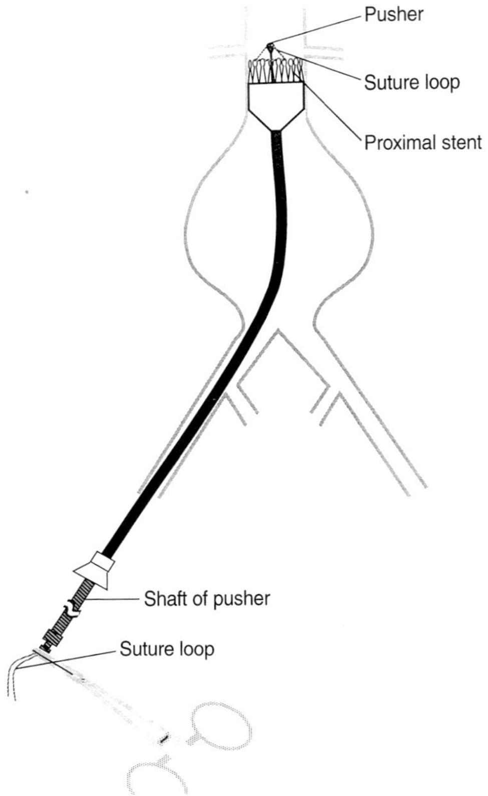

Fig. 11.2 Deployment of the proximal stent, guided by serial angiography.

14. The guidewire is replaced before delivery system removal (Fig. 11.3), to facilitate subsequent instrumentation of the stent–graft.
15. Completion angiography is performed to look for perigraft leak and to assess stent–graft position and patency. Subsequent adjunctive manoeuvres depend mainly on angiographic findings. Angiographic assessment is sometimes supplemented by intravascular ultrasonography, although we have yet to base any clinical decisions on this additional information.
16. The delivery system for the contralateral iliac artery occluder is inserted through a longitudinal femoral arteriotomy, and advanced over a guidewire into the common iliac artery.

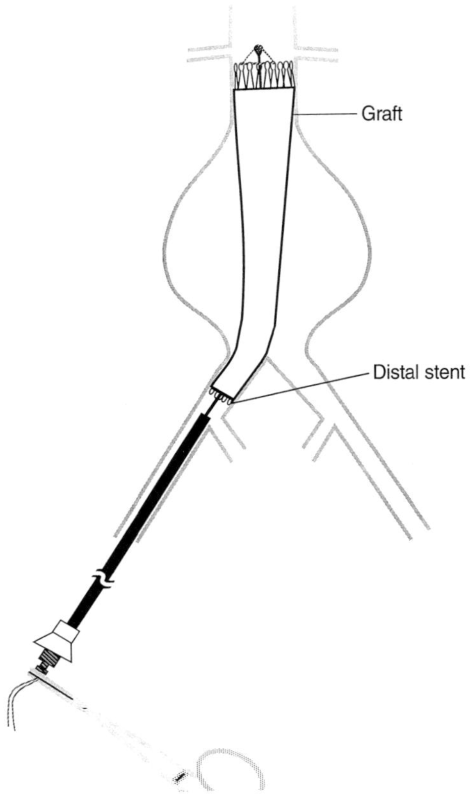

Fig. 11.3 Removal of the delivery system.

17. The dilator is removed to permit insertion of the occluder, which is advanced through the sheath into the common iliac artery.
18. Contrast is injected through the sheath to assess the completeness of iliac artery occlusion and the patency of the external to internal iliac artery pathway.
19. The longitudinal arteriotomies are joined by constructing a conventional femorofemoral bypass (Fig. 11.4).
20. Assessment of the short-term result also includes contrast enhanced spiral CT, within 1 week of stent–graft insertion. Any contrast seen outside the lumen of the graft on CT is interpreted as 'persistent perigraft perfusion'. This is further investigated angiographically, and treated depending on the cause.[10]

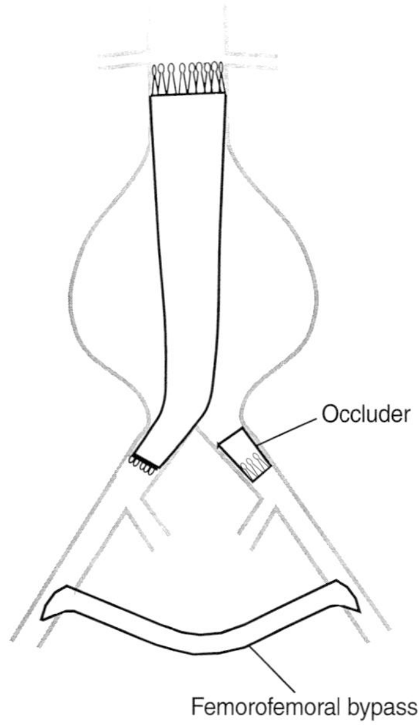

Fig. 11.4 Completion of the procedure with insertion of a contralateral common iliac artery occluder and femorofemoral bypass.

Complications and management

Between November 1993 and November 1995, 30 patients underwent elective abdominal aortic aneurysm exclusion using the Ivancev–Malmö system. These are divided into three groups of ten patients each, to show the effects of accumulating experience. The same trend towards improved results is apparent throughout the results. The procedure has become quicker, the blood loss less (Table 11.1), the

Table 11.1 Mean duration and estimated blood loss for the first, second and third groups of ten patients to undergo endovascular aneurysm exclusion.

	First 10	*Second 10*	*Third 10*
Duration (min)	242	240	225
Blood loss (ml)	1806	867	525

Table 11.2 Complications occurring in the first, second and third groups of ten patients to undergo endovascular aneurysm exclusion.

	First 10	*Second 10*	*Third 10*
Immediate conversion	5	0	0
Late conversion	1	0	0
Renal artery occlusion	1	0	1
Haemorrhage	1	0	0
Perigraft leak	1	0	1
Kink	4	3	0
Iliac artery dissection	0	2	1

complications less frequent (Table 11.2), the morbidity lower, and successful endovascular aneurysm exclusion more common (Table 11.3).

Short-term success is defined as exclusion of the aneurysm by CT criteria. Morbidity rates (Table 11.3) include all patients who suffered complications with clinical manifestations or who were returned to the operating room for any reason. Not included are cases of immediate conversion to open repair in which the recovery was uncomplicated, cases listed as mortalities, and those involving only percutaneous procedures after operation. The artificial distinctions between return to the operating room and treatment in the angiography suite, between clinical and silent (radiographically diagnosed) complications, and between immediate and subsequent conversion, all illustrate the difficulty in applying the reporting standards of conventional surgery to endovascular procedures. However, cases in which an additional procedure was performed percutaneously in the angiography suite are listed as complications in Table 11.2.

Some of the apparent progression up the 'learning curve' resulted from increasing skill with the device and improved patient selection.

Table 11.3 Results in the first, second and third groups of ten patients to undergo endovascular aneurysm exclusion.

	First 10	*Second 10*	*Third 10*
Mortality	1	2	1
Morbidity	4	1	1
Success	4	8	9

Another factor was the development of adjunctive manoeuvres to treat potential problems. These include:

1. Reorientation of the proximal stent with valvulotomy balloons to correct proximal perigraft leak (performed on four occasions).
2. Insertion of a second stent–graft above the first to correct proximal perigraft leak (performed on three occasions).
3. Retroperitoneal exposure of the iliac arteries, to assist in delivery system insertion or to exclude flow to common iliac artery aneurysms (performed on five occasions).
4. Routine Wallstent (Schneider) insertion to correct kinking.

Follow-up

Angiography and spiral CT with intra-arterial contrast are performed routinely at 1, 6, 12, 18 and 24 months after the initial procedure. Mean follow-up is now more than 1 year for both groups. Of note, there have been no cases of graft infection, persistent perigraft leaks, or late leaks. A single case of graft thrombosis was associated with proximal stent disruption and migration, shortly after an open operation to correct distal leakage. The structural failure of this stent was attributed to the application of vascular clamps. However, there are two other cases in which distal migration of the prosthesis produced kinking severe enough to warrant additional Wallstent insertion.

Serial CT scans have demonstrated several interesting changes in aneurysm morphology. The change in aneurysm diameter has been variable. In no case has an excluded aneurysm enlarged. Most have declined in size, and some are back within the normal range of aortic dimensions (Fig. 11.5). Two cases of inflammatory aneurysm have shown progressive thinning of the inflammatory mantle.

Summary: advantages and disadvantages of the Ivancev–Malmö system

The principal advantages of this system are its simplicity and the ready availability of the components. We have found its limitations to be predictable consequences of individual arterial anatomy. Some patients simply lack the anatomic substrate for successful endovascular repair with this system. For example, we know that the Gianturco Z

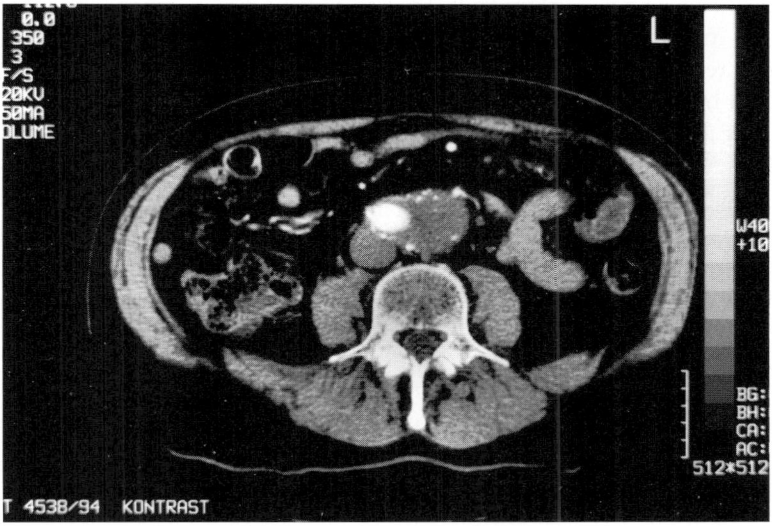

(a)

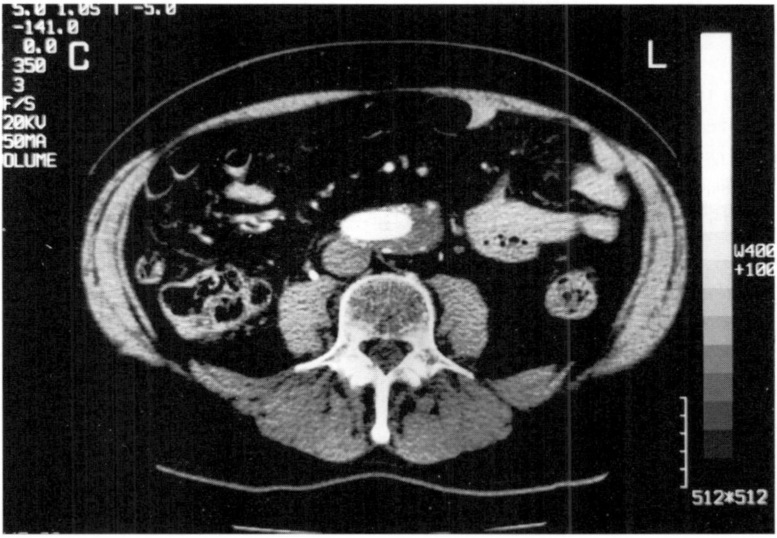

(b)

Fig. 11.5 CT scan (a) 1 month and (b) 12 months after endovascular aneurysm exclusion showing reduced aneurysm diameter following the procedure.

stent used in this system will not produce secure haemostatic attachment in a short, angulated, conical, thrombus-lined neck, even in the short term. However, it is doubtful whether any of the current systems could be applied in such a case.

The prosthesis used in the current version of this system has only two stents, one at each end. To prevent kinking we have found it necessary to insert a third stent (Wallstent). It would probably be better if this were incorporated in the original prosthesis, as it is in some systems, such as the Stentor (Mintec). In addition to kink resistance, a fully stented prosthesis may have other advantages, such as a more stable position.

The lack of any mechanism for the implantation of bifurcated prostheses represents another limitation of the Ivancev–Malmö system. Aortoaortic implantation of a straight prosthesis is usually not feasible, because of the paucity of the distal implantation site in most cases.[11] The aortouni-iliac prosthesis is effective and versatile, but it cannot work without femorofemoral bypass and contralateral common iliac artery occlusion.

Femorofemoral bypass is a standard technique with known patency rates, which are generally inferior to the rates achieved by conventional aortofemoral bypass performed for occlusive disease, although it remains to be seen whether these rates apply when femorofemoral bypass is performed as an adjunct to endovascular aneurysm repair. The presence of graft in the base of the groin wound is another potential source of long-term morbidity.

We believe that the optimal common iliac artery occlusion device has yet to be developed. The one we use works well when the vessel is straight and of uniform caliber, but when the iliac artery is irregular, angulated, or aneurysmal, we find that additional coils, stents, or balloons are often required to achieve complete occlusion.

A bifurcated aortobi-iliac prosthesis is subject to neither of these potential limitations. However, a bifurcated prosthesis lacks some of the versatility of the uni-iliac configuration, because it requires suitable implantation sites in both iliac arteries.

References

1. Lawrence DD Jr, Charnsangavej C, Wright KC *et al.* Percutaneously endovascular graft: experimental evaluation. *Radiology* 1987; **163**: 357–60.
2. Mirich D, Wright KC, Wallace S *et al.* Percutaneously placed endovascular grafts for aortic aneurysms: feasibility study. *Radiology* 1989; **170**: 1033–7.

3. Dake MD, Miller DC, Semba CP, Mitchell RS, Walker PJ, Liddell RP. Transluminal placement of endovascular stent–grafts for the treatment of descending thoracic aortic aneurysms. *N Engl J Med* 1994; **331**: 1729–34.
4. Chuter TAM, Ivancev K, Lindblad B, Brunkwall J, Aren C, Risberg B. Case report: Endovascular stent–graft exclusion of an aortobronchial fistula. *J Vasc Intervention Radiol* (in press).
5. Lindblad B, Ivancev K, Chuter TAM *et al.* Case report: Endovascular exclusion of juxtarenal anastomotic pseudoaneurysm. *J Eur Vasc Endovasc Surg* (in press).
6. Parodi JC. Endovascular repair of abdominal aortic aneurysms and other arterial lesions. *J Vasc Surg* 1995; **21**: 549–57.
7. Marin ML, Veith FL, Cynamon J *et al.* Initial experience with transluminally placed endovascular grafts for the treatment of complex vascular lesions. *Ann Surg* 1995; **222**: 449–69.
8. May J, White G, Waugh R, Yu W, Harris J. Treatment of complex abdominal aortic aneurysms by a combination of endoluminal and extraluminal aortofemoral grafts. *J Vasc Surg* 1994; **19**: 924–33.
9. Yusuf SW, Baker DM, Hind RE *et al.* Endoluminal transfemoral abdominal aortic aneurysm repair with aorto-uni-iliac graft and femorofemoral bypass. *Br J Surg* 1995; **82**: 916.
10. Ivancev K, Chuter TAM, Lindblad B, Lindh M, Brunkwall J, Risberg B. Endovascular treatment of perigraft perfusion following transfemoral aneurysm repair. *World J Surg* (in press).
11. Chuter TAM, Green RM, Ouriel K, DeWeese JA. Infrarenal aortic aneurysm morphology: implications for transfemoral repair. *J Vasc Surg* 1994; **20**: 44–50.

12

The Parodi system

Juan Carlos Parodi, Claudio Schonholz and Ricardo La Mura

Department of Vascular Surgery, Instituto Cardiovascular de Buenos Aires, Mercedes 4255, Cap. Fed., Buenos Aires, Argentina

Based on the concept of endoluminal aneurysm exclusion, we began to develop a plan for endovascular treatment for abdominal aortic aneurysms (AAAs) in 1976. Two prototypes were developed and were marked by a high failure rate.[1]

The first was a thin fabric graft mounted on a metallic cage-like structure composed of a self-expandable mesh with a zig-zag configuration. The apparatus was compressed inside a tubular sheath, which acted as a vessel introducer and carrier. Experiments in normal canine aortas led to the abandonment of this prototype due to an inconsistent deployment of the metallic cage. The radial expansion properties of the cage were difficult to control and predict. Over-expansion resulted in aortic wall injury and subsequent rupture. Conversely, under-expansion led to leakage of blood between the apparatus and the host aorta, with subsequent device migrations. The second prototype involved a Dacron graft fitted on a Silastic bag with a cylindrical lumen, which could be distended by injection of silicone into the bag. Unfortunately, this method was associated with prompt graft thrombosis of the aorta in all animal studies. Both prototypes were eventually abandoned because of the discouraging results.[2,3] With the stent technology emerging in the field of endovascular treatment, we reinitiated our project in 1988, using balloon-expandable stents.

Our current approach is based on the concept that stents may be used in place of sutures to secure the proximal and distal ends of the fabric graft within the lumen of the aneurysm. With the use of a stent–graft combination, it is possible to treat patients with AAA by transfemoral placement of a prosthetic graft.

This chapter details the endoluminal treatment of AAAs in 88 patients and of thoracic aneurysms in three.

Animal feasibility studies

To test the concept of intraluminal graft implantation, a canine aneurysm model was used. A 6-cm segment of the infrarenal aorta was resected and replaced with a fusiform conduit made of crimped woven Dacron, measuring 8 cm in length. Histologic studies demonstrated endothelium graft coverage of the experimental aneurysm neck, coupled with mural thrombus formation in the body of the aneurysm. Both of these changes were regularly encountered within 1 month after implantation of the aneurysmal graft. Six weeks later the aneurysms were bypassed using endoluminal graft deployment techniques. A non-crimped knitted Dacron tube of an appropriate diameter and length was attached to carefully selected stents (Palmaz; Johnson & Johnson Interventional Systems). Two-thirds of each stent was covered by graft material, but one-third was left exposed to anchor the graft to the aortic wall. The graft was folded clockwise in two folds, mounted on a balloon catheter, placed over a guidewire and loaded into a 14-Fr Teflon sheath. The right femoral artery was chosen for vascular access. Under fluoroscopic guidance the leading stent was advanced over the guidewire into the neck of the aneurysm, below the renal orifices and above the body of the aneurysm. Following the proper positioning of the device, the introducer sheath was withdrawn and balloon inflation used to secure the graft by deploying either one or two stents. In one group of dogs only a proximal stent was used, but in a second, larger, group a distal stent was added to achieve total aneurysm exclusion. Angiography was then used to confirm correct stent–graft deployment and verify that the aneurysm was successfully bypassed.

We operated on a total of 43 dogs, in most cases to evaluate different models for experimental aneurysms or to test a variety of balloons and replacement grafts. In the last group of dogs, we performed 6-month evaluations, obtaining colour Doppler ultrasonographic (duplex) scans in some cases and complete pathologic studies in all animals. Using both optical and electronic microscopy, we found that both ends of stented grafts were covered by endothelium and that the shaft of the graft within the mural thrombus of the experimental AAA was covered by a fibrin platelet barrier. Once we were satisfied that a Dacron graft could be delivered through a catheter and fixed firmly in place by balloon-expandable stents, we obtained the permission of our institution's ethics committee to perform a pilot clinical study with a small group of patients who were fully informed regarding the nature of the work and were subsequently followed very carefully.

Clinical experience

Device components

The first component of the device is a super-stiff guidewire with a diameter of 0.038 inches. This facilitates introduction of the device through tortuous iliac arteries, keeps the axis of our device parallel to that of the aorta, and by minimizing manipulations prevents disruption of laminated thrombus that lines atherosclerotic aneurysms.

The balloon-expandable stent is a cylindrical tube with longitudinal slots that adopt a diamond shape when expanded. This design, initially described by Palmaz *et al.*,[4,5] permits the stent to expand from a diameter of only 5 mm when collapsed to more than 30 mm when expanded. The stent is 3.5 cm in length, and its metallic component represents only 20% of its surface area after deployment.

The knitted Dacron graft has a wall thickness of 0.2 mm and is fabricated using strong yarns with tensile and bursting strengths comparable with those of commercially available grafts. The compliance of the shaft of the graft (15%) is also similar to that of standard knitted Dacron grafts, but the compliance of the segment overlapping the stent is 45% in order to adapt to its expansion. Between these two segments, a transitional zone of intermediate compliance is interposed in an attempt to avoid abrupt changes in the diameter of the graft that could eventually produce deleterious friction between the stent and the shaft of the graft itself. The diameter and length of each graft is tailored to fit the individual patient, but the grafts we have employed most often are 18–20 mm in diameter and 8–12 cm in length (Fig. 12.1).

A thin gold wire marker is knitted to each graft. This permits radiographic identification of both ends and the sides of the graft so that torsion can be corrected during implantation. The balloon catheters have a shaft constructed of polyvinylchloride with a 9-Fr diameter, and they contain either two or three channels depending on the number of low-profile, non-elastomeric polyethylene balloons affixed to them. If two balloons are used, the caudal one has a cylindrical configuration leading into a 30° angle in the catheter shaft immediately below it in order to accommodate the typical angle of origin taken by the iliac arteries at the level of the aortic bifurcation. We generally use just two balloon diameters that adapt to an inflated diameter of 18–30 mm. The last piece of the device is a Teflon sheath which has a diameter of 21 Fr and a haemostatic valve at the proximal end (Fig. 12.2).

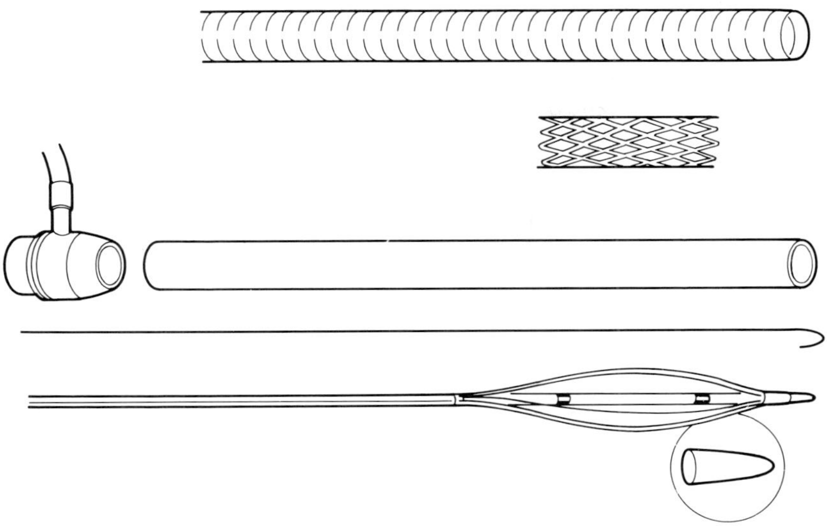

Fig. 12.1 The elements comprising the endovascular device.

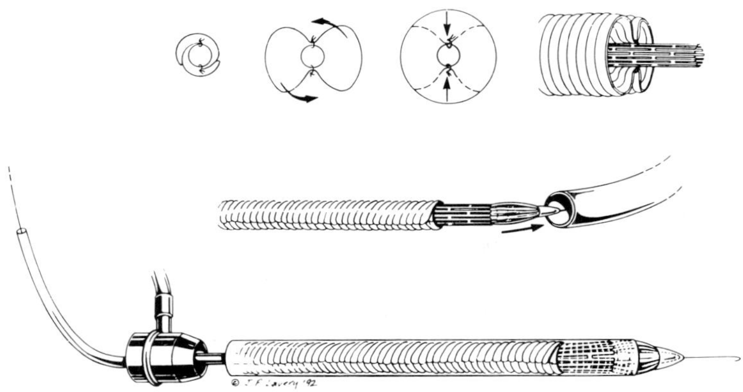

Fig. 12.2 The graft–stent combination is mounted on a valvuloplasty balloon and placed under fluoroscopic control through a sheath introduced through femoral arteriotomy.

Procedure

Details of the procedure have been published before.[3,5] In summary they are as follows.

Under local or epidural anaesthesia the patient is prepared and draped as for a standard AAA resection. A small incision is developed over the chosen common femoral artery; usually the straight and wider artery is selected for access (Fig. 12.3). A soft-tipped guidewire is advanced in the aorta up to the level of the diaphragm; over the guidewire a pigtail diagnostic catheter is placed inside the lumen of the aorta with the tip located proximal to the renal arteries. The first injection of 30 ml contrast medium is performed. The pigtail catheter is coded with a radiopaque marker, which is engraved on its surface

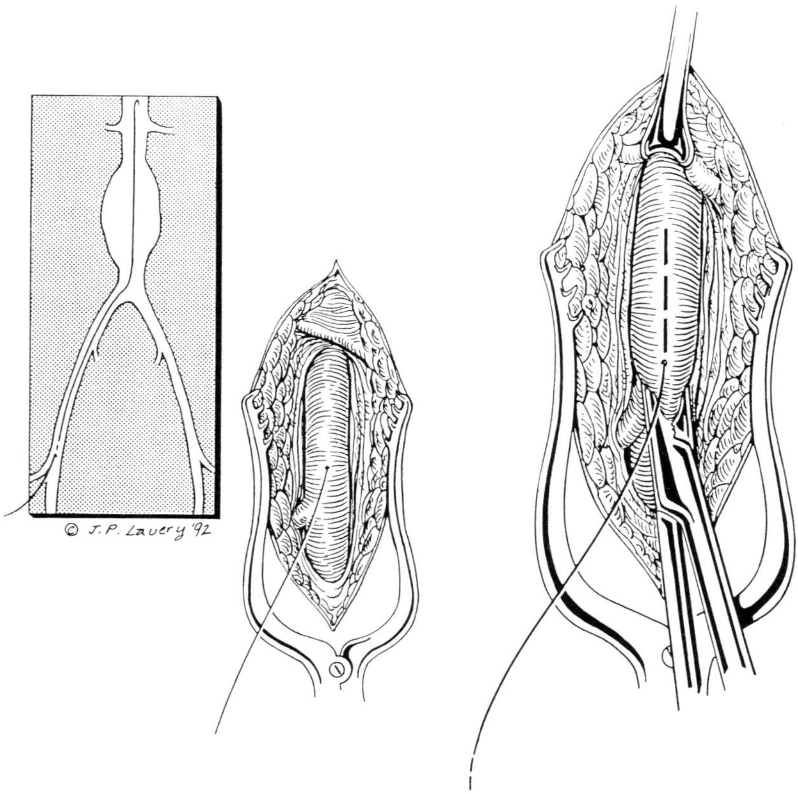

Fig. 12.3 A small incision is made over the femoral artery and a soft-tipped guidewire is placed in the aorta.

every 2 cm to facilitate length and diameter measurements. With a previously obtained angiogram and computed tomography (CT) scan, and in conjunction with the new angiogram, target areas are defined. They could be the proximal neck of the aneurysm and distal cuff when this latter exists, or the common iliac artery in the case of absence of the distal cuff.

The preloaded sheath containing the stent and graft mounted on a balloon is placed inside the lumen of the aneurysm under fluoroscopic guidance (Fig. 12.4). Once in place, the sheath is removed and the cranial balloon is inflated with a diluted solution of ionic contrast medium and saline. The balloon is kept inflated for 1 min and then gently deflated. Before proceeding with balloon inflation the mean blood pressure is dropped using nitroglycerin solution. Pressure is kept in 70 mmHg during balloon inflation. The size of the balloon is selected beforehand according to the diameter of the neck of the aneurysm measured in the previous angiogram and CT scan.

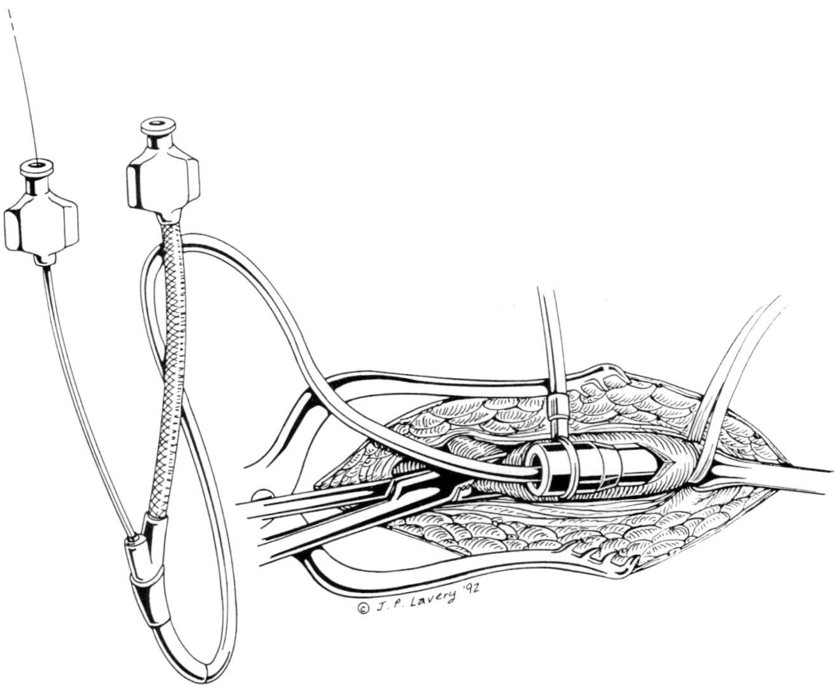

Fig. 12.4 The preloaded sheath containing the device is advanced and a femoral incision is made.

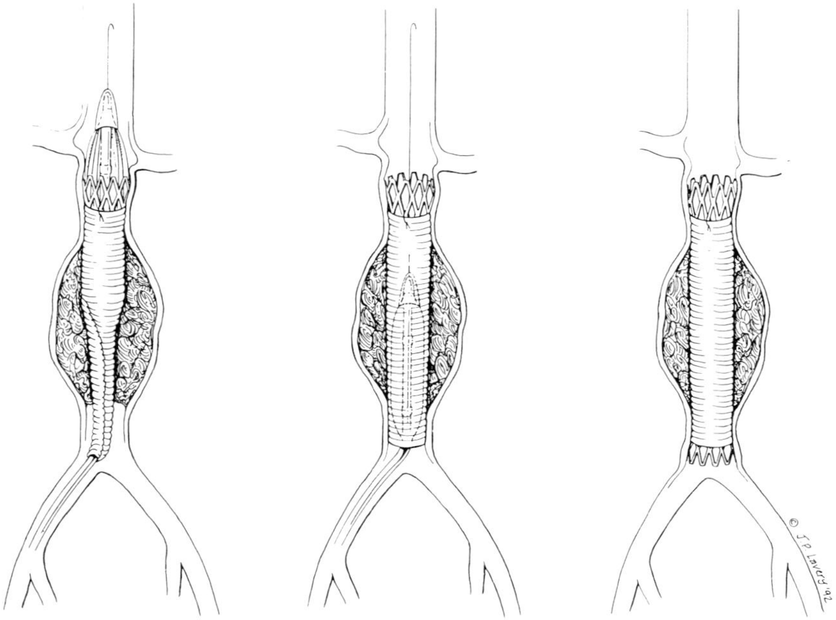

Fig. 12.5 Device deployment sequence.

After securing the proximal stent, the second stent is placed. In some cases in which a double-balloon device is used, the second balloon (either aortic or iliac) is positioned at the appropriate level and inflated, deploying the second stent (Fig. 12.5). A final angiogram is obtained. In the case that an aortoiliac graft is placed, the procedure is finished by performing a femorofemoral bypass and balloon or stent occlusion of the contralateral common iliac artery.

When a complex procedure is anticipated, blood loss from the field is saved and retransfused after being filtered. Blood loss occurs when sheaths of different diameter have to be changed and additional procedures, such as implanting a covered stent, are necessary.

The duration of the procedure varies according to the complexity of the case: between 25 min and 3 hours.

Patient selection

Patients considered potential candidates for endoluminal aneurysm bypass have to be evaluated as if they are to undergo conventional operative repair. Contrast-enhanced CT of the abdominal aorta is performed at 1-cm intervals, with added views across the proximal and distal ends of the aneurysm. The CT scan can give an estimate of the proximal neck, the distance between the renal arteries and the beginning of the body of the aneurysm, and the diameter of the aorta at the upper and lower ends of the aortic aneurysm. Also, the distance from the renal arteries to the aortic bifurcation can be calculated and used to predict the graft length that will be needed.

In addition, a biplanar abdominal aortogram is obtained in every patient, as it provides further detail concerning the visceral branches, the patency of the inferior mesenteric and lumbar arteries, and the course and diameter of the iliac arteries. Angiography is performed with a pigtail catheter having gold calibrations at 2-cm intervals and with a radiopaque ruler positioned vertically behind the patient to obtain accurate measurements.

Both the angiographic features and the CT data should complement each other. If substantial differences are encountered, the data must be reviewed before device assembly. Minor differences are not uncommon, with the CT scan sometimes overestimating the intraluminal diameter of the aorta by a factor of 1–4 mm, as the axial sections may not provide a true axial section of an angulated aorta. Once all the dimensions have been determined and agreed on, the implantation device can be designed.

Clinical results

As stated above, initially only those patients with serious associated pathologic conditions, implying a high surgical risk with conventional repair, were selected for endoluminal bypass. However, after initial clinical success, few patients who were suitable candidates for standard operative repair have been treated by endoluminal bypass. The following anatomic criteria are desirable for the endoluminal placement of an aortoaortic tube graft:

1. Both the proximal and distal necks of the aortic aneurysm have to measure at least 2 cm in length.
2. At least one of the iliac arteries has to be patent and sufficiently straight to allow delivery of the device and carrier. An external iliac diameter of at least 7 mm is desirable for a common femoral approach.

Eighty-eight patients with abdominal aortic aneurysms were treated from September 1990 to June 1995. Five patients were admitted to the clinic with pain probably related to their aneurysm, but none was ruptured. One patient was admitted as an emergency for a rapidly growing aortic dilatation caused by infrarenal aortic dissection. Two patients were admitted with the diagnosis of blue-toe syndrome in which the source of the emboli was an AAA.

The size of aneurysm at the time of treatment was more than 5 cm in diameter in most cases. Two patients had small aneurysms that caused microembolization and one patient with an aneurysm of less than 5 cm had bilateral carotid endarterectomy and coronary bypass surgery in the same year, and decided to have his 4.5-cm AAA treated by the endoluminal method.

Seventy-six men and 12 women were treated. The average age was 73 (range 57–87) years; ten patients were more than 80 years of age.

Table 12.1 Procedures performed in 88 patients.

Procedure	*No. performed*
Aortoaortic graft with one stent (proximal)	8
Aortoaortic graft with two stents (both ends)	37
Aortoiliac stent–graft	38
Aortobi-iliac stent–graft	2
Thoracic stent–graft	3
Total	88

Table 12.2 Associated pathologic conditions.

Condition	*No. of patients*
Severe chronic heart disease	53
Recent myocardial infarction	23
Severe pulmonary insufficiency	26
Renal insufficiency	5
Acute cerebral infarction	1
Two or more previous strokes	10
Hostile abdomen	2
Hepatic failure	2
Mild pulmonary insufficiency	12
Intermittent claudication	33
Disseminated intravascular coagulation	1

Forty-five of 88 patients underwent aortic tube graft replacement, with eight patients having only proximal stent placement (Table 12.1). All patients had at least one associated morbid condition. Associated pathologic conditions are given in Table 12.2.

Results

Of the 88 procedures for AAA exclusion, 75% aortoiliac and 84% aortoaortic procedures were considered an initial success. The definition of a successful procedure includes complete exclusion of the aneurysm with restoration of normal blood flow. The stent–graft should be in contact with the aortic wall, as sealing when the stent graft is deployed in an area covered with laminated thrombus proved to be incomplete and temporary. Patients with successful procedures recovered rapidly, had breakfast the next morning, and walked within 24–48 hours after the procedure. Typically they were discharged from hospital after 3 or 4 days (Figs 12.6 and 12.7).

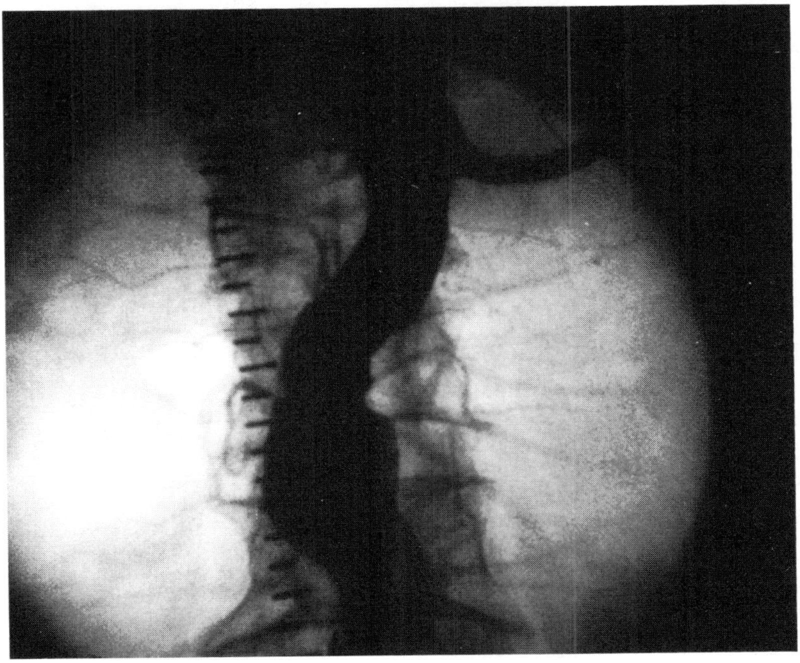

Fig. 12.6 Aortogram showing aortic aneurysms with both necks.

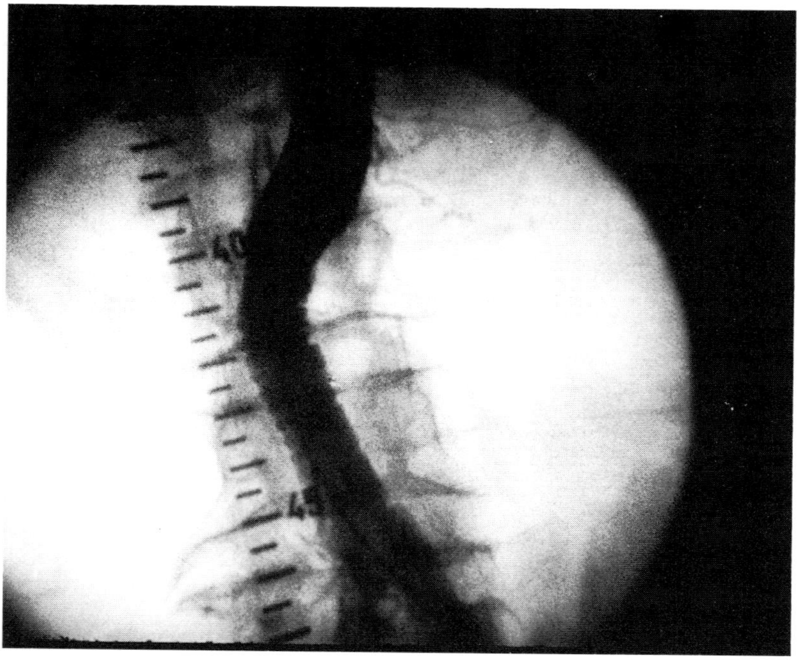

Fig. 12.7 Aortogram following deployment of an endovascular graft.

Of the 88 procedures, 18 (20%) were considered as initial failures. Four of the 18 failures were correctable by means of endoluminal treatment, but, because of the prohibitive risk in this group of patients, additional treatment was not attempted at that time.

Failures

There was one case of misplacement of the proximal stent, which was treated by standard surgical procedure. The patient survived and did well. There were three cases of proximal leak. In one patient with minimal leak, the size of the aneurysm decreased in spite of the leak, and the leak disappeared in a few weeks. This patient died from an unrelated cause 6 months after the procedure. The other two patients had a significant leak: one died after 7 months from cardiac insufficiency, and the other died from a ruptured aneurysm 2 months after the procedure. We consider every case of leak as a failure.

One case of incomplete deployment of the proximal stent resulted in migration of the graft. Because of the failure, the patient was treated by standard AAA resection. Liver cirrhosis, ascites, and gastrointestinal bleeding were the indications for endoluminal treatment. The patient survived the operation but died from abnormal bleeding the next day.

Two patients had a distal leak. One leak lasted for 3 weeks and then subsided. The second leak was minimal but persistent and the patient died from pulmonary and cardiac insufficiency 8 months later. Two patients had massive microembolization after difficult procedures applied in large and tortuous aneurysms. The procedures ended with massive microembolization and the patients died after developing disseminated intravascular coagulation and multiple organ failure.

One other patient died suddenly after 2 days. At autopsy macroscopic examination disclosed findings of intestinal ischaemia, which was considered to be related to embolization during the procedure. Microscopic examination, however, did not show occlusion of the superior mesenteric artery or its branches. A diagnosis of nonocclusive mesenteric ischaemia was therefore established. The operative mortality rate (within 30 days) was 8%.

Complications

In addition to the above-mentioned complications associated with failures, there were others that could be solved at the time of occurrence (see Table 12.3). In six of the 88 aortic procedures, both renal artery ostia were covered with the stent; the graft attached to the stent was placed distally to the renal arteries. None of these patients developed renal insufficiency. Colour duplex scans of the renal arteries were normal, and they are repeated every 6 months. Three balloon dilatations of the iliac arteries were performed in the series. Before inserting the stent–graft device, two common femoral aneurysms were corrected surgically at the same time as the procedure, and four

Table 12.3 Complications.

Complication	*No. of patients*
Groin haematoma	2
Proximal leak (treated with a covered stent)	1
Injury to the external iliac artery (sutured)	1
Minimal distal microembolism treated by intra-arterial injection of prostaglandin	1
Distal leak (treated with covered stent)	1

common iliac temporary conduits with a 10-mm tubular Dacron graft were constructed to permit access to the aorta in the presence of very tortuous and stenotic iliac arteries.

Long-term results

All patients were followed by clinical examination, colour duplex studies every 6 months, and CT once a year. Angiography was performed in some patients, and in every patient in whom the colour duplex or CT scans indicated or suggested any sign of leak, dilatation, or any change when compared with the study performed immediately after the procedure.

The average follow-up period was 16 (range 1–43) months. One patient developed a distal aortic dilatation 18 months after the initial procedure. The distal stent was placed high above the aortic bifurcation within the mural thrombus and not in contact with the normal aortic wall. The complication was corrected by adding a short segment of graft and performing a surgical anastomosis between the old graft and the aortic bifurcation. The patient recovered uneventfully. Three patients who had only the proximal stent deployed developed a distal reflux with shrinkage of the graft 8, 18, and 24 months after the procedure. Of these three patients, two were treated by insertion of a covered stent at the distal end. One patient died 13 months after the procedure from carcinoma of the colon. Another patient died after being admitted to the clinic because of cardiac failure and respiratory insufficiency 8 months after the initial procedure. Two patients died from cardiac insufficiency 6 and 7 months after the procedure. One patient with proximal leak (failure) died from a ruptured AAA 2 months after an unsuccessful procedure. One patient was readmitted to the clinic 3 months after the initial procedure with pulmonary oedema and was discharged after 1 week. Of the patients in the initial group, 70% of the primary procedures remain satisfactory at the time of the last follow-up or, in some cases, at the time of the death from an unrelated cause. Most of the complications were correctable by additional endoluminal procedures.

Discussion

After 88 procedures for the treatment of aneurysms some preliminary conclusions are possible. There are more problems than were initially anticipated. The procedure is simple in theory, but several details should be attended to before moving ahead with the widespread use of the method. First, measurements of diameters and lengths are crucial. We learned with great effort how to obtain reliable data using enhanced CT scans, quantitative angiography, and three-dimensional reconstruction by means of magnetic resonance imaging or CT. Scan images, intraluminal measurement, and some geometric calculations helped us to obtain reasonably reliable data. Understanding that elongation occurs as dilatation of the aorta develops, and also that elongation occurs in different planes, allowed us to calculate more accurately the actual length of the artery.

Second, access problems accounted for several puzzles we had to work out. Narrow, stenotic, and tortuous iliac arteries were responsible for these difficulties. The rigid stent and the large diameter of the sheath needed for the implantation were drawbacks from the beginning. We overcame some of these problems by modifying the device and using different manoeuvres during the procedure. Reducing the diameter of the sheath to 18 Fr was a remarkable advance toward the ideal device.

The use of an extra-stiff wire, the 'pull-down' manoeuvre, and sometimes implantation of a temporary conduit on the common iliac artery were also useful resources to overcome some of the problems. The pull-down manoeuvre consists of dissecting free the common femoral and external iliac arteries, lifting the inguinal ligament up, and using blunt dissection to reach the iliac bifurcation from the groin. Small branches should be divided between suture ligatures. When the arteries are free, by pulling the artery gently toward the feet of the patient, the tortuous artery becomes straighter, making the introduction of the sheath possible (Fig. 12.8). When the distal aortic cuff is not present, an aortobi-iliac graft has to be used as advocated by Chuter.[6] In addition, when the angle between the iliac arteries become larger than 90°, an aortoiliac graft should be used, placing a femorofemoral bypass.

Third, balloon-expandable stents, because of their high radial force, appear to provide secure anchoring mechanisms. We had one problem when the stent was incompletely deployed (one case of stent migration). Intraluminal ultrasonography is the ideal way to check the completeness of stent deployment.

Fourth, microembolization is what we consider to be the main and most dreadful problem with this procedure. Microembolization occurred three times in our experience, and two of the three cases

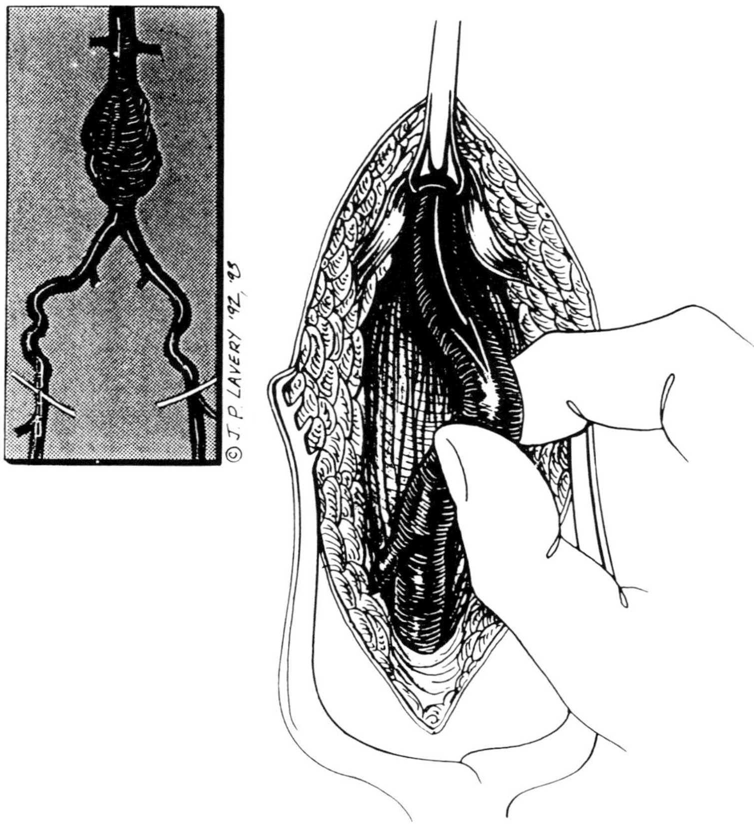

Fig. 12.8 The 'pull-down' manoeuvre.

resulted in death. In the remaining case discrete microembolization of the right foot was successfully treated with intra-arterial administration of prostaglandin E_1. The two cases that resulted in massive microembolization were technically difficult procedures in patients with large aneurysms. In one case visceral ischaemia was found at autopsy. In this last case technical problems occurred during the procedure in relation to inappropriate balloon sizing. Microscopic examination, however, disclosed a nonocclusive intestinal infarction, and embolization was ruled out in this case. A mild, reversible case of microembolization occurred on the side of the implantation of an occluding stent after an aortoiliac graft implantation with the addition of a femorofemoral bypass and was caused by incomplete deployment of the stent. Reviewing our cases of embolization, it appears very clear that large and tortuous aneurysms pose an increased risk of embolization. This is probably due to the following: on advancing the guidewire from the femoral artery into the aorta and then into the proximal neck, the operator will negotiate it inside a large and tortuous chamber coated with friable material. Sometimes it is very difficult to get the guidewire inside the proximal neck, because from within the cavity of the aneurysm the orifice of the proximal neck is often very small. It may be advisable in such cases to insert the guidewire percutaneously from the brachial artery.

Miscalculation of the length of the aneurysm often created the necessity to change the device or to use complementary procedures such as implanting a further covered stent to increase the length of the device or to cover a leak. The more intravascular manipulations we perform, the more the risk of dislodging particles from the aortic wall.

What can we do to prevent microembolization? (1) In large aneurysms with large lumens, the guidewire can be introduced from the brachial artery and recovered in the common femoral artery that has been chosen in advance. (2) Care should be taken to measure precisely the length and diameters of the arteries and to perform a simple well-planned procedure. (3) Experience of treating successfully patients who were admitted for spontaneous visceral and distal embolization, allows us to state that, even in the presence of friable thrombus in the lumen of the AAA, the endoluminal procedure can be performed safely.

References

1. Parodi JC. Endovascular repair of abdominal aortic aneurysms. *Adv Vasc Surg* 1993; **1**: 85–106.
2. Parodi JC, Palmaz JC, Barone HD *et al.* Tratamiento endoluminal de los aneurismas de aorta abdominal – estudio experimental. Presented at the second Convencion de cirujanos Vasculares de Habla Hispana, 13 October, 1990, Buenos Aires.
3. Parodi JC, Palmaz JC, Baroneh D *et al.* Transfemoral intraluminal graft implantation for abdominal aortic aneurysms. *Ann Vasc Surg* 1991; **5**: 491–9.
4. Palmaz JC, Richter GM, Noeldge G *et al.* Intraluminal stents in atherosclerotic iliac artery stenosis: preliminary report of multicenter study. *Radiology* 1988; **168**: 727–31.
5. Rees CR, Palmaz JC, Garcia O *et al.* Angioplasty and stenting of completely occluded iliac arteries. *Radiology* 1989; **172**: 953–9.
6. Chuter T. Bifurcated endovascular graft insertion for abdominal aortic aneurysms. In: Greenhalgh RM, ed. *Vascular and Endovascular Surgical Techniques*. Philadelphia, PA: WB Saunders, 1994: 92.

13

Endovascular repair of thoracic aneurysm

Michael D. Dake and Charles P. Semba

Section of Cardiovascular and Interventional Radiology, Department of Radiology, Stanford University Medical Center, Stanford, CA 94305, USA

Introduction

Over the past 30 years, surgical therapy for thoracic aortic aneurysms has advanced greatly. Despite important improvements in the management of these aneurysms by surgical resection and graft replacement, significant perioperative morbidity and mortality still occur, particularly in patients who have significant coexisting medical illness or who have previously undergone one or more operations for treatment of intrathoracic disease.[1–7] In light of these persistent clinical challenges, a less invasive approach is desirable, especially for patients considered at high risk for surgery because of pre-existing severe neurologic, cardiovascular, pulmonary, or renal dysfunction, some of whom may not tolerate general anaesthesia or extracorporeal bypass. The development of endovascular stent–grafts provides a less invasive alternative that may offer a lower risk and less expensive treatment than traditional operative therapy.

This chapter describes our initial clinical experience with transluminally placed, self-expanding stent–grafts for the treatment of thoracic aortic aneurysm. This preliminary experience suggests that endovascular stent–grafts may provide a safe and effective therapy to manage highly selected patients with aneurysm of the descending thoracic aorta.

Background

Dotter initially conceived the concept of a transluminally placed endovascular stent–graft in a 1969 report describing his experience with metallic coil-spring tubes placed in canine popliteal arteries.[8] His work did not strictly explore combinations of stents and prosthetic graft material as currently implanted, but it did propose the insertion of endovascular grafts through remote arterial access sites to treat vascular lesions without the extensive incision or dissection necessary to expose the diseased segments directly. Shortly thereafter, a number of investigators developed prototype endovascular stent–grafts and performed feasibility studies using experimental animal models of abdominal aortic aneurysms.[9–15] Recently, the clinical application of endovascular stent–grafts has been reported for the management of a wide variety of vascular diseases including abdominal aortic aneurysm,[16–23] descending thoracic aortic aneurysm,[24,25] subclavian artery aneurysm,[26,27] iliac artery aneurysm,[28,29] popliteal artery aneurysm,[30] arteriovenous fistula,[31,32] and peripheral occlusive disease.[33–35] These initial reports describe the challenges of applying new techniques using essentially prototypical devices for the treatment of complex vascular lesions. Despite the obvious need for further development of these primitive devices, early results support the concept and suggest that stent–grafts will play an increasingly significant role in the future management of vascular disease.

Thoracic aortic aneurysm

Natural history studies that describe the fate of untreated thoracic aortic aneurysm estimate a survival rate of 50% at 5 years and of 30% at 10 years.[36] The 5-year survival rate for these patients is worse than that reported for patients with untreated abdominal aortic aneurysm.[37,38] In cases of thoracic aortic aneurysm, rupture is responsible for 33–50% of the mortality.[1,37] Other causes of death are usually related to coexisting medical disease, particularly diffuse cardiovascular pathology often related to the presence of hypertension.

The development of thoracic aortic aneurysm is commonly an asymptomatic process, usually attracting clinical attention only upon its identification as an unsuspected abnormality on routine chest radiography. If symptoms are experienced, they often reflect progressive enlargement of the aneurysm with impingement upon adjacent structures or rupture.

In terms of aetiology, a retrospective study of 107 patients with thoracic aortic aneurysm estimated atherosclerosis as the cause in 78% of cases.[36] The atherosclerotic process is associated with degeneration and progressive weakening of the aortic wall with resultant dilatation.

The aneurysmal dilatation has a fusiform configuration in approximately 80% of cases.[36] In the other 20%, a saccular aneurysm shape is evident. In cases of saccular thoracic aortic aneurysm, 75% are noted in either the ascending aorta or transverse arch. Aneurysms with a fusiform configuration, however, are located in the ascending or transverse arch in 50% of cases, and identified in the descending thoracic aorta in the other 50%.

Materials and methods

Patient selection

Since July 1992 we have placed endovascular stent–grafts in 72 patients with 76 descending thoracic aortic aneurysms. Of these 76 aneurysms, 68 originated distal to the left subclavian artery and ended above the celiac axis. In seven cases the aneurysm involved or originated less than 1.5 cm distal to the left subclavian artery origin. In these cases, antecedent transposition of the left subclavian artery to the left carotid artery, or graft placement from the left carotid to the left subclavian artery, was performed immediately before stent–graft placement under the same general anaesthesia. In one case where the aneurysm extended to include the origin of the celiac trunk, but did not involve the superior mesenteric or renal artery origins, transcatheter coil embolization of the proximal celiac trunk was performed before stent–graft placement over its ostium. All patients were at relatively high risk for traditional surgical repair because of severe co-morbid medical and surgical illness, and most had undergone previous cardiac or aortic surgery. The aneurysms were due to a variety of aetiologies, including trauma ($n = 5$), dissection ($n = 5$), anastomosis ($n = 4$), and mycosis ($n = 2$); however, atherosclerosis was responsible for 60 of the 76 lesions. Some 52 of the cases were considered to be true aneurysms and 24 false aneurysms. The mean age of the patients was 66 (range 35–88) years.

Each case has its own unique anatomic considerations and, consequently, all the stent–graft prostheses are custom fabricated. The unique morphology and dimensions of each patient's aorta are defined by preprocedural imaging using spiral computed tomography (CT) with axial and three-dimensional reconstructions, as well as conventional arteriography. This preprocedural imaging protocol is the key to determine the anatomic suitability of an individual aneurysm for stent–graft repair, including the adequacy of proximal and distal necks. The spiral CT data allow measurement of the dimensions necessary to custom-build the stent–graft, including the diameter of the device based on the caliber of the adjacent normal aorta, and the overall length required to bridge the aneurysm. Aortography is performed to define precisely the anatomic relationships between the aneurysm, its necks, and the left subclavian and celiac arteries, configuration and relative degree of the aortic arch curvature, number and size of patent intercostal arteries, presence of an anterior spinal or medullary artery, and to assess the size, tortuosity, and any abnormalities of the abdominal aortic, iliac, and femoral arteries.

Optimally, a discrete neck of at least 15–20 mm should exist between the distal aspect of the left subclavian artery origin and the aneurysm to avert inadvertent placement of a stent–graft across this artery. If the proximal neck is less than ideal, a longer proximal neck may be artificially created by surgically transposing the left subclavian artery on to the left common carotid artery or by placing a bypass graft between the left common carotid artery and the left subclavian artery before stent–graft placement. The overall length of the device is calculated to extend only 15–20 mm of stent–graft into both the proximal and distal necks to avoid unnecessary occlusion of patent intercostal arteries adjacent to the aneurysm. In some cases, the iliac and common femoral arteries are not of sufficient diameter to accommodate the stent–graft delivery system. In these situations, where the pelvic conduit arteries do not provide an adequate access route to the aorta, an alternative surgical approach for stent–graft introduction via the distal infrarenal abdominal aorta is used. This access is commonly obtained by using a left retroperitoneal exposure and was necessary in seven cases because of insufficient iliac or common femoral arteries.

Stents

A stent is a lattice-like framework designed to buttress tissue in a desired configuration. In a stent–graft application, the stent provides a sutureless means of securing graft material at the proximal and distal necks of an aneurysm. Stents are usually manufactured from stainless steel, nitinol, or tantalum. Based on the mechanism of deployment, stents are often categorized into two basic designs: balloon expandable and self-expanding. The stents used in our clinical experience to date are self-expanding and composed of 0.020-inch surgical-grade stainless steel wire formed into a series of Z-shaped bends (Fig. 13.1).

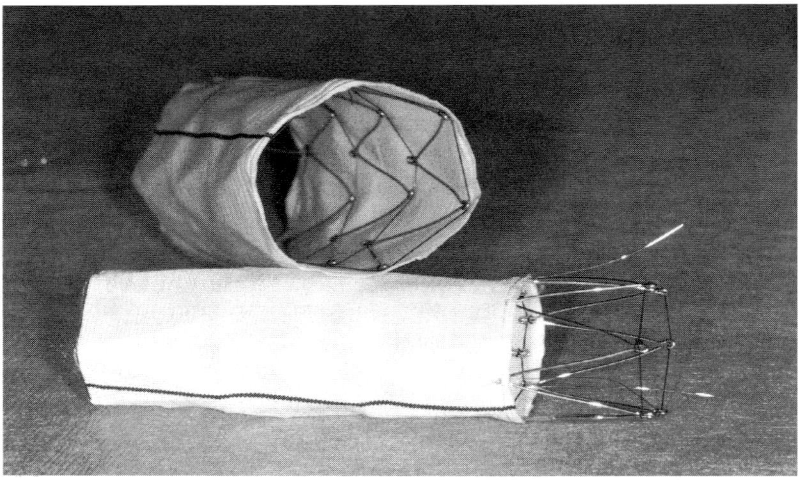

Fig. 13.1 Vascular stent–graft used for treatment of thoracic aortic aneurysms. The underlying stent is composed of individual stainless steel Z-shaped stent bodies combined together with polypropylene suture. The stent framework is covered with a skin of woven polyester graft material that is attached at its ends with interrupted polypropylene sutures.

Individual stent bodies are 2.5 cm in length with variable diameters ranging from 24 to 45 mm. In our clinical series, the mean diameter of the stent–grafts used is 35 mm. Several stent bodies may be combined to obtain the necessary total length determined by spiral CT measurements. Attachment together of individual stent bodies is achieved with 2–0 polypropylene suture. The mean length of stent–graft devices in our experience is 10 cm.

The metallic Z stent endoskeleton acts as a frame to support the entire length of graft material required to bridge the aneurysm from proximal to distal neck and to prevent kinking, buckling, or collapse of the graft within the aneurysm. Slight oversizing of the Z stent–graft diameter by 5–8% above the CT measurements provides sufficient radial force to anchor the graft material into position and seal it snugly against the aneurysm necks. No hooks or anchoring wires are used to prevent migration.

Graft material

The graft material used in our thoracic stent–grafts is woven polyester (Cooley Veri-Soft; Meadox Medical, Oakland, NJ, USA). Woven polyester material is selected because it is resistant to radial stretch, relatively nonporous, and thin. It has been used for many years as a prosthetic graft for the surgical treatment of thoracic aortic aneurysms without unacceptable dilatation or degeneration. In preparation of the graft material for attachment to the underlying stent, the crimps are ironed out with a hand iron to reduce the overall diameter of the device. A single piece of the ironed tubular graft material is cut to the appropriate length and secured to the Z stent framework with multiple interrupted 5–0 polypropylene sutures (Fig. 13.1). The cut edges of the graft material are heat sealed to prevent fraying during handling and insertion. After fabrication, the device is gas sterilized by means of an ethylene oxide treatment.

Delivery system

The delivery system used for the introduction and deployment of our thoracic stent–graft is quite simple and composed of four components: a Teflon delivery sheath of variable diameter depending on the size of the stent–graft, with an external haemostatic valve; a gradually tapered single-piece obturator to facilitate sheath introduction and advancement over a 0.035-inch extra stiff guidewire; a loading cartridge of equal diameter to the delivery sheath to facilitate stent–graft introduction through the valve and into the sheath; and a solid mandrel pusher with a blunt end to advance the stent–graft through the delivery sheath.

Endovascular procedure

All candidates for thoracic stent–graft placement are evaluated by both the Cardiothoracic Surgery and Interventional Radiology teams before providing informed consent for both conventional surgical and stent–graft procedures. All procedures are performed in the operating rooms of Stanford University Hospital with the patient supine or in a right lateral decubitus position under general anaesthesia on a radiolucent table. The operative field is prepared in anticipation of an open procedure. A portable fluoroscopic C-arm image intensifier capable of video playback and hard-copy image archiving is utilized in association with a mechanical contrast media injector to facilitate intraprocedural arteriorography. After surgical dissection and isolation of the most favourable femoral artery based on pelvic vascular anatomy, the

Seldinger technique is used to introduce a 5-Fr angiographic pigtail catheter to perform a preliminary thoracic aortogram. Once the ideal projection for identification of the proximal and distal necks has been determined, the pigtail catheter is removed over an exchange-length (260 cm) 0.035-inch extra stiff guidewire and anticoagulation with heparin (300 IU/kg) is administered. Typically, the delivery sheath and coaxial dilator are introduced through a transverse arteriotomy and advanced over the wire under fluoroscopic guidance. Once the delivery sheath has been placed across the aneurysm into the proximal neck, the dilator and guidewire are withdrawn. The stent–graft is advanced from its loading cartridge using the pusher and advanced through the sheath until it bridges the aneurysm. After the device has been appropriately located proximal to the aneurysm, the arterial blood pressure is lowered to a mean of 50–60 mmHg using an intravenous infusion of sodium nitroprusside. This reduction in blood pressure just before deployment of the device reduces the risk of downstream migration of the stent–graft during initial deployment due to arterial flow contacting the partially expanded covered prosthesis. After a final fluoroscopic check of the stent–graft position, the stent–graft is deployed by holding the pusher stationary and rapidly withdrawing the sheath. Immediately after stent–graft placement, the nitroprusside infusion is discontinued to allow the blood pressure to normalize. A completion aortogram is performed and in some cases transoesophageal ultrasonographic imaging is used to look for arteriographically occult perigraft leak and filling of the aneurysm sac. If the stent–graft does not completely cover the entire length of the aneurysm, a second device may be placed in a similar manner. If there is no perigraft leak evident on the completion aortogram or ultrasonographic imaging, the delivery sheath is removed, the anticoagulant effects of the heparin reversed with protamine sulphate and the common femoral artery repaired.

Patients typically spend the first 12–24 hours after the procedure in the intensive care unit until they are extubated and haemodynamically stable. Further recuperation on a nonmonitored ward for 1–2 days is the usual routine before hospital discharge. No postprocedural anticoagulation is administered. Before discharge, all patients undergo a repeat aortogram and spiral CT examination to evaluate the immediate results of stent–graft treatment. Subsequently, they undergo a repeat spiral CT examination 6 months after stent–graft placement and yearly thereafter.

Results

In the 72 cases of descending thoracic aortic aneurysm treated by endovascular stent–graft placement, the mean diameter of the aneurysm treated was 6.2 (range 5–11) cm. The stent–graft was successfully deployed in all cases; however, in 23 patients placement of more than one device was necessary to bridge the aneurysm completely and to exclude flow to the aneurysm sac. In 45 patients, the stent–graft was successfully introduced through the femoral artery approach. In nine patients with small and/or diseased pelvic arteries which could not accommodate the delivery system, the sheath and dilator were inserted via direct puncture of the infrarenal abdominal aorta ($n = 6$) or the common iliac artery above the inadequate arterial segment ($n = 3$). In 17 cases, the stent–graft was delivered in conjunction with standard surgical repair of an abdominal aortic aneurysm. In eight patients requiring placement of an aortic tube graft, the delivery system was introduced via a 10-mm polyester side-arm graft attached to the aortic tube graft segment after its insertion. In a further eight cases, the thoracic stent–graft was advanced via one limb of a bifurcated graft after anastomosis of the proximal graft to the aorta, and of the contralateral limb to the iliac or common femoral artery. In one case, endovascular stent–graft placement was performed for treatment of both a descending thoracic aortic aneurysm and an abdominal aortic aneurysm associated with a complex type B aortic dissection. The only other access route for stent–graft introduction in this series involves placement of the device via the ascending aorta in a patient undergoing a circulatory arrest procedure for standard operative repair of a transverse aortic arch aneurysm.

Complete thrombosis of the aneurysm sac surrounding the thoracic stent–graft (Fig. 13.2) was achieved in 68 of the 72 patients. Major complications were identified in 11 patients treated by stent–graft placement. Four patients died within 30 days of the procedure and a further three succumbed during a prolonged postprocedural hospital stay. Two of the four early deaths occurred within the first 48 hours immediately after stent–graft deployment. One death was related to complications associated with an iliac artery rupture that occurred during introduction of the delivery sheath, and another patient died 36 hours after stent–graft placement as a result of massive cerebral haemorrhage. The cause of death in this case was probably related to the anticoagulation required during the procedure to prevent throm-

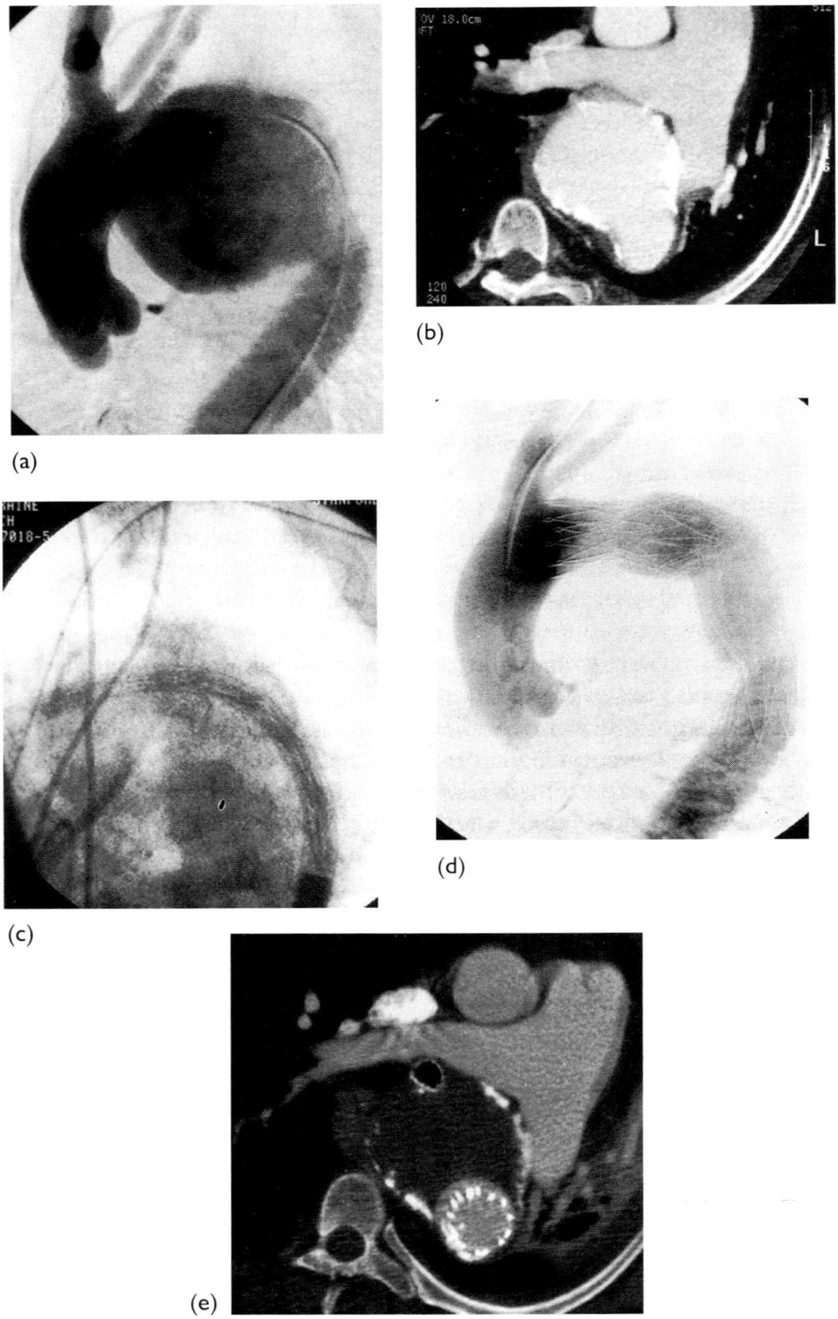

(a) (b) (c) (d) (e)

bosis formation within the large delivery sheath. The other two early deaths were an 83-year-old man who died 27 days after the procedure, following aspiration and development of bilateral pneumonia and respiratory failure, and a 72-year-old woman who died 19 days after the procedure from multiorgan failure associated with sepsis. This woman had a nonhealing groin wound associated with prolonged steroid administration for chronic pulmonary disease.

Three patients developed paraplegia (4%); one of these died 31 days after the procedure. This patient and one other with persistent moderate distal lower-extremity paraparesis had thoracic stent–graft placement in conjunction with standard surgical repair of an abdominal aortic aneurysm. A further patient became paraplegic after a procedure performed exclusively for stent–graft treatment of a long thoracic aortic aneurysm. This patient had previously undergone aortobifemoral bypass graft placement for treatment of an abdominal aortic aneurysm. Four cases of stroke (6%) occurred. Two resulted in death at 36 hours and 42 days after the procedure. One patient had sudden onset of left hemiparesis 9 hours after the procedure. This 72-year-old woman had multiple bilateral old cerebral infarctions identified on a CT scan without evidence of an acute abnormality. Three months after the stent–graft procedure, she exhibited mild residual left-sided strength deficits. The last case of stroke occurred in a 66-year-old woman who underwent combined surgical repair of a transverse aortic arch aneurysm under circulatory arrest and subsequent stent–graft treatment of a descending thoracic aortic aneurysm via the ascending aorta. After the procedure, a large left occipital infarct was identified during neurologic investigations. There have been no cases requiring immediate or late surgical conversion. There have been no instances of embolization distal to the stent–graft or stent–graft infection. One

Fig. 13.2 (a) Arch aortogram demonstrates a large post-traumatic aneurysm of the proximal descending thoracic aorta distal to the left subclavian artery. (b) Axial CT scan through the level of the aneurysm demonstrates a calcified wall without evidence of mural thrombus lining the aneurysm sac. (c) Stent–graft within its delivery sheath before deployment across the aneurysm. (d) Completion aortogram following stent–graft placement demonstrates a good position of the stent–graft without evidence of perigraft leakage of contrast media or persistent filling of the aneurysm sac. (e) Postprocedure CT scan at the same level as the pre-stent–graft image shows thrombosis of the aneurysm sac surrounding a patent prosthesis.

patient sustained a non-Q wave myocardial infarction without significant clinical sequelae.

Thrombosis of the aneurysm occurred in 68 of the 72 patients. The mean follow-up time for this group is 12.4 (range 1–43) months. Three late out-of-hospital deaths occurred at 3, 4.5, and 14 months after stent–graft placement. In two of these cases, the cause of death is unknown. In one case, however, a previously thrombosed aneurysm following stent–graft placement in a 79-year-old man apparently recanalized 4.5 months after the procedure via a penetrating ulcer of the oesophagus located distal to the device. The patient died after the aneurysm eroded into the oesophagus.

The thoracic stent–graft procedure does not employ specific neuroprotective measures and clearly does not allow reimplantation of intercostal arteries once they have been isolated. The incidence of paraplegia (4%) in our series, however, is not significantly different from that reported by Svensson *et al.*[7] (5%) in a review of 832 patients treated surgically for descending thoracic aorta pathology. The vast majority of cases in their series were aneurysms managed by operative graft replacement. Although we do not routinely search for the anterior spinal or medullary artery during preprocedural arteriography, whenever possible we try to limit the length of the stent–graft to avoid unnecessary occlusion of patent intercostal arteries. In our experience, no patient was excluded from consideration for stent–graft treatment on the basis of intercostal or spinal artery anatomy.

It should be noted that, during the initial phase of stent–graft development for the treatment of descending thoracic aortic aneurysm, a number of device-related as well as clinical complications will occur (Fig. 12.2). In our experience, stent–graft procedures may require adjunctive percutaneous manoeuvres after deployment of the initial prosthesis to ensure exclusion of the aneurysm. These include transcatheter coil embolization of small perigraft leaks (five patients), balloon dilatation of the devices, deployment of additional stent–grafts, and placement of uncovered stents. In this regard, the relative frequency of 'rescue' techniques currently required underscores the need for considerable experience in catheter techniques before any team attempts these procedures.

The initial morbidity and mortality rates encountered in our 72 patients compare favourably with results from large contemporary surgical series; however, long-term rigorous follow-up is clearly necessary to evaluate persistent aneurysm thrombosis, extension of the aneurysm to adjacent aortic segments, intragraft thrombosis, distal embolization, infection, stent breakage, graft degeneration, and evolution of the aneurysm size. If these data eventually prove acceptable, possible benefits of stent–graft placement for the treatment of selected thoracic aortic aneurysms include a reduction in procedure time, blood loss, length of intubation, intensive care requirement, total hospital stay, overall complications, and even death in patients who are considered to be at high risk for operative repair.

References

1. Pressler V, McNamara JJ. Thoracic aortic aneurysm: natural history and treatment. *J Thorac Cardiovasc Surg* 1980; **79**: 489–98.
2. DeBakey ME, McCollum CH, Graham JM. Surgical treatment of aneurysms of the descending thoracic aorta: long-term results in 500 patients. *J Cardiovasc Surg* 1978; **19**: 571–6.
3. Moreno-Cabral CE, Miller DC, Mitchell RS *et al.* Degenerative and atherosclerotic aneurysms of the thoracic aorta: determinants of early and late surgical outcome. *J Thorac Cardiovasc Surg* 1984; **88**: 1020–32.
4. Desanctis RW, Doroghazi RM, Austen WG *et al.* Aortic dissection. *N Engl J Med* 1987; **317**: 1060–7.
5. Miller DC, Mitchell RS, Oyer PE *et al.* Independent determinants of operative mortality for patients with aortic dissections. *Circulation* 1984; **70**: 153–64.
6. Ergin MA, Galla JD, Lansman S *et al.* Acute dissection of the aorta: current surgical treatment. *Surg Clin North Am* 1985; **65**: 721–41.
7. Svensson LG, Crawford ES, Hess KR *et al.* Variables predictive of outcome in 832 patients undergoing repairs of the descending thoracic aorta. *Chest* 1993; **104**: 1248–53.
8. Dotter CT. Transluminally placed coil spring endarterial tube grafts: long-term patency in canine popliteal artery. *Invest Radiol* 1969; **4**: 329–32.
9. Balko A, Piansecki CJ, Shah DM, Carney WI, Hopkins RW, Jackson BT. Transfemoral placement of intraluminal polyurethane prosthesis for abdominal aortic aneurysms. *J Surg Res* 1986; **40**: 305–9.
10. Lawrence DD, Charnsangavej C, Wright KC, Gianturco C, Wallace S. Percutaneous endovascular graft: experimental evaluation. *Radiology* 1987; **163**: 357–60.
11. Yoshioka T, Wright KC, Wallace S, Lawrence DD, Gianturco C. Self-expanding endovascular graft: an experimental study in dogs. *AJR Am J Roentgenol* 1988; **151**: 673–6.
12. Mirich D, Wright KC, Wallace S *et al.* Percutaneously placed endovascular grafts for aortic aneurysms: feasibility study. *Radiology* 1989; **170**: 1033–7.
13. Laborde JC, Parodi JC, Clem MF *et al.* Intraluminal bypass of abdominal aortic aneurysm: feasibility study. *Radiology* 1992; **184**: 185–90.
14. Chuter TAM, Green RM, Ouriel K, Fiore W, DeWeese JA. Transfemoral graft placement. *J Vasc Surg* 1993; **18**: 185–97.
15. Palmaz JC, Tio FO, Laborde JC *et al.* Use of stents covered with polytetrafluoroethylene in experimental abdominal aortic aneurysm. *JVIR* 1955; **6**: 879–85.

16. Parodi JC, Palmaz JC, Barone HD. Transfemoral intraluminal graft implantation for the abdominal aortic aneurysms. *Ann Vasc Surg* 1991; **5**: 491–9.
17. Moore WS, Vecera CL. Repair of abdominal aortic aneurysm by transfemoral endovascular graft placement. *Ann Surg* 1994; **220**: 331–41.
18. May J, White GH, Waugh R *et al.* Treatment of complex abdominal aortic aneurysms by combination of endoluminal and extraluminal aortofemoral grafts. *J Vasc Surg* 1994; **19**: 924–33.
19. May J, Whit GH, Yu W *et al.* Endoluminal grafting of abdominal aortic aneurysms: causes of failure and their prevention. *J Endovasc Surg* 1994; **1**: 44–52.
20. Parodi JC. Endovascular repair of abdominal aortic aneurysms and other arterial lesions. *J Vasc Surg* 1995; **21**: 549–57.
21. Scott RAP, Chuter TAM. Clinical endovascular placement of bifurcated graft in abdominal aortic aneurysm with laparotomy. *Lancet* 1994; **343**: 413.
22. Yusuf SW, Baker DM, Chuter TAM, Whitaker SC, Wenham PW, Hopkinson BR. Transfemoral endoluminal repair of abdominal aortic aneurysm with bifurcated graft. *Lancet* 1994; **344**: 350–1.
23. Marin ML, Veith FJ, Cynamon J *et al.* Initial experience with transluminally placed endovascular grafts for the treatment of complex vascular lesions. *Ann Surg* 1995; **222**: 449–69.
24. Dake MD, Miller DC, Semba CP *et al.* Transluminal placement of endovascular stent–grafts for the treatment of descending thoracic aortic aneurysms. *N Engl J Med* 1994; **331**: 1729–34.
25. Fann JI, Dake MD, Semba CP, Liddell RP, Pfeffer TA, Miller DC. Endovascular stent–grafting after arch aneurysm repair using the 'elephant trunk'. *Ann Thorac Surg* 1995; **60**: 1102–5.
26. May J, White G, Waugh R *et al.* Transluminal placement of a prosthetic graft–stent device for treatment of subclavian artery aneurysm. *J Vasc Surg* 1993; **18**: 1056–9.
27. Schmitter SP, Marx M, Bernstein R, Wack J, Semba CP, Dake MD. Angioplasty-induced subclavian artery dissection in a patient with internal mammary artery graft: treatment with endovascular stent and stent–graft. *AJR Am J Roentgenol* 1995; **165**: 449–51.
28. Razavi MK, Dake MD, Semba CP, Nyman URO, Liddell RP. Percutaneous endoluminal placement of stent–grafts for the treatment of isolated iliac artery aneurysms. *Radiology* 1995; **197**: 801–4.
29. Marin ML, Veith FJ, Lyon RT *et al.* Transfemoral endovascular repair of iliac artery aneurysms. *Am J Surg* 1995; **170**: 179–82.
30. Marin ML, Veith FJ, Panetta TF *et al.* Transfemoral endoluminal stented graft repair of a popliteal artery aneurysm. *J Vasc Surg* 1994; **19**: 754–7.
31. Marin ML, Veith FJ, Panetta TF *et al.* Percutaneous transfemoral insertion of a stented graft to repair a traumatic femoral arteriovenous fistula. *J Vasc Surg* 1993; **18**: 229–302.
32. Marin ML, Veith FJ, Panetta TF *et al.* Transluminally placed endovascular stented graft repair for arterial trauma. *J Vasc Surg* 1994; **20**: 466–73.
33. Cragg AH, Dake MD. Percutaneous femoropopliteal graft placement. *Radiology* 1993; **187**: 643–8.
34. Marin ML, Veith FJ, Cynamon J *et al.* Transfemoral endovascular stented graft treatment of aorto-iliac and femoropopliteal occlusive disease for limb salvage. *Am J Surg* 1994; **168**: 156–62.

35. Sanchez LA, Marin ML, Veith FJ *et al.* Placement of endovascular stented grafts via remote access sites: a new approach to the treatment of failed aortoiliofemoral reconstructions. *Ann Vasc Surg* 1995; **9**: 1–8.
36. Joyce JW, Fairbairn JF II, Kincaid OW *et al.* Aneurysms of the thoracic aorta: a clinical study with special reference to prognosis. *Circulation* 1964; **29**: 176–81.
37. Bickerstaff LK, Pairolero PC, Hollier LH *et al.* Thoracic aortic aneurysms: a population-based study. *Surgery* 1982; **92**: 1103–8.
38. Estes JE Jr. Abdominal aortic aneurysm: a study of 102 cases. *Circulation* 1950; **2**: 258–64.

14

Endovascular repair of iliac artery and other peripheral aneurysms

Michael L. Marin and Frank J. Veith

Division of Vascular Surgery, Department of Surgery, Montefiore Medical Center, The University Hospital for the Albert Einstein College of Medicine, 111 East 210th Street, New York, NY 10467, USA

Introduction

Isolated aneurysms of the iliac arteries are relatively uncommon, accounting for only 2–7% of atherosclerotic aneurysms of the aorto-iliac segment.[1–4] Similar to abdominal aortic aneurysms, iliac aneurysms may rupture, embolize, thrombose, or produce symptoms related to pressure on adjacent structures. Mortality rates following sudden rupture and emergency surgery for iliac artery aneurysms have been reported to be high, approximately 33%.[5] However, because of the infrequent nature of these lesions, management guidelines have not been well defined for the asymptomatic patient.[4] Furthermore, the technical complexities of operating on vessels deep within the pelvis, especially after previous aortic surgery, have made standard elective surgical management of iliac aneurysms more difficult than for aortic aneurysms.[3] Alternative therapies using simple aneurysm ligation, coil embolization, or the placement of porous intravascular stents have been attempted to treat these aneurysms.[6–8] While technical exclusion of flow from within aneurysms has been demonstrated, continued growth and rupture of thrombosed and excluded lesions are well documented.[9–12]

Another recently developed, less invasive, approach for aneurysm exclusion involves the use of endovascular grafts. These devices may be composed of prosthetic grafts coupled to anchoring stents which are placed within the lumen of the vessels directly across an aneurysm. Endovascular grafts have been successfully used to treat infrarenal aortic aneurysms, thoracic aortic aneurysms, occlusive vascular disease, and vascular trauma.[13–17] This chapter reviews the Montefiore experience with endovascular grafts for treating iliac artery and other peripheral artery aneurysms.

Methods

Endovascular graft device

All endovascular grafts used in this study were composed of 6-mm thin-walled polytetrafluoroethylene (PTFE) grafts (W.L. Gore and Associates, Flagstaff, AZ, USA). Each graft was sewn to a Palmaz balloon-expandable stent (P308 or P294; Johnson and Johnson Interventional Systems, Warren, NJ, USA) at the cephalad end of the graft (Fig. 14.1). To localize the caudal end of each graft and to facilitate placement of a second (distal) anchoring stent, radiopaque markers consisting of gold thread (24 K, 0.01 inch) were placed at the distal

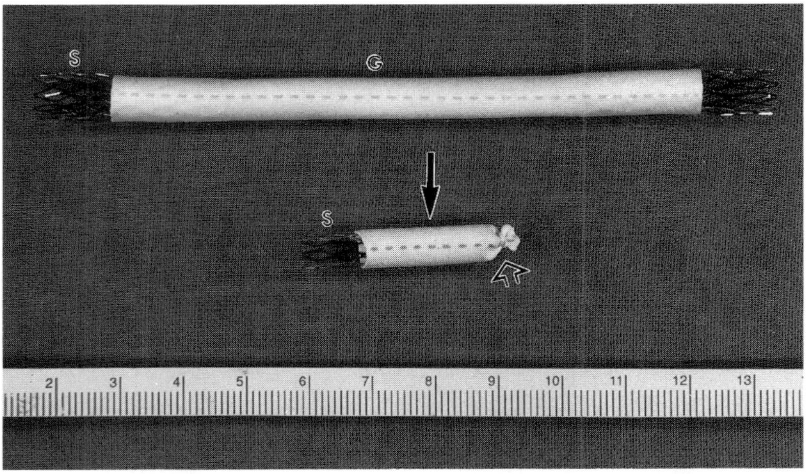

Fig. 14.1 Top: Photograph of an endovascular stented graft constructed from a balloon-expandable stent (S) and a 6-mm polytetrafluoroethylene (PTFE) graft (G). Bottom: Photograph of an occluding stent composed of a Palmaz iliac stent sutured to a 6-mm PTFE graft. The distal end of the graft protrudes like a 'windsock' from the end of the stent (solid arrow). A purse-string suture is applied to occlude the end of the graft (open arrow). (Reprinted by permission of the publisher from Marin ML, Veith FJ, Lyon RT *et al.* Transfemoral endovascular repair of iliac artery aneurysms. *Am J Surg* 1995; **170**: 179–82. Copyright © 1995 by Excerpta Medica.)

end of each graft. The endovascular grafts were then coaxially loaded on to appropriately sized balloon angioplasty catheters and inserted into 14-Fr introducer sheaths fashioned with a second tapered balloon tip and a proximal haemostatic valve. The length of the endovascular grafts ranged from 7 to 32 (mean 20) cm. For popliteal aneurysm repair the grafts were fabricated so the marker was on the proximal portion of the graft and the stent was sutured to the distal end of the prosthesis. Two such grafts were inserted, of 17 and 23 cm in length.

Mechanism of repair

Each patient with an iliac artery aneurysm underwent repair using a choice of one of six different techniques (Fig. 14.2). Selection of the

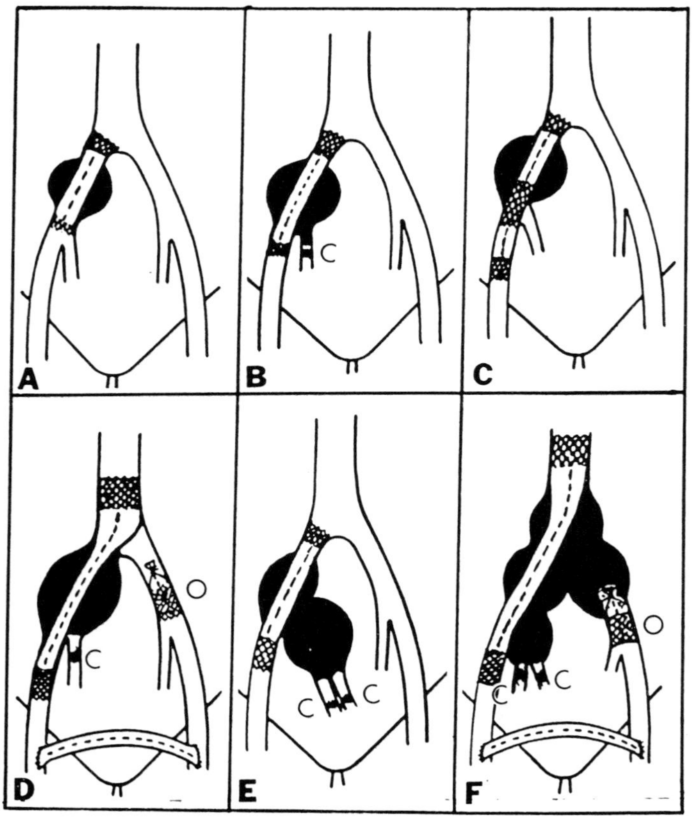

Fig. 14.2

appropriate repair technique was based on the morphology of the aneurysm as displayed on preoperative computed tomography (CT) scan and angiography.

In cases in which backflow from the internal iliac artery and its branches was a concern, Gianturco coils (Cook, Bloomington, IN, USA) were placed to thrombose and occlude this vessel (techniques B,

Fig. 14. 2 Techniques for the endoluminal repair of iliac artery aneurysms. (A) Localized common iliac artery aneurysm treated with stents anchoring the endovascular graft proximal and distal to the aneurysm. (B) If the aneurysm of the common iliac artery extends to the hypogastric vessel, an occlusion coil (c) is usually placed at the internal iliac artery orifice before endovascular stent grafting to prevent retrograde flow from the hypogastric artery into the iliac aneurysm. (C) Alternatively, retrograde flow into the aneurysm may be prevented by expansion of the graft across the hypogastric orifice or placement of an additional balloon-expandable stent within the lumen of the graft, securing the graft material across the hypogastric artery orifice. (D) When no aneurysmal neck (normal iliac artery) is present within the cephalad portion of the aneurysm, the stented graft may be anchored to a normal portion of the distal aorta. A coil (c) may be placed in the proximal hypogastric artery to prevent retrograde flow from this vessel into the aneurysm. A covered 'occluding' stent (o) is then positioned in the contralateral common iliac artery. A femorofemoral bypass is placed to re-establish vascular continuity. (E) If a wide mouth opening of a hypogastric artery aneurysm is present, the anterior and posterior divisions of the hypogastric artery are individually coil embolized (c) and the endovascular graft is secured with a stent above and below the origin of the aneurysmal artery, functionally excluding it from the circulation. (F) When the aorta and iliac arteries are involved in the aneurysmal process, all three aneurysms can be treated by modification of the type F reconstruction. The branches of the aneurysmal iliac arteries are embolized before operation with coils. The proximal portion of the endovascular stented graft is then positioned immediately below the renal arteries. The distal part of the graft is brought down one iliac artery to below the most distal extent of the aneurysms. The contralateral iliac artery is then occluded with an 'occluding' stent (o) and a femorofemoral bypass is done to perfuse the opposite leg. In reconstruction techniques B–E, the second stent is responsible for fixing the distal portion of the graft to the arterial wall. The distal stent in these reconstructions may be eliminated by extending the endovascular graft to the common femoral artery (site of device insertion) and performing an endoluminal anastomosis[14] before closure of the arteriotomy. (Reprinted by permission of the publisher from Marin ML, Veith FJ, Lyon RT *et al.* Transfemoral endovascular repair of iliac artery aneurysms. *Am J Surg* 1995; **170**: 179–82. Copyright © 1995 by Excerpta Medica.)

D, and E; Fig. 14.2). In instances in which occlusion of the contralateral common iliac artery was required (technique F; Fig. 14.2), a stent covered with a PTFE graft sealed at its cephalic end by a purse-string suture was used (see Fig. 14.1). All procedures were performed in the operating room under fluoroscopic guidance.

Three patients with popliteal aneurysms and one with a subclavian artery aneurysm occurring as a complication of thoracic outlet syndrome were treated with simple stent–graft–stent repairs.

Patients

The 22 patients in this series were all men with an age range of 56–89 (mean 74) years. Seven had undergone previous surgery for an aortic aneurysm 6–26 years before the endovascular grafting procedure. Sixteen patients had coronary artery disease with clinical evidence of previous myocardial infarction; eight had chronic obstructive pulmonary disease; eight had diabetes; and three had chronic renal failure (serum creatinine level greater than 3.0 mg/dl), one of whom required chronic maintenance haemodialysis. The distribution of the arterial lesions is outlined in Table 14.1.

Results

Iliac grafts were successfully placed in all 19 patients who underwent endovascular repair (Table 14.1; Fig. 14.3). Fourteen patients had the

Fig. 14.3 Transfemoral repair of a right internal iliac artery aneurysm 5 years after a bifurcated graft repair of aortic and common iliac artery aneurysms. (a) CT documents the presence of the right internal iliac artery aneurysm (arrow). (b) The two limbs of the bifurcated graft can be identified. (c) Transfemoral arteriography documents filling of the aneurysm before coil embolization of the anterior and posterior divisions of the vessel. (Note aneurysmal wall calcification (small arrows).) (d) Following endovascular graft repair, the aneurysm has thrombosed. Contrast can be identified within the endovascular graft (arrow). (e) This CT scan documents fixation of the Palmaz stent (arrow) within the old bifurcated graft. (f) Postoperative digital arteriogram shows the anchoring stents (arrows) and coils in the posterior and anterior divisions of the vessel to prevent retrograde flow (large arrow). Inset: Drawing of the completed repair. (Reprinted by permission of the publisher from Marin ML, Veith FJ, Cynamon J *et al.* Initial experience with transluminally placed endovascular grafts for the treatment of complex vascular lesions. *Ann Surg* 1995; **222**: 449–69.)

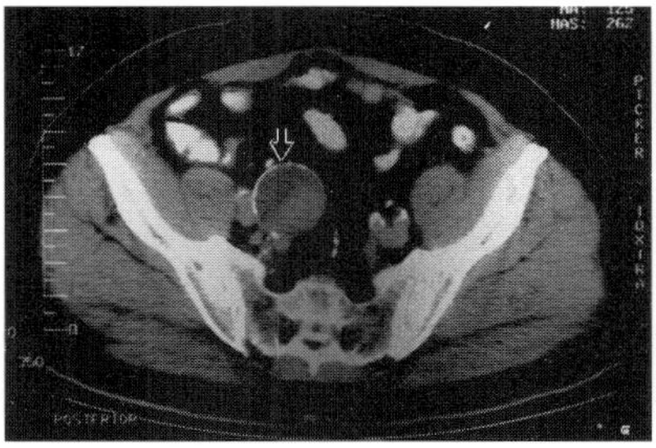

(a)

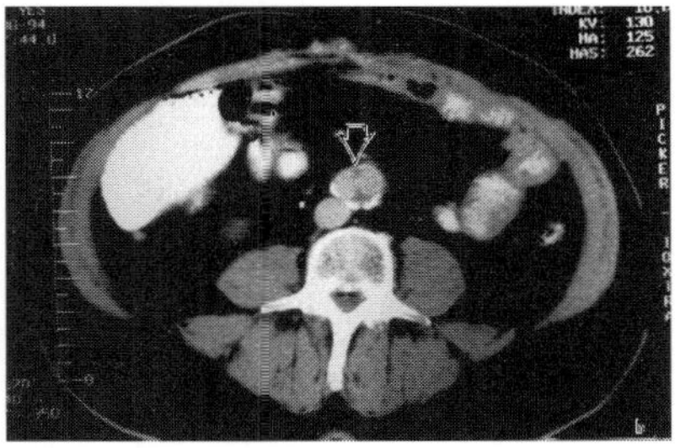

(b)

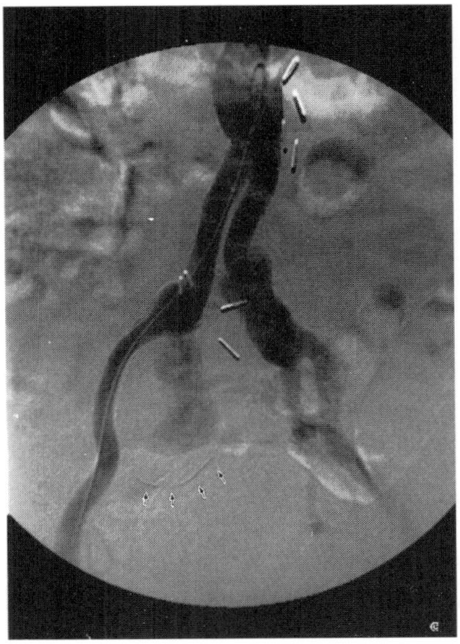

(c)

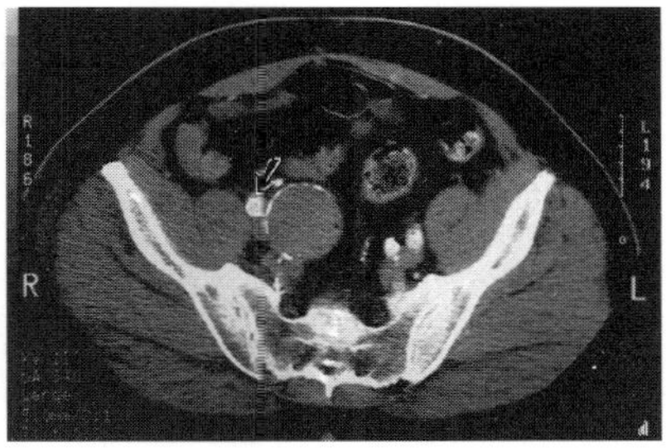

(d)

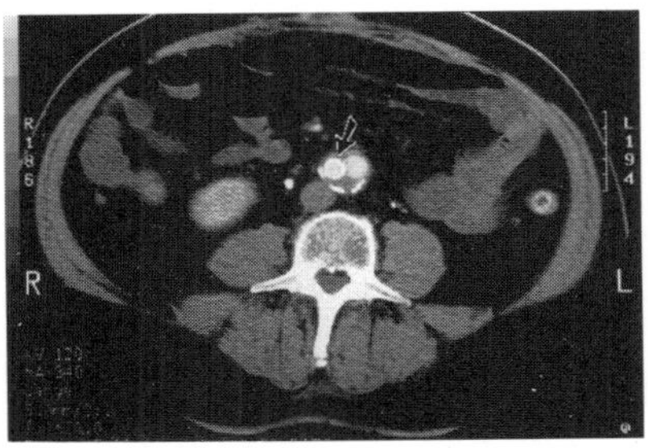

(e)

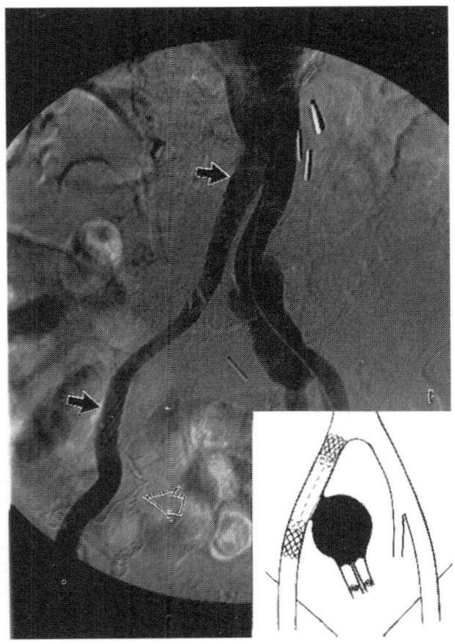

(f)

Table 14.1 Endovascular repair of iliac, popliteal, and subclavian artery aneurysms.

Aneurysm location	*Iliac reconstruction technique**	*Aneurysm size (cm)*		*Complications*	*Length of hospital stay (days)*	*Duration of follow-up (months)*
		preop.	*postop.*			
Left CIA	A	4.2	4.2		12‡	23§
Right CIA†	F	3.0	3.0		13‡	29
Right CIA	A	3.6	3.4		2	26
Right IAA	E	5.2	5.0		4	21
Right CIA		3.2	3.2			
Right CIA	D	5.2	5.2	Transient colonic ischemia	12	20
Right CIA†	F	5.0	4.9	Groin lymphocele	10‡	18
Left CIA		9.0	8.9			
Right CIA	C	2.9	2.9		5	17
Right CIA	C	3.4	3.4	Distal embolization; graft kink requiring stent	12	17
Left CIA	B	4.6	4.5		3	16
Right CIA	D	8.2	7.2		3	16
Right IAA	E	4.7	4.5		2	16
Right CIA		3.0	2.9			

Right CIA	D	10.0	8.5		5	16
Right CIA	E	3.0	3.0		2	14
Right IIA		6.0	5.5			
Left IIA	E	5.5	4.0		2	4
Left CIA	A	4.0	3.0	Haematoma	4	4
Right CIA	B	3.5	3.5		2	4
Right CIA	B	4.0	4.0		3	2
Right CIA	A	8.0	6.0		2	2
Left CIA	B	4.5	4.5		3	2
Left subclavian	—	3.0	3.0	Thrombosed at 6 weeks	2	13¶
Left popliteal	—	4.0	4.0	Thrombosis at 6 days	—	12#
Left popliteal	—	3.5	3.0		5	36

CIA, common iliac artery; IAA, internal iliac artery; EIA, external iliac artery.
*Techniques: see Figure 14.2.
†Concomitant abdominal aortic aneurysm.
‡Extended hospital stay for additional therapy for unrelated medical illness.
§Died from metastatic colonic cancer with a patent graft.
¶Graft closed 6 weeks postprocedure without limb-threatening consequences.
#Graft closed 6 days postprocedure and was converted to an open repair.

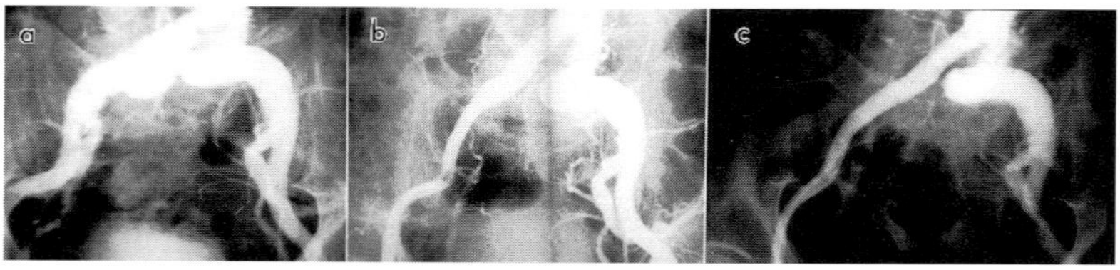

Fig. 14.4 Transfemoral arteriography of a patient with a right common iliac artery aneurysm. (a) Preoperative arteriogram demonstrates a large common iliac aneurysm. (b) Following insertion of an endovascular graft, the common iliac artery aneurysm is excluded; however, a stenosis was detected in the body of the graft that was flow limiting. (c) After insertion of a Palmaz balloon-expandable stent, the stenosis was corrected. (Reprinted by permission of the publisher from Marin ML, Veith FJ, Lyon RT *et al.* Transfemoral endovascular repair of iliac artery aneurysms. *Am J Surg* 1995; **170**: 179–82. Copyright © by Excerpta Medica.)

grafts inserted under epidural, three under local, and two under general anaesthesia. Intraoperative blood loss ranged from 50 to 2800 (mean 330) ml. Operating time ranged from 2 to 6 (mean 3) hours. No procedure-related deaths occurred. No acute graft thromboses occurred. In one patient a postoperative arteriogram demonstrated a kink in the endovascular graft, which was treated by the percutaneous insertion of a balloon expandable stent (Fig. 14.4). One patient was treated for contralateral distal ischaemia secondary to embolization from a plaque in a diseased infrarenal aorta. Postprocedural colonoscopy in an asymptomatic patient who had sacrifice of the right internal iliac artery was consistent with mild colonic mucosal ischaemia, which resolved without intervention. The length of hospital stay for patients with iliac aneurysms ranged from 2 to 13 days. Three patients had attempted endovascular grafting for popliteal aneurysms (Fig. 14.5). One patient had a failed procedure due to technical problems introducing the graft. The second patient had successful grafting, but the conduit thrombosed on day 6 after operation, necessitating successful conversion to standard bypass surgery. A third patient has had a functioning superficial femoral to below-knee popliteal bypass for over 3 years. Another patient had an endovascular stented graft placed to repair a subclavian artery aneurysm which occurred 2 years after surgical correction of thoracic outlet syndrome. Six weeks after successful grafting, the conduit thrombosed without limb-threatening consequences. No further treatment was used.

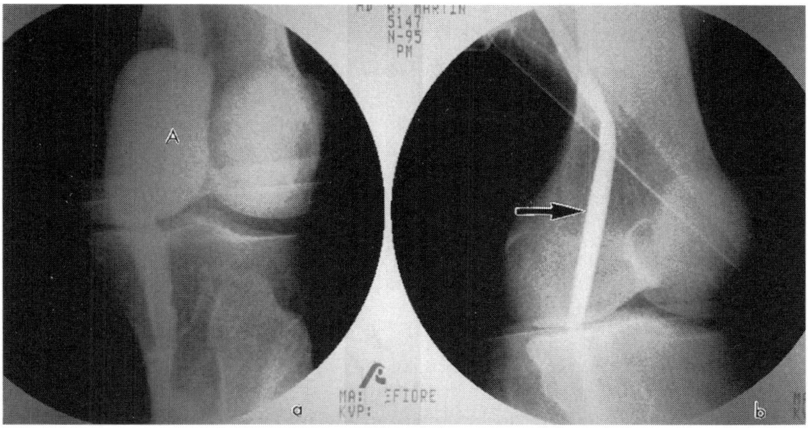

Fig. 14.5 Transluminal repair of a popliteal artery aneurysm. (a) A transfemoral digital arteriogram demonstrates a large popliteal artery aneurysm (A). (b) Following insertion of an endovascular graft (arrow) fixed to the below-knee popliteal artery with a 1-cm Palmaz stent, the popliteal artery aneurysm is excluded. (Reprinted by permission of the publisher from Marin ML, Veith FJ, Cynamon J *et al.* Initial experience with transluminally placed endovascular grafts for the treatment of complex vascular lesions. *Ann Surg* 1995; **222**: 449–69.)

Summary

This report evaluates the application of transfemoral endovascular repair of iliac artery and other peripheral artery aneurysms. Over a 29-month period, 19 patients with significant co-morbid illnesses and a total of 23 iliac artery aneurysms (two patients with popliteal aneurysms and one with a subclavian aneurysm) were treated with endovascular grafts composed of PTFE combined with balloon-expandable stents. Endovascular iliac grafts were successfully placed in 18 patients. No procedural deaths occurred. Follow-up ranged from 2 to 29 months. Two graft thromboses occurred.

Transluminally placed endovascular stented grafts can be used successfully to exclude peripheral artery aneurysms from the circulation while maintaining distal arterial perfusion. However, longer follow-up in more patients is necessary to confirm the efficacy of this technique.

References

1. Nachbur BH, Inderbitzi RG, Bar W. Isolated iliac aneurysms. *Eur J Vasc Surg* 1991; **5**: 375–81.
2. McCready RA, Pairolero PC, Gilmore JC, Kazmier FJ, Cherry KJ Jr, Hollier LH. Isolated iliac artery aneurysms. *Surgery* 1983; **93**: 688–93.
3. Lowry SF, Kraft RO. Isolated aneurysms of the iliac artery. *Arch Surg* 1978; **113**: 1289–93.
4. Sacks NPM, Huddy SPJ, Wegner T, Giddings AEB. Management of solitary iliac aneurysms. *J Cardiovasc Surg* 1992; **33**: 679–83.
5. Richardson JW, Greenfield LJ. Natural history of management of iliac aneurysms. *J Vasc Surg* 1988; **8**: 165–71.
6. Reuter SR, Carson SN. Thrombosis of a common iliac artery aneurysm by selective embolization and extraanatomic bypass. *Am J Radiol* 1980; **134**: 1248–50.
7. Michaels JA, McWhinnie D, Hands LJ, Collin J, Fletcher EWL. Iliac aneurysm treated by percutaneous occlusion and femorofemoral crossover grafting. *Br J Surg* 1994; **81**: 37–8.
8. Vorwerk D, Gunther RW, Wendt G, Schurmann K. Ulcerated plaques and focal aneurysms of iliac arteries: treatment with noncovered, self-expanding stents. *Am J Radiol* 1994; **162**: 1421–4.
9. Deb B, Benjamin M, Comerota AJ. Delayed rupture of an internal iliac artery aneurysm following proximal ligation for abdominal aortic aneurysm repair. *Ann Vasc Surg* 1992; **6**: 537–40.
10. Kwaan JHM, Dahl RK. Fatal rupture after successful surgical thrombosis of an abdominal aortic aneurysm. *Surgery* 1984; **95**: 235–7.
11. Schanzer H, Papa MC, Miller CM. Rupture of surgically thrombosed abdominal aortic aneurysm. *J Vasc Surg* 1985; **2**: 278–80.
12. Cho SI, Johnson WC, Bush HL Jr, Widrich WC, Huse JB, Nasbeth DC. Lethal complications associated with nonrestrictive treatment of abdominal aortic aneurysms. *Arch Surg* 1982; **117**: 1214–17.
13. Parodi JC, Palmaz JC, Barone HD. Transfemoral intraluminal graft implantation for abdominal aortic aneurysms. *Ann Vasc Surg* 1991; **5**: 491–9.
14. Dake MD, Miller DC, Semba CP *et al.* Transluminal placement of endovascular stent–grafts for the treatment of descending thoracic aortic aneurysms. *N Engl J Med* 1994; **331**: 1729–34.
15. Marin ML, Veith FJ, Panetta TF *et al.* Transfemoral endoluminal stented graft repair of a popliteal artery aneurysm. *J Vasc Surg* 1994; **19**: 754–7.
16. Marin ML, Veith FJ, Cynamon J *et al.* Transfemoral endovascular stented graft treatment of aorto-iliac and femoropopliteal occlusive disease for limb salvage. *Am J Surg* 1994; **168**: 156–62.
17. Marin ML, Veith FJ, Panetta TF *et al.* Transluminally placed endovascular stented graft repair for arterial trauma. *J Vasc Surg* 1994; **20**: 466–73.

15

Endovascular stented grafts for the management of acute arterial injuries

Michael L. Marin and Frank J. Veith

Division of Vascular Surgery, Department of Surgery, Montefiore Medical Center, The University Hospital for the Albert Einstein College of Medicine, 111 East 210th Street, New York, NY 10467, USA

Introduction

An increase in civilian trauma over the past decade is clearly linked to an overall rise in handgun-associated injuries. Penetrating trauma to the vascular system from these high-velocity missiles may lead to the formation of arterial occlusions, pseudoaneurysms and arteriovenous fistulas. Over the past 30 years, the optimal management of these vascular lesions has been reviewed for both military and civilian trauma experiences.[1–6] These injuries, demonstrating pulse deficits in association with severe limb or organ ischaemia, expanding arterial haematomas or active haemorrhage from the injured vessel, mandate urgent surgical exploration and arterial repair. The direct surgical repair of these vascular injuries may be complicated by several factors, including inaccessibility of the vascular lesion when trauma occurs to central vessels. In addition, false aneurysms and arteriovenous fistulas may markedly distort local anatomy and induce significant venous hypertension, further increasing the challenge of a standard surgical repair, often at a cost of considerable blood loss.

Alternative treatments using catheter directed techniques may reduce procedural risks and improve outcome in patients who are stable after a vascular injury. One such therapy employs endovascular stented grafts directly to repair the injured vessel from the luminal surface.[7–11] These devices permit minimally invasive arterial repairs to be performed from readily accessible sites in the vasculature which are remote from the area of arterial trauma.

This chapter describes the development and clinical experience at the Montefiore Medical Center with the placement of stented grafts for the treatment of arterial pseudoaneurysms and arteriovenous fistulas.

Techniques and devices

Transluminally placed stented grafts for treating traumatic arterial lesions were conceptualized by Dotter[12] in 1969, and one of the first clinical applications of this technology was performed by Volodos *et al.*[13] using a Dacron graft and a self-expanding stent. Experimental and clinical experience to date has demonstrated success with several different devices for treating traumatic arterial lesions[7,8,14] (Fig. 15.1). The ideal composition of the external covering on the stent or the best mechanism for stent deployment has not yet been identified in the treatment of traumatic lesions.

At the Montefiore Medical Center, we have predominantly used the Palmaz balloon-expandable stent in conjunction with thin-walled polytetrafluoroethylene (PTFE) graft material to perform arterial repairs of pseudoaneurysms and arteriovenous fistulas (Fig. 15.2). The stents varied between 2 and 3 cm in length and were fixed inside 6-mm GORE-TEX grafts (W.L. Gore and Associates, Flagstaff, AZ, USA) by two 'U' stitches (Fig. 15.3a). The stented graft was then mounted on to a balloon angioplasty catheter which had a tapered dilator tip (Fig. 15.3b). The entire device was loaded into a 12-Fr delivery catheter for over-the-wire insertion either percutaneously or through an arterial cut-down.

Recently we have begun a Phase I Food and Drug Administration trial of the Corvita stent–graft device for arterial trauma (Corvita Corporation, Miami, FL, USA). This device is fabricated from a self-expanding stent of braided wire similar in construction to the Wallstent (Schneider Corporation, Minneapolis, MN, USA). The stent is covered with polyurethane fibre (see Fig. 15.1d). The stent–graft is cut to the desired size with a wire-cutting shears in the operating room and then loaded into a specially designed delivery sheath (see Fig. 15.1e).

Results

As shown in Table 15.1, 11 patients received 11 stented grafts to treat traumatic arterial lesions. The age range was 18–85 years; nine patients were men. Seven injuries occurred as a result of gunshot

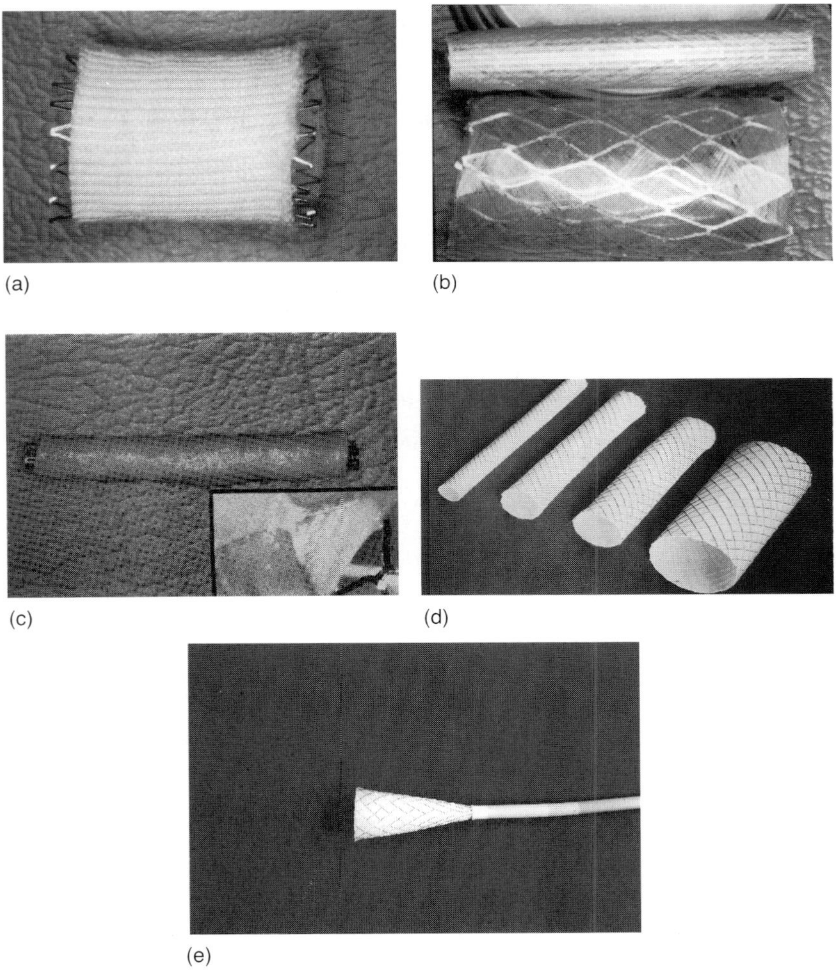

Fig. 15.1 Endovascular covered stents. (a) Dacron graft material may be used to cover the balloon-expandable stents. These devices have been used by Parodi[7] to treat traumatic lesions. (b) Polyurethane can be fabricated directly on to a stent. This material has 'elastic' properties, permitting a closed stent to remain well covered following deployment. (c) Autogenous vein can be used to cover stents, creating biological stented grafts. The collapsed stent–graft assumes a small profile following deployment, the vein which effectively covers the struts of the stent (inset). (d) Corvita endovascular stented graft for arterial trauma. This polyurethane-covered stent structurally resembles the Wallstent. (e) Delivery catheter system for the Corvita stent graft. A central 'pusher' catheter ejects the self-expanding device from the distal end of the catheter.

Table 15.1 Stented grafts for arterial trauma.

Patient No.	*Sex*	*Age (years)*	*Mechanism of injury*	*Vessels(s) involved*	*Pseudo-aneurysm*	*Arteriovenous fistula*	*Anaesthesia*
1	M	20	Bullet	Left SFA Left SFV	Yes	Yes	General
2	M	28	Bullet	Right SFA	Yes	No	Local
3	M	22	Bullet	Left SFA	Yes	No	Local
4	M	24	Knife	Left ASA	Yes	No	General
5	M	35	Bullet	Right ASA	Yes	No	Local
6	F	78	Catheterization	Right SA	Yes	No	Local
7	M	78	Catheterization	Left CIA	Yes	No	Epidural
8	M	18	Bullet	Right SA	Yes	Yes	Local
9	M	18	Bullet	Right ASA	Yes	No	Local
10	M	22	Bullet	Right ASA	Yes	No	Local
11	F	85	Surgical trauma	Right CIA	Yes	Yes	Local

Associated injuries	Injury to repair time interval	Stent–graft length (cm)	Access	Hospital stay (days)	Patency (months)	Complications
Soft tissue buttock	36 h	3	Left SFA percutaneous	5	38	
Left open femur fracture	12 h	3	Right SFA arteriotomy	9	36	
Soft tissue right thigh; left deep venous thrombosis	12 h	3	Left SFA arteriotomy	6	2*	
Pneumothorax; haemothorax	4 h	3	Left brachial arteriotomy	7	33	Stent compression
Brachial plexus	3 weeks	3	Right brachial arteriotomy	4	29	
Haemothorax	24 h	3	Right brachial arteriotomy	8 weeks†	28	
None	4 months	2	Left CFA arteriotomy	2	28	
Haemothorax	48 h	3	Right brachial artery	4	21	
None	6 h	3	Right brachial artery	3	12	
Haemothorax	3 h	3	Right brachial artery	6	12	
None	8 years	5‡	Left CFA percutaneous	4	3	Distal emboli (treated with catheter suction thrombectomy)

SFV, superficial femoral vein; SFA, superficial femoral artery; SA, subclavian artery; CIA, common iliac artery; ASA, axillary subclavian artery; CFA, common femoral artery.
*Died 2 months postprocedure (homicide).
†Hospitalized for multiple medical problems.
‡Corvita stent–graft.

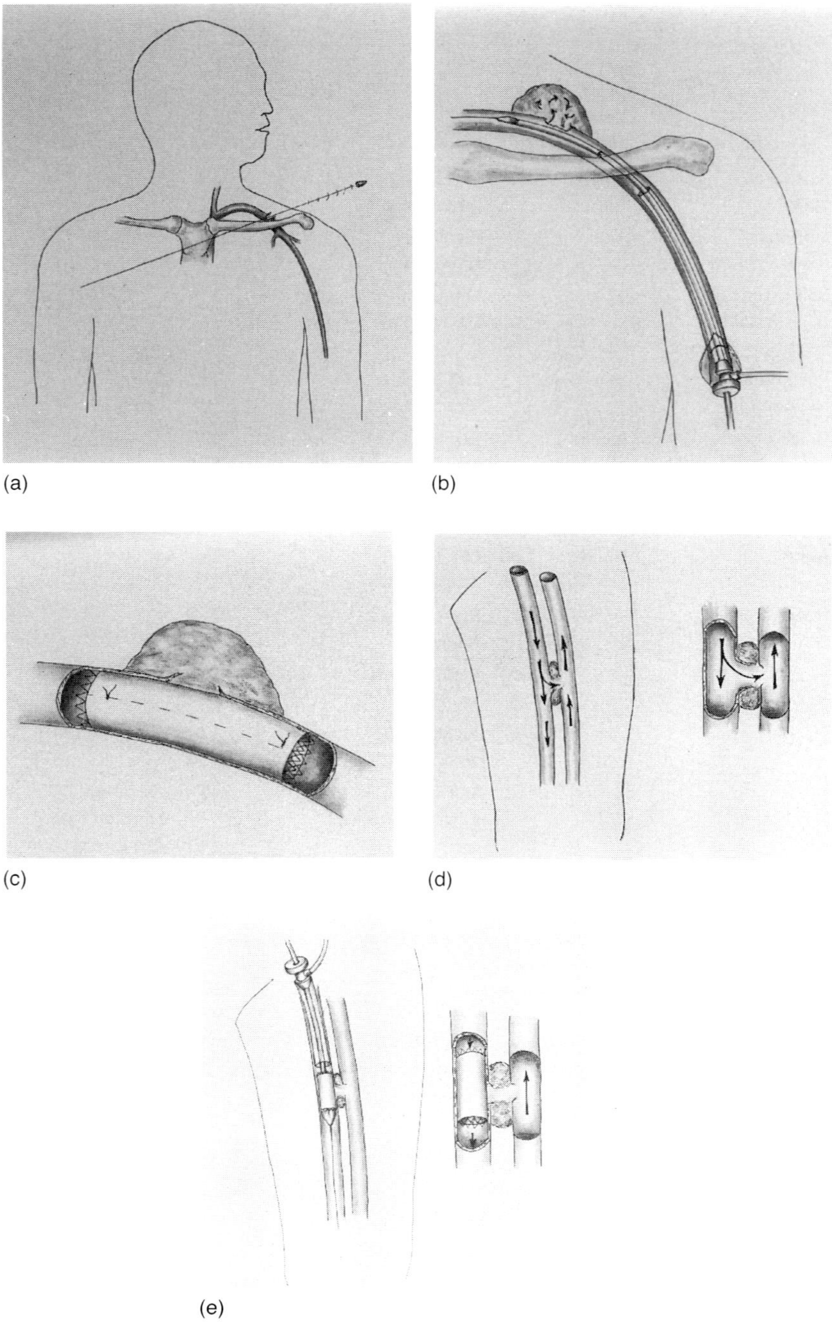

(a) (b) (c) (d) (e)

wounds (Fig. 15.4). One knife wound, two iatrogenic needle catheterization injuries and one patient who had arterial trauma at the time of gynaecological surgery constituted the remaining patients (Figs. 15.5 and 15.6). All injuries were associated with a surrounding pseudoaneurysm. In three instances the arterial injury formed a fistula to an injured adjacent vein. Associated injuries were present in seven patients with arterial trauma and in one patient with an iatrogenic arterial injury (Table 15.1). With these stented graft repairs, in-hospital stay averaged 5 days (excluding patient number 6 who had a protracted hospital stay secondary to pre-existing co-morbid medical conditions). Stented graft patency was 100% with no early or late graft occlusions at up to 38 months. One patient with a left axillary subclavian stent–graft developed compression of the stent at 12 months which was treated by balloon angioplasty. This problem was detected again 3 months later. This compressed device did not thrombose with careful follow-up over 2 years. Mean follow-up was 24 (range 3–38) months. One patient who had an axillary pseudoaneurysm repaired with a stented graft required a vein patch of a small brachial artery at the catheter insertion site at the conclusion of the procedure.

Discussion

Prompt diagnosis and treatment of penetrating vascular trauma are required to avoid the delayed sequelae that may occur when significant injuries to arteries are left untreated.[15–18] Traumatic arteriovenous fistulas and pseudoaneurysms involving nonessential vessels, such as

---

Fig. 15.2 Schematic drawing of stented graft repair of an arterial injury. (a) A bullet wound partially disrupts the wall of the vessel. (b) The stent–graft device is delivered to the site of injury via a remote arteriotomy. (c) Once deployed, the stented graft covers the hole in the vessel. (d) When an arteriovenous fistula forms following a vascular injury, the same principles apply for stented graft repair. In this example, the stent–graft device is inserted in the superficial femoral artery at a site remote from the arterial injury. (e) Following deployment, the stented graft occludes the arteriovenous fistula. (Reprinted by permission of the publisher from Marin ML, Veith FJ, Panetta TF *et al.* Transluminally placed endovascular stented graft repair for arterial trauma. *J Vasc Surg* 1994; **20**: 466–73.)

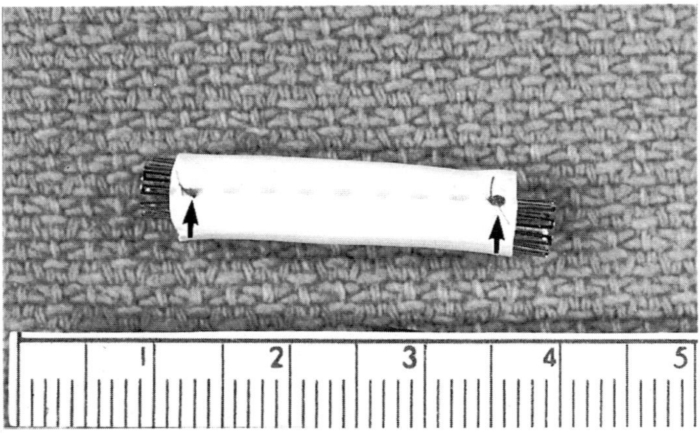

(a)

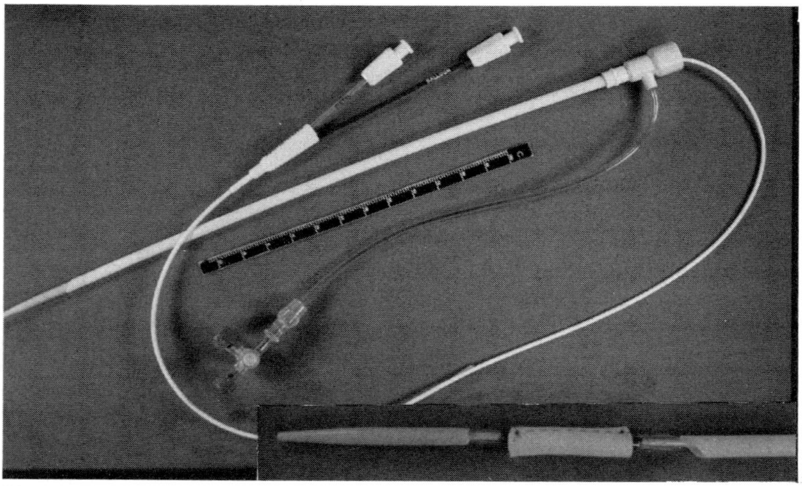

(b)

Fig. 15.3 (a) An endovascular stented graft. A segment of PTFE is attached to a stainless steel-slotted balloon-expandable (Palmaz) stent using two 5–0 polypropylene 'U' stitches (arrows). (Reprinted by permission of the publisher from Marin ML, Veith FJ, Panetta TF *et al.* Transluminally placed endovascular stented graft repair for arterial trauma. *J Vasc Surg* 1994; **20**: 466–73.) (b) The stent–graft is mounted on an angioplasty balloon and placed into a sheath before insertion. Note the presence of a dilator tip at the end of the balloon catheter which provides a smooth taper within the catheter (inset).

branches of the hypogastric or deep femoral arteries, can be treated effectively by catheter-directed arterial embolization.[19,20] Long-term follow-up of coil-treated lesions has been favourable. Small anatomically favourable groin pseudoaneurysms secondary to catheterization injuries may be treated effectively with ultrasonographically guided compression. Other injuries to vital arteries traditionally have required direct surgical repair of the damaged vessel employing either lateral repairs or replacement vascular conduits to restore critical arterial flow and to avoid delayed complications.

Endovascular methods are rapidly evolving to treat a variety of vascular problems, including arterial trauma.[20] Endovascular therapy with balloon angioplasty of large vessels such as the iliac arteries appears to be a safe and effective alternative to surgery for some forms of stenotic and occlusive vascular disease.[21] This form of therapy may be successfully extended to more complex lesions by the use of intra-arterial stents.[22] The blending of intravascular stent and prosthetic graft technologies has resulted in the evolution of new devices (stented grafts) with a wide range of potential applications in the vascular system. Early feasibility studies of these devices have shown them to be technically capable of excluding experimentally created arterial aneurysms with the potential for treating other lesions.[23–25] Clinical experience with stented grafts for trauma has been reported by several investigators.[7–9]

This chapter reviews the preliminary experience at the Montefiore Medical Center with stented grafts for the treatment of traumatic arterial lesions. Follow-up of these patients extends to 38 months. In this series, device insertion was accomplished with uniform technical success and a satisfactory repair of the arterial lesion has been maintained in all cases, with preservation of the arterial flow through the injured critical segment. Distal embolization occurred in one patient, which was managed by catheter-based suction thrombectomy of a small plaque embolism in the superficial femoral artery.

Endovascular stented grafts inserted from a remote site in the arterial tree have several advantages over conventional repairs. Compared with standard operative repair of similar lesions, stented grafts appear to be associated with less blood loss and a reduced requirement for anaesthesia and dissection in the traumatized field. These advantages would be particularly important in patients with large, central vessel injuries or truncal arteriovenous fistulas with venous hypertension. Standard surgical repair of such lesions is notoriously difficult and associated with significant blood loss. Stented graft repair of these

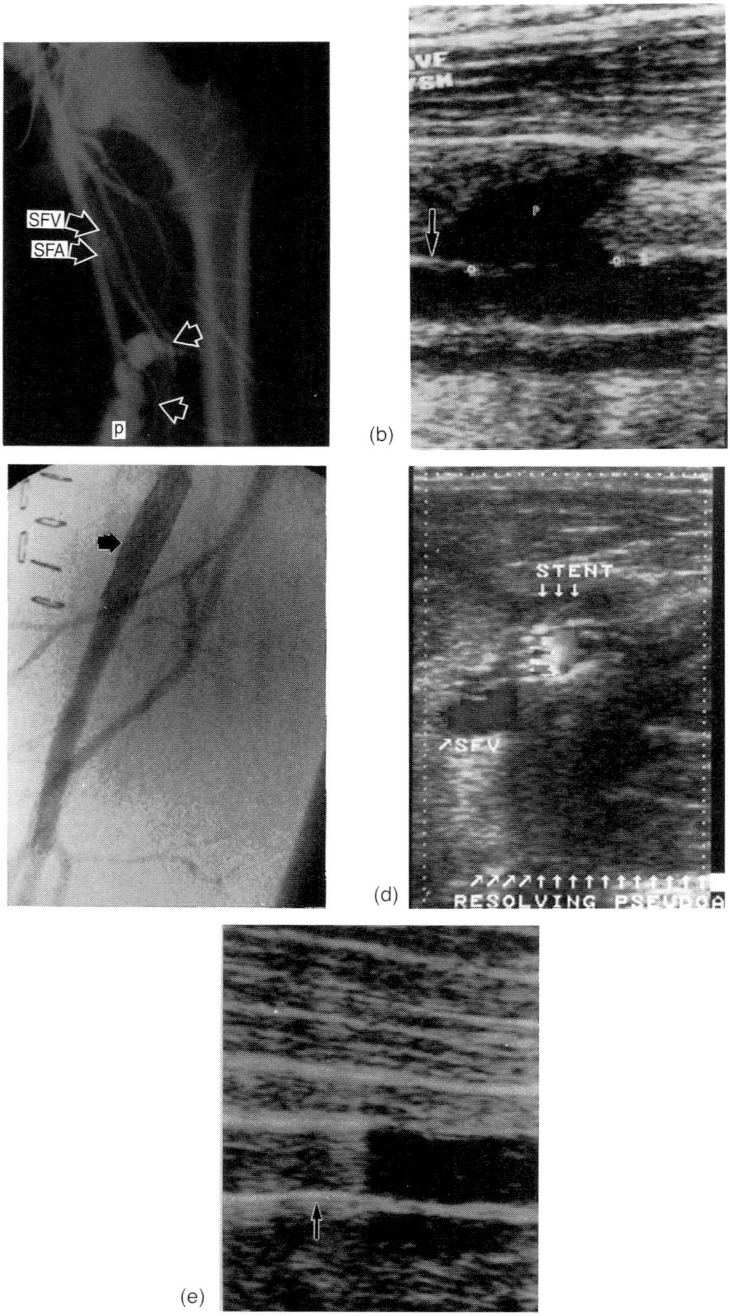

(a) (b) (c) (d) (e)

central or truncal artery false aneurysms avoids the need for extensive operations through major body cavities. These advantages are also important in patients who are critically ill from coexisting traumatic injuries or underlying major medical co-morbidities. With these dire circumstances, the use of stented grafts already appears justified to treat some traumatic lesions of major critical arteries.

Controversy presently exists regarding the best conduit for management of extremity arterial trauma distal to the subclavian and common femoral vessels, and this concern would be expected to extend to the use of prosthetic stented grafts. Autogenous vein is preferred by most surgeons, with excellent early and late patency rates.[26] Autogenous veins have also been used to fashion stented grafts for the treatment of arterial trauma in infected fields as well as to repair arterial injuries located in the carotid circulation where mural thrombosis would present the greatest risk for embolization. Alternatively, others have achieved satisfactory results with conventional surgery using prosthetic grafts for extremity arterial wounds.[27] While long autogenous grafts for arteriosclerotic ischaemia have been associated with better patency than arterial reconstructions performed with prosthetics, it is likely

---

Fig. 15.4 (a) Femoral arteriogram after gunshot wound to left thigh. An arteriovenous fistula associated with a large pseudoaneurysm is seen between the left superficial femoral artery (SFA) and the superficial femoral vein (SFV). Selective catheterization of the deep femoral artery (1) and the SFA branch (2) showed that these vessels were not injured. p, Pseudoaneurysm. (b) Duplex ultrasonographic image of the SFA depicted in (a). Loss of the intimal stripe (arrow) and associated pseudoaneurysm (p) are seen. The arterial defect measures approximately 13 mm (distance between stars). (c) Completion arteriogram demonstrates patency of the SFA, proper positioning of the stented graft (arrow), and no evidence of the arteriovenous fistula or extravasation. Metal clips were placed in the skin before the procedure to facilitate fluoroscopic localization of the arteriovenous fistula and proper placement of the stented graft. (d) Transverse and longitudinal duplex ultrasonographic images of stented graft repair of the SFA after 3 months. (d) Transverse image of artery and vein at the level of the stent can be identified, with evidence of normal flow in both vessels. (e) Longitudinal duplex ultrasonogram identifies stented graft within artery (arrow). Minimal changes in peak systolic velocities are appreciated between the native SFA and the portion of the vessel that is covered by the stented graft. (Reprinted by permission of the publisher from Marin ML, Veith FJ, Panetta TF *et al.* Percutaneous transfemoral insertion of a stented graft to repair a traumatic femoral arteriovenous fistula. *J Vasc Surg* 1993; **18**: 299–302.)

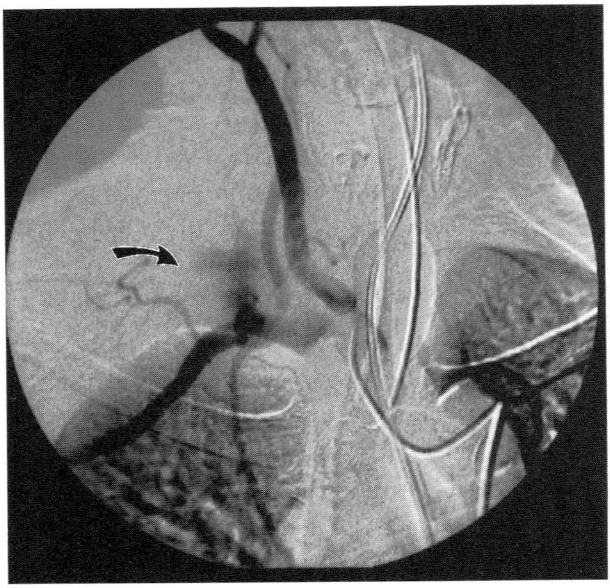

(a)

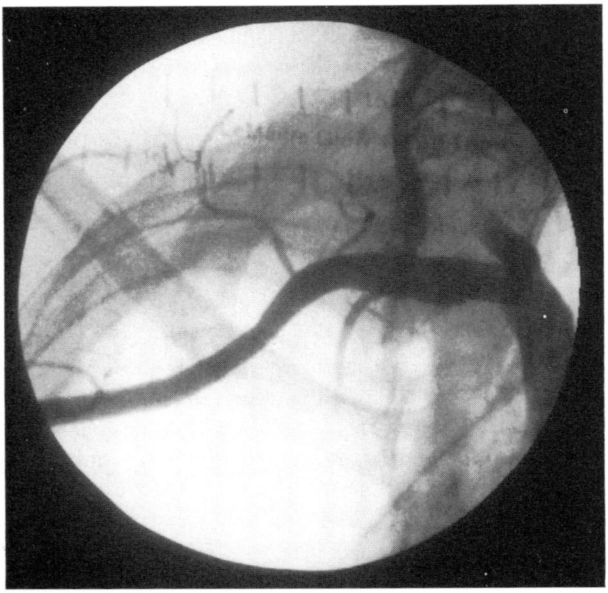

(b)

Fig. 15.5 (a) Arteriogram showing a large pseudoaneurysm of the right subclavian artery (arrow) just distal to the vertebral artery which occurred after attempted insertion of a subclavian vein catheter. (b) Following stented graft placement through the right brachial artery, the pseudoaneurysm was excluded. Vertebral artery flow was maintained. (Reprinted by permission of the publisher from Marin ML, Veith FJ, Panetta TF *et al.* Transluminally placed endovascular stented graft repair for arterial trauma. *J Vasc Surg* 1994; **20**: 466–73.)

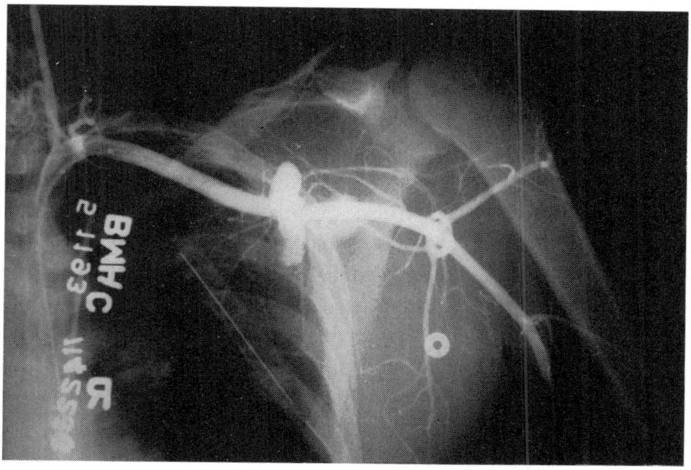

(a)

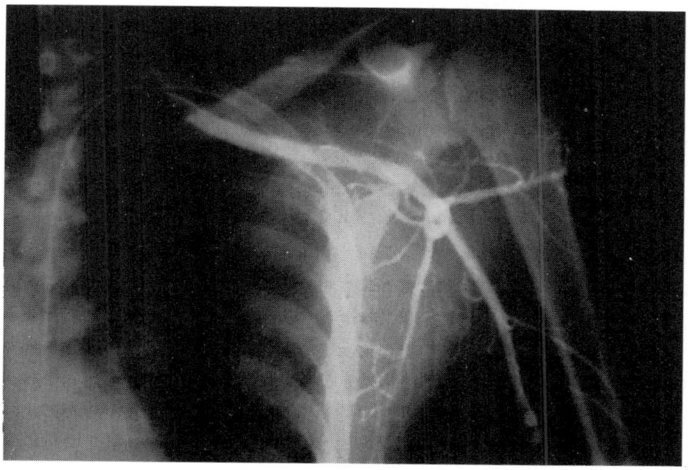

(b)

Fig. 15.6 (a) Axillary subclavian artery arteriogram of a patient with a large pseudoaneurysm after a stab wound to the chest resulting in a haemopneumothorax. (b) Following transluminal insertion of the stent graft device, the pseudoaneurysm was repaired and flow was restored. (Reprinted by permission of the publisher from Marin ML, Veith FJ, Panetta TF *et al.* Transluminally placed endovascular stented graft repair for arterial trauma. *J Vasc Surg* 1994; **20**: 466–73.)

that short (3 cm or less) prosthetic graft segments will function satisfactorily in the axillary and superficial femoral arteries. However, this premise remains to be proven by longer patient follow-up. Even if late failure of stent grafts in these locations occurs, percutaneous transluminal angioplasty or a subsequent elective vein graft bypass could then be performed in a field free of traumatized tissue and contamination, and when the status of the venous circulation is known. Obviously, if the function of prosthetic stented grafts in the superficial femoral and axillary arteries is poor, an autogenous vein-covered stent device could be considered as an alternative.

One theoretical problem with stented graft repairs involves the potential for stimulating intimal hyperplasia at the stent–graft arterial junction. While any form of traumatic injury to an artery may induce hyperplastic activity in the cells that compose the arterial wall, the Palmaz intra-arterial stent has been shown to cause a relatively limited intimal hyperplastic response in experimental studies as well as in the treatment of stenotic or occluded iliac arteries in patients.[22] In the latter setting, prolonged patency has been the rule.

Despite the potential disadvantages of using a thrombogenic stented graft device that could stimulate intimal hyperplasia to treat a traumatic lesion of the axillary or femoral arteries, the advantages of minimally invasive deployment, decreased blood loss, and the ability to insert stented grafts under local anaesthesia through remote sites make this endovascular technique for repair of penetrating vascular injuries a potentially important tool to be considered for more widespread use. This is already true for multiple trauma and critically ill patients with central artery injuries. Long-term follow-up of these repairs will be necessary to evaluate fully the safety and efficacy of these devices in extremity arteries and in other less critical circumstances.

Summary

Intravascular stents have become important tools for the management of vascular lesions; however, stents in combination with vascular grafts have only recently been applied clinically. This chapter describes an experience with stented grafts for the treatment of penetrating arterial trauma. The use of stented grafts appears to be associated with decreased blood loss, a less invasive insertion procedure, reduced requirements for anaesthesia, and a limited need for extensive dissection in the traumatized field. These advantages are especially important in patients with central arteriovenous fistulas or false aneurysms, particularly those who are critically ill from other coexisting injuries or medical co-morbidities. The use of stented grafts already appears justified to treat traumatic arterial lesions in these circumstances. Although the early results are encouraging, documentation of long-term effectiveness must be obtained before these devices can be recommended for widespread or generalized use in the treatment of major arterial injuries.

References

1. Drapanas T, Hewitt RL, Weichert RF, Smith AD. Civilian vascular injuries: a critical appraisal of three decades of management. *Ann Surg* 1970; **172**: 351–60.
2. Burnett HF, Parnell CL, Williams GD, Campbell GS. Peripheral arterial injuries: a reassessment. *Ann Surg* 1976; **183**: 701–9.
3. Perry MO, Thal ER, Shires GT. Management of arterial injuries. *Ann Surg* 1971; **173**: 403–8.
4. Feliciano DV, Bitondo CG, Mattox KL *et al.* Civilian trauma in the 1980s. A 1-year experience with 456 vascular and cardiac injuries. *Ann Surg* 1984; **199**: 717–24.
5. Jahnke EJ Jr, Seeley SF. Acute vascular injuries in the Korean war: an analysis of 77 consecutive cases. *Ann Surg* 1953; **138**: 158–77.
6. Rich NM, Spencer FC. *Vascular Trauma*. Philadelphia, PA: WB Saunders, 1978.
7. Parodi JC. Endovascular repair of abdominal aortic aneurysms and other arterial lesions. *J Vasc Surg* 1995; **21**: 549–57.
8. Marin ML, Veith FJ, Panetta TF *et al.* Transluminally placed endovascular stented graft repair for arterial trauma. *J Vasc Surg* 1994; **20**: 466–73.
9. Becker GJ, Benenati JF, Zemel G *et al.* Percutaneous placement of a balloon-expandable intraluminal graft for life threatening subclavian arterial hemorrhage. *J Vasc Intervent Radiol* 1991; **2**: 225–9.
10. May J, White G, Waugh R, Yu W, Harris J. Transluminal placement of a prosthetic graft–stent device for treatment of subclavian artery aneurysm. *J Vasc Surg* 1993; **18**: 1056–9.
11. Schmitter SP, Marx M, Bernstein R *et al.* Angioplasty-induced subclavian artery dissection in a patient with internal mammary artery graft: treatment with endovascular stent and stent–graft. *Am J Roentgenol* 1995; **165**: 449–51.
12. Dotter CT. Transluminally-placed coilspring endarterial tube grafts. Long-term patency in canine popliteal artery. *Invest Radiol* 1969; **4**: 329–32.
13. Volodos NL, Karpovich IP, Troyan VI *et al.* Clinical experience of the use of self-fixing synthetic prostheses for remote endoprosthetics of the thoracic and the abdominal aorta and iliac arteries through the femoral artery and as intraoperative endoprosthesis for aorta reconstruction. *Vasa Suppl* 1991; **33**: 93–5.
14. Rivera FJ, Palmaz JC, Encarnacion CE *et al.* Aneurysm and pseudoaneurysm balloon expandable stent/graft bypass: clinical experience. *J Vasc Intervent Radiol* 1994; **5**: 19 (abstract).
15. Feliciano DV, Cruse PA, Burch JM, Bitondo CG. Delayed diagnosis of arterial injuries. *Am J Surg* 1987; **154**: 579–84.

16. Richardson JD, Vitale GC, Flint LM Jr. Penetrating arterial trauma: analysis of missed vascular injuries. *Arch Surg* 1987; **122**: 678–83.
17. Ben-Menachem Y. Vascular injuries of the extremities: hazards of unnecessary delays in diagnosis. *Orthopedics* 1986; **9**: 333–8.
18. Escobar GA, Escobar SC, Marquez L *et al.* Vascular trauma: late sequelae and treatment. *J Cardiovasc Surg* 1980; **21**: 35–40.
19. Rosch J, Dotter CT, Brown MJ. Selective arterial embolization. A new method for control of acute gastrointestinal bleeding. *Radiology* 1972; **102**: 303–6.
20. Panetta TF, Sclafani SJA, Goldstein AS, Phillips TF. Percutaneous transcatheter embolization for arterial trauma. *J Vasc Surg* 1985; **2**: 54–64.
21. Johnston KW, Rae M, Hogg-Johnston SA *et al.* 5-Year results of a prospective study of percutaneous transluminal angioplasty. *Ann Surg* 1987; **206**: 403–13.
22. Palmaz JC, Laborde JC, Rivera FJ, Encarnacion CE, Lutz JD, Moss JG. Stenting of the iliac arteries with the Palmaz stent: experience from a multicenter trial. *Cardiovasc Intervent Radiol* 1992; **15**: 291–7.
23. Mirich D, Wright KC, Wallace S *et al.* Percutaneously placed endovascular grafts for aortic aneurysms: feasibility study. *Radiology* 1989; **170**: 1033–7.
24. Laborde JC, Parodi JC, Clem MF *et al.* Intraluminal bypass of abdominal aortic aneurysm: feasibility study. *Radiology* 1992; **184**: 185–90.
25. Balko A, Piasecki GJ, Shah DM, Carney WI, Hopkins RW, Jackson BT. Transfemoral placement of intraluminal polyurethane prosthesis for abdominal aortic aneurysm. *J Surg Res* 1986; **40**: 305–9.
26. Keen RR, Meyer JP, Durham JR *et al.* Autogenous vein graft repair of injured extremity arteries: early and late results with 134 consecutive patients. *J Vasc Surg* 1991; **13**: 664–8.
27. Feliciano DV, Mattox KL, Graham JM, Bitondo CG. Five-year experience with PTFE grafts in vascular wounds. *J Trauma* 1985; **25**: 71–82.

16

The Nottingham experience

Waquar Yusuf, Peter W. Wenham and Brian R. Hopkinson

Department of Vascular Surgery, University Hospital, Queen's Medical Centre, Nottingham NG7 2UH, UK

Introduction

In Nottingham the study on endovascular abdominal aortic aneurysm (AAA) repair commenced in March 1994. Studies in our unit have focused on the physiological effects of endovascular surgery,[1,2] the development of methods to enable endovascular treatment of the majority of patients with infrarenal AAA[3] and the feasibility of endovascular repair of leaking AAAs.[4] In this chapter the technical aspects of endovascular repair and clinical outcome are discussed.

Patients and methods

Preoperative assessment of aneurysm suitability for endovascular repair is carried out with spiral computed tomography (CT) and calibrated angiography as detailed in Chapter 2. So far, 70 patients have undergone endovascular repair of infrarenal AAA in our unit. The median age was 69 (range 52–86) years. Of these 70 patients, two underwent repair with an aortoaortic graft, 14 with a bifurcated graft with the Chuter–Gianturco system[5] and the majority (54 of 70) with an aortouni-iliac graft with femorofemoral bypass and contralateral iliac occlusion,[6] using the Chuter delivery system in three and the Ivancev–Malmö system in the rest. Elective endovascular repair was undertaken in 66 cases and urgent endovascular repair for contained rupture was undertaken in four. Of the 66 patients undergoing elective repair, 30 (45%) were considered to be at high risk from conventional surgery; 18 (60%) of these 30 patients had been referred to us by vascular surgeons from other hospitals (Table 16.1). Of four patients with leaking aneurysms, three had additional risk factors. The diam-

Table 16.1 High surgical risk cases.

	No. of patients
Poor left ventricular function	7
With renal transplant	1
With thrombocytopenia (platelet count 60×10^9/l)	1
With renal impairment (creatinine 160 μmol/l	1
Aortic stenosis (58 mm gradient), left ventricular hypertrophy	1
Age >85 years	3
Creatinine >200 μmol/l	4
With horseshoe kidney and angina	1
Severe chronic obstructive airway disease	2
Recent myocardial infarction and/or unstable angina	2
Thrombocytopenia (platelet count $<60 \times 10^9$/l)	2
Cirrhosis	1
Hostile abdomen	
Inflammatory aneurysm	2
Periaortic lymphoma	1
Periduodenal abscess	1

eter of the aneurysm, length of neck and diameter of neck are shown in Fig. 16.1.

The design of the bifurcated graft and its delivery system (Chuter–Gianturco) is described in Chapter 7 and the Ivancev–Malmö delivery system is described in Chapter 11.

Components used in the endoprosthesis

The aortouni-iliac prosthesis consists of: (a) Gianturco stent (William Cook, Europe) with a resting diameter of 45 mm with four cranially projecting hooks and four caudally pointing spikes for securing the prosthesis within the aneurysm neck; (b) Gianturco stents without hooks and spikes with a resting diameter of 16, 20 or 30 mm for securing the graft within the iliac artery; (c) uncorrugated thin-walled Dacron graft, tapered from a diameter of 18–34 to 12–24 mm. The endoprosthesis is assembled from these components for each individual case. A Gianturco stent of suitable size covered with Dacron is used to occlude the contralateral common iliac artery.

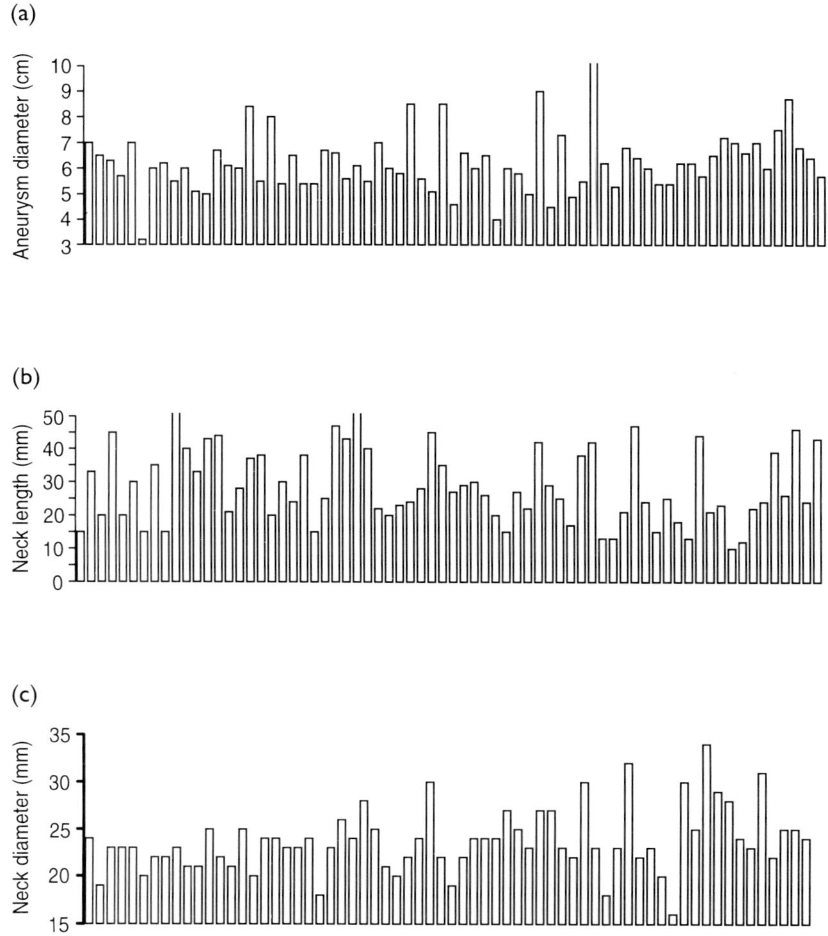

Fig. 16.1 Distribution of (a) aneurysmal diameter, (b) neck length and (c) neck diameter in 70 patients undergoing endovascular abdominal aortic aneurysm repair.

Procedure

The technique of bifurcated graft deployment is presented in detail in Chapter 7. The technique of aortouni-iliac is similar to that described in Chapter 11. However, certain modifications required in individual situations are presented. In the presence of significant neck angulation or tortuosity it may be difficult to introduce the delivery system. In addition, there is a risk of upper end graft kinking. Provided other aspects of anatomy are favourable, a brachiofemoral guidewire is used to facilitate introduction of the delivery system and two Gianturco stents in series are used to prevent graft kinking. If both the common iliacs are unsuitable for graft limb implantation and other features are favourable, the graft limb can be implanted in the external iliac artery, provided it is of adequate size. Embolization of the internal iliac artery may be required to prevent retrograde perigraft perfusion of the aneurysm. Accessory or lower pole renal artery may be sacrificed by implanting the endoprosthesis across their origin, provided renal function is normal and there is adequate renal reserve.

The uncorrugated thin-walled graft is susceptible to twisting or kinking, and additional support with Wallstents is often required. We have pursued a policy of selective use of Wallstents for the aortouni-iliac grafts. Images are obtained in both anteroposterior and lateral views before femorofemoral bypass to look for any narrowing or twist in the graft and to assess the need for a Wallstent. Completion angiography is performed at the end to assess the following: (a) the seal around the proximal stent; (b) graft patency; (c) the seal around the iliac stent; (d) patency of internal iliacs; (e) effective occlusion of the contralateral common iliac; and (f) patency of the femorofemoral bypass graft. Any leakage around the proximal stent at the end of the procedure is not acceptable and two approaches have been used to deal with this problem. In the early part of our experience a laparotomy was carried out to apply periaortic ligatures of nylon tape around the proximal stent. Later, this problem was dealt with by balloon dilatation of the proximal stent with a 30-mm angioplasty (valvuloplasty) balloon, which seems to expand the stent–graft fully and perhaps reorient the stent along the true axis of the aneurysm neck. The last stage of the procedure includes occlusion of the contralateral common iliac artery with a covered Gianturco stent and a traditional femorofemoral bypass. If the common iliac artery is too short or tortuous for accurate deployment of the occluding stent, ligation of the common iliac artery via an extraperitoneal approach is preferred in order to avoid the risk of internal iliac occlusion.

Results

The endovascular approach alone with bilateral common femoral artery exposure or occasional extraperitoneal exposure of the common iliac artery was used in 62 (89%) of the 70 cases. Additional surgical intervention was required in eight patients. Of these eight cases, removal of the endoprosthesis and replacement with a conventional inlay graft was carried out in one patient, closure of the infrarenal aorta and axillobifemoral bypass in one, anastomosis of distal end of the graft to common iliac in one, and laparotomy for periaortic ligatures in four. In one patient with a particularly tortuous, wide and thrombus-lined aneurysmal neck, the endoprosthesis failed to achieve a seal but further intervention was considered too hazardous because of significant pre-existing cardiac problems.

The median duration of the successful endovascular procedure was 140 (range 70–480) min; median blood loss was 500 (range 500–1200) ml. At a median follow-up of 9 (range 0–24, interquartile range 5–16) months, 58 (83%) of 70 endovascular grafts remained in satisfactory condition according to the criteria shown in Table 16.2. Two patients died with satisfactory grafts during the second and fourth postoperative months, one from pneumonia and one from dialysis line sepsis. No aneurysm has increased significantly in size and most aneurysms underwent a reduction in size after the first year following repair. The reasons for eight grafts being in an unsatisfactory state is shown in Table 16.3.

Table 16.2 Criteria for satisfactory endovascular repair on follow-up CT scan.

No evidence of stent migration
No evidence of graft kink or occlusion
No flow of contrast into the aneurysm sac
No increase of aneurysm size

Table 16.3 Reasons for endoprosthesis being unsatisfactory.

	No. of patients
Occlusion of left limb of a bifurcated graft at 3 months	1
Leak around iliac occlusion device	2
Localized inflow via lumbars	2
Leak around distal aortic stent	1
Displacement of distal aortic stent	1
Follow-up radiological information not available in maldeployed graft	1
Graft thrombosis following open cholecystectomy 3 months after endovascular repair	1

Leaking aortic aneurysm

Endovascular repair was attempted in four haemodynamically stable patients with aneurysm leak contained within the retroperitoneum. Three patients were treated within 24 hours of onset of symptoms and one 4 days after onset. One patient had a second myocardial infarction within 3 weeks of the time of presentation, and another had severe chronic obstructive airway disease and obesity. All these repairs were carried out with an aortouni-iliac graft. All patients underwent contrast-enhanced spiral CT scan before the procedure. Endovascular exclusion of aneurysm was successfully achieved in all cases; however, an 84-year-old patient died from renal failure 2 weeks after operation. The other three remain alive and well at 3, 5 and 18 months after surgery.

Secondary interventions

The insertion of a Wallstent within 24 hours of the procedure to deal with the occlusion of grafts not supported with Wallstents was required in two cases. Ligation of common iliac artery in the presence of persistent aneurysm perfusion around the iliac occluding device was required in one patient at 7 months after operation. Axillobisuperficial femoral bypass following removal of an infected femorofemoral bypass graft was required in one patient at 3 weeks. Thrombectomy of an endovascular graft was required 3 months after implantation. This occurred in the early postoperative period following an open cholecystectomy for complicated cholelithiasis. Femorofemoral bypass was required to deal with occlusion of a limb of a bifurcated graft 3 months after implantation.

Complications and management

Local and systemic complications are shown in Table 16.4. Management of some of the local complications are presented here. Renal artery embolus probably occurred as a result of clot formation within the delivery sheath due to inadequate anticoagulation. However, it is possible for embolization to occur from the aneurysm sac due to flow turbulence in the aorta during the procedure. This was treated by a combination of intraoperative thrombolysis with three boluses of 5 mg recombinant tissue-type plasminogen activator (Boehringer Ingleheim), clot aspiration and Fogarty balloon embolectomy via a

Table 16.4 Complications.

Local	*No. of patients*
Superficial wound infection	3
Iliac artery rupture	1
Aortic laceration	1
Renal artery embolus	1
Disarticulation of delivery system	1
Femorofemoral graft infection	1
Lymph leakage	1
Haemorrhage from iliac arteriotomy	1
Systemic	
Renal impairment	5
Myocardial infarction	2
Quadrant anopia	2
Pneumonia	2
Jaundice	1
Atrial fibrillation	1
Colonic ischaemia	1
Dialysis fistula thrombosis	1

8-Fr guiding catheter (Cordis). A disarticulated delivery system was removed with the help of an intravascular retrieval basket (William Cook, Europe). The infected femorofemoral graft had to be removed, and an axillobisuperficial femoral bypass via a lateral approach was performed. One lymph leakage resolved after excision of the lymphocoele. The overall 30-day mortality rate was 8 of 70 (11%); the mortality rate for patients considered to be at unacceptably high risk for conventional surgery was 7 of 30 (24%) and 1 of 41 (2%) for the subgroup of patients considered to have acceptable risk for surgery.

Discussion

The technique of aortouni-iliac with femorofemoral bypass was developed by several groups[7–9] to overcome the limitations of an aorto-aortic graft. According to studies carried out in our unit, endovascular repair with a tubular aortoaortic graft is rarely feasible and a minority of patients are suitable for endovascular repair using the bifurcated grafts currently undergoing evaluation.[10] Our experience with the aortoaortic graft is limited to two cases as we have been unable to find more patients with a suitable distal aortic neck. However, in one case a localized leak developed around the distal stent at 3 months, and the distal stent migrated upwards in the other at 6 months. In both cases the completion angiograms were satisfactory and the distal stent had been deployed in an optimum position. With the aortouni-iliac graft we can treat aneurysms with a neck diameter 30 mm or more and a common iliac diameter of 24 mm or greater. Other technical modifications have enabled us to deal with considerable neck and iliac angulations, which had previously precluded endovascular repair. Overall, nearly 60% of patients referred to our unit with AAA can undergo endovascular repair with the aortouni-iliac graft. As the only absolute anatomical prerequisite that need to be established before this type of repair is the presence of a suitable neck below the renal artery, aortouni-iliac repair is at present the most appropriate approach for urgent or emergency repair of leaking AAA. A femorofemoral crossover bypass, required with aortouni-iliac repair, adds to the potential early and long-term complications. It would certainly be desirable to have a purely endovascular approach that would be suitable for the majority of substantial aneurysms, and this is an important area for future research and development.

References

1. Baxendale B, Baker DM, Hind R *et al*. Haemodynamic changes during endovascular graft insertion for aortic aneurysms. *Int Angiol* 1995; **14**(Suppl 1): 247.
2. El-Marasy NM, Yusuf SW, Lonsdale RJ *et al*. Study of the effect of endovascular aneurysm repair on colonic perfusion. *J Endovasc Surg* 1996; **3**: 80–122.
3. Yusuf SW, Whitaker SC, Baker DM, Hind RE, Chuter TAM, Gregson RHS. Endoluminal repair may be possible in the majority of aneurysms. *Br J Surg* 1995; **82**: 561.
4. Yusuf SW, Whitaker SC, Chuter TAM, Wenham PW, Hopkinson BR. Emergency endovascular repair of leaking aortic aneurysm. *Lancet* 1994; **344**: 1645.
5. Yusuf SW, Baker DM, Chuter TAM, Whitaker SC, Wenham PW, Hopkinson BR. Transfemoral endoluminal repair of abdominal aortic aneurysm with bifurcated graft. *Lancet* 1994; **344**: 650–1.
6. Yusuf SW, Baker DM, Hind RE *et al*. Endoluminal transfemoral abdominal aortic aneurysm repair with aortouni-iliac graft and femorofemoral crossover. *Br J Surg* 1995; **82**: 916.
7. May J, White G, Waugh RC, Yu W, Harris JP. Treatment of complex abdominal aortic aneurysms by a combination of endoluminal and extraluminal aortofemoral grafts. *J Vasc Surg* 1994; **19**: 924–33.
8. Parodi JC. Endovascular repair of abdominal aortic aneurysms and other arterial lesions. *J Vasc Surg* 1995; **21**: 549–57.

9. Marin ML, Veith FJ, Cynamon J. Initial experience with transluminally placed endovascular grafts for the treatment of complex vascular lesions. *Ann Surg* 1995; **22**: 449–69.
10. Armon MP, Yusuf SW, Lateif K *et al.* Anatomical suitability of aortic aneurysms for endovascular repair. *Br J Surg* (in press).

17

The Perth bifurcated system

Shane T.R. MacSweeney and
Michael M.D. Lawrence-Brown

Department of Vascular Surgery, University Hospital, Queens Medical Centre, Nottingham NG7 2UH, UK

Department of Vascular Surgery, Royal Perth Hospital, GPO 2213, Perth 6001, Australia

Introduction

The potential benefits of an endovascular approach to the repair of abdominal aortic aneurysm are clear. However, the feasibility of aortoaortic grafting, as pioneered by Parodi *et al.*,[1] is limited by several factors. The most important of these is lack of a distal aneurysm neck in which to fix the distal end of an aortic tube graft.[2,3] This problem can be overcome by inserting an endovascular aortoiliac graft in combination with a surgical femorofemoral crossover graft.[4,5] This approach, whilst undoubtedly effective, is in some respects a compromise. The alternative of a unitary endovascular bifurcated system has its own difficulties.[6] Successful orientation and deployment of a bifurcated graft is a more complex process than deployment of an aortoaortic or aortoiliac system. The potential for technical failure including twisting and kinking of a bifurcated system is increased because of the spiral configuration of the iliac arteries. Passage of a graft–stent system along the spiral during insertion may cause it to rotate.[7] The degree of rotation depends on the tortuosity of the vessel. An ideal endovascular system would combine the relative technical simplicity of deployment of an aortoaortic or aortouni-iliac system with the versatility of a bifurcated system. A modular bifurcated graft developed to overcome these limitations is described in this chapter.

Design of the delivery system and endoprosthesis

The device is a modular system consisting of two sections. The main section comprises a standard woven non-crimped Dacron bifurcation graft with one iliac limb cut short. This is deployed initially in a similar fashion to an aortouni-iliac system with the short limb being oriented so as to overlie the contralateral iliac artery origin. The main piece is held securely at top and bottom so that it can easily be rotated to ensure correct orientation. An extension stent–graft made up with the excised iliac limb is then inserted from the opposite groin into the short limb of the main component, thereby reconstituting the original aortobi-iliac graft. The extension piece is symmetrical and therefore rotation is relatively unimportant.

Proximal fixation is provided by a Gianturco Z stent (WA Cook); this projects beyond the Dacron-covered part of the graft. In addition the entire system is lined with self-expanding stainless steel Z stents which contribute to the seal at the proximal neck. The Z stents reduce any tendency to kinking and provide torsional rigidity as well as stable fixation at the junction of the main piece and extension piece, and at the distal limbs. Each graft–stent system is tailor made for the individual patient. A Dacron cuff is sewn to the proximal end of the bifurcation graft and the Gianturco Z stent is sewn into this. This allows the system to be designed to fit exactly the diameter of the proximal neck. If the aortic and iliac dimensions correspond to a standard sized bifurcation graft, then the top stent is sewn directly into the bifurcation graft and no further modification is required. Similar modifications can be carried out to the iliac limb and extension piece as necessary (Fig. 17.1).

Patient selection criteria

Patients were considered to be suitable for endovascular repair when open surgery was unduly hazardous, the risk of death from rupture was considered to be greater than the risk of death from intercurrent disease and they had a good quality of life (Table 17.1). Preoperative assessment included spiral computed tomography (CT) with reconstruction in sagittal and coronal planes from which the dimensions of the graft were calculated, and angiography to assess the internal dimensions and tortuosity of the iliac vessels. A length of normal-calibre aorta between renal arteries and the aneurysm of less than 1 cm and the need to exclude both internal iliac arteries to deal with bilateral iliac aneurysms were considered contraindications to endovascular repair. Informed consent and ethical approval were obtained.

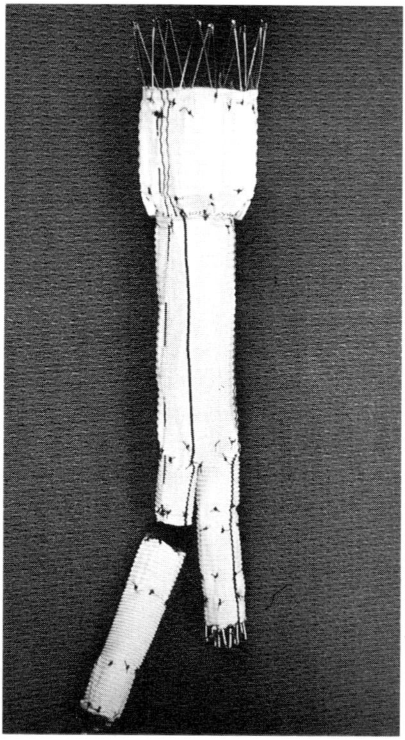

Fig. 17.1 The bifurcate system before loading into the delivery sheath. The Gianturco stent can be seen projecting beyond the top of the graft. In this patient, who had an ectatic aorta, the stent is mounted on a cuff of Dacron to accommodate to the non-standard aortic diameter. The extension piece lies to the bottom left of the picture.

Table 17.1 Characteristics and indications for endovascular surgery in 21 patients.

Median (range) age (years)	74 (60–86)
Sex ratio (M : F)	18 : 3
Median (range) aneurysm diameter (cm)	6.5 (5.0–9.5)
Severe ischaemic or valvular heart disease	13
Severe respiratory disease	7
Hostile abdomen	5
Renal failure	5
Malignant disease	3
Age over 80 years	4
Morbid obesity	2

Procedure

The procedure is performed under epidural or general anaesthesia with the patient draped to allow rapid conversion to open repair. Both common femoral arteries are surgically exposed. A guidewire is passed from the left femoral artery into the aorta and angiography performed to delineate the renal artery origins and the aortic bifurcation. Radio-opaque markers are placed at these reference points to reduce the need for repeated angiography. A 20-Fr sheath mounted on a Coon's dilator (WA Cook, Australia) is passed over an Amplatz super-stiff guidewire (WA Cook, Australia) into the femoral artery without an arteriotomy. This ensures that the artery fits snugly around the sheath and reduces blood loss. The sheath is advanced into the aorta.

The graft assembly is soaked in a saline solution containing heparin 100 000 units/l. Some 5000 units heparin is given intravenously before deployment.

To reduce the bulk of the delivery system, the compressed loaded graft–stent assembly is transferred from a loading sheath into the 20-Fr sheath via a specially designed haemostatic valve, avoiding the need to place one sheath inside the other. Each end of the graft is securely held by a cap; premature release of the caps is prevented by a safety catch (Fig. 17.2). This allows the graft to be advanced into the aorta via the sheath and the entire system to be rotated or moved proximally or distally even after the system has been partially deployed by withdrawal of the delivery sheath. Final deployment is effected by removing the caps after triggering the safety catch.

The Dacron-covered portion of the stent-graft is positioned just below the renal arteries. The uncovered Gianturco stent is usually deployed proximal to this, extending across the renal artery origins into the normal-calibre suprarenal aorta. This uses the maximum possible length of normal-calibre aorta proximal to the aneurysm to ensure secure fixation and a haemostatic seal. It is essential to avoid parallax error to ensure accurate deployment and avoid covering the renal artery orifices with Dacron. The short limb is then cannulated from the opposite groin by a guidewire. This is straightforward provided the short limb has been positioned accurately, overlying the common iliac artery origin. A 14-Fr delivery sheath mounted on a Coon's dilator is passed over the guidewire into the short limb of the main body of the graft. The dilator is removed and the extension piece pushed upwards. When positioning is satisfactory the extension piece is deployed by withdrawing the sheath. Completion angiography is

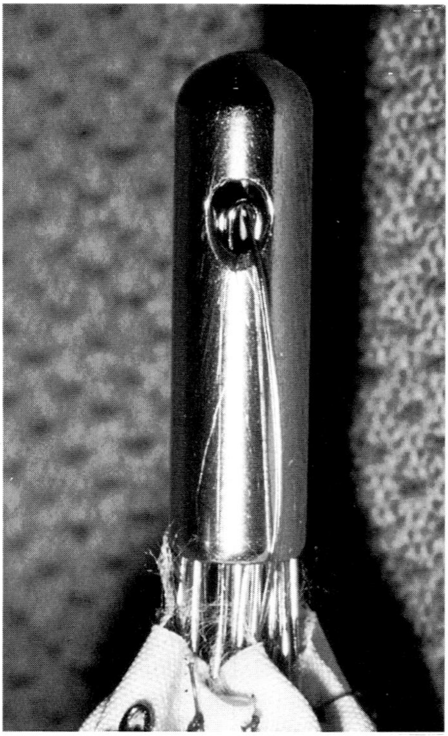

Fig. 17.2 The Gianturco stent loaded into the top cap. Withdrawal of the wire (safety catch) allows the top cap to be pushed off the graft, deploying the stent.

performed to confirm exclusion of the aneurysm and the groins are closed (Fig. 17.3).

Complications and management

Complications are shown in Table 17.2.

The aneurysm appeared to have been excluded in 20 of 21 patients at completion. In three of these patients a leak was noted at postprocedure angiography but was thought to have been sealed successfully by balloon dilatation; however, at follow-up all three leaks were found to have persisted. One patient was known to have a leak that was impossible to balloon dilate owing to tortuosity of the iliac arteries. The aneurysm was successfully excluded in 17 (81%) of 21 patients.

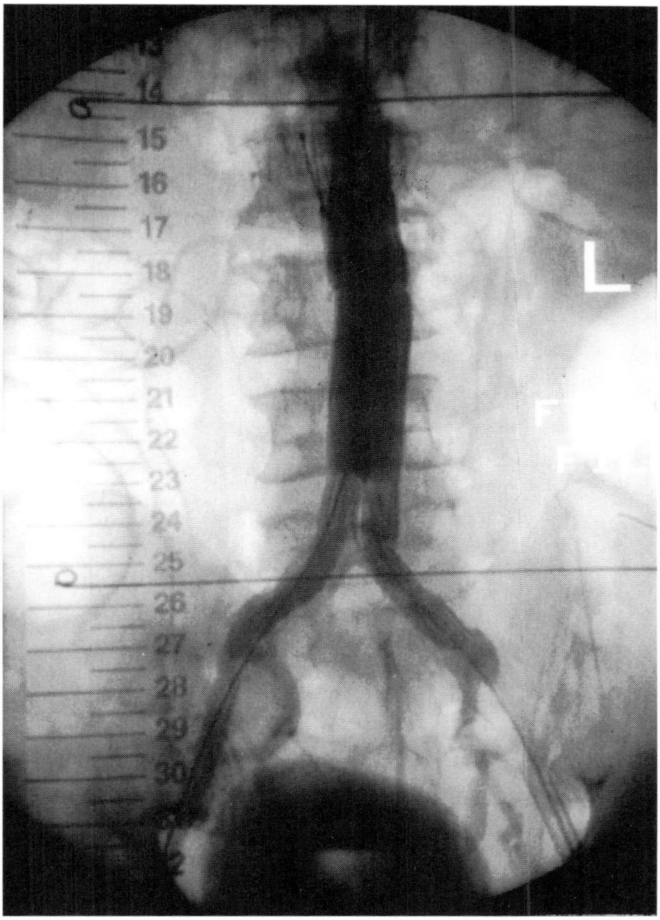

Fig. 17.3 Completion angiogram showing satisfactory exclusion of the aneurysm. The outlines of the Gianturco and Z stents can be seen. The radio-opaque markers showing the positions of the renal arteries (top) and aortic bifurcation can be seen.

Two of the leaks were around the proximal end of the graft, one at the distal limbs and one at the junction of the extension piece with the graft. One of the patients with a proximal leak went on to rupture the aneurysm 3 days after surgery, accounting for one perioperative death. The other aneurysms remain unchanged in diameter; the leak at the junction of the extension piece and the graft had sealed spontaneously

Table 17.2 Complications

	No of patients ($n = 21$)
Major	
Death	1(5)
Stroke	1(5)
Leaks	
Proximal	2(10)
Distal	1(5)
Graft-to-graft interface	1(5)
Late	
Unilateral graft occlusion	2(10)
Bilateral graft occlusion	1(5)
Minor	
Wound haematoma	3(14)
Wound infection	1(5)
Chest infection	1(5)
Urinary infection	1(5)
Atrial fibrillation	1(5)

Values in parentheses are percentages.

by 6 months postprocedure, the others remain unchanged. Two patients went on to occlude one iliac limb of the graft within a few weeks of the procedure and one was discovered incidentally to have occluded both at 6-month follow-up CT. None has undergone surgical intervention.

Follow-up

All 17 aneurysms that were excluded initially remained excluded on follow-up CT at a medium follow-up of 30 (range 4–60) weeks (Fig. 17.4). Deployment of the uncovered Gianturco stent across the renal artery origins was performed in 18 patients (86%). This has not been associated with either renal artery occlusion, either at the time of the procedure or subsequently, or deterioration in renal function (median preoperative serum creatinine concentration 113.5 (range 74–1096) versus 116.5 (range 75–960) μmol/l at a median follow-up of 30 (range 4–60) weeks after operation.

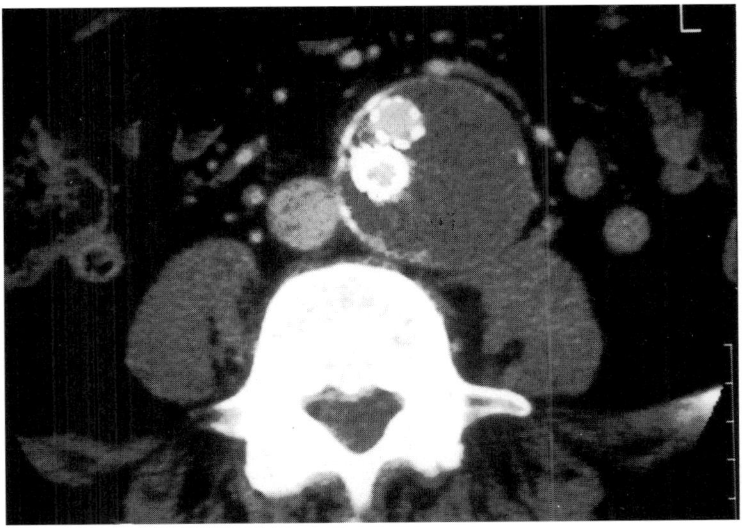

(a)

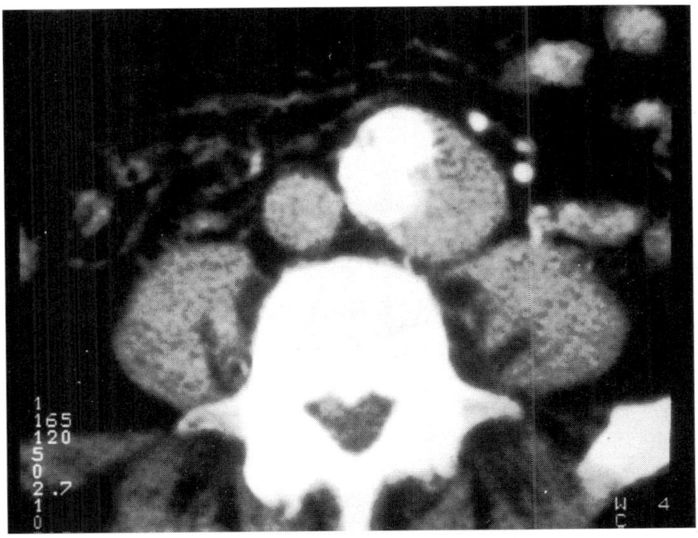

(b)

Fig. 17.4 Follow-up contrast-enhanced CT scans at (a) 3 months and (b) 9 months following the procedure. The aneurysm remains excluded and has decreased in diameter.

Summary

The Perth bifurcated system provides a satisfactory method of endovascular repair of abdominal aortic aneurysm in the short and medium term. The long-term results on which success or failure will depend remain to be established. Many of the technical difficulties encountered during the early experience have been overcome by modifications in design or technique. For example, stenting the graft throughout has largely prevented kinking of the graft limbs, which occurred in some of the early grafts that were stented at top and bottom alone; some of these kinked limbs went on to occlude. Similarly the ‘pull-down’ technique, as described by Parodi[8], has been helpful in overcoming difficulties associated with iliac tortuosity. The appreciation of the need to angle the image intensifier as necessary to provide a true perpendicular image when stenting an angulated proximal aneurysm neck with scrupulous avoidance of parallax error has improved the accuracy of graft deployment. Deployment of the proximal Gianturco stent across the renal artery origins appears to provide secure fixation, with no case of stent–graft migration, and appears to be safe in the short and medium term. This should not be extrapolated to other types of stent which have wires placed more closely together, and may serve as a framework for the development of thrombus or neointimal hyperplasia. Completion angiography has limitations in the detection of leaks that may be of major clinical significance[9]. Early postoperative colour duplex scanning may facilitate early recognition of this problem. A proximal leak is a potentially life-threatening complication and should be regarded as an indication for urgent intervention by either further endovascular manoeuvres or conversion to open repair. Distal leaks appear to be less serious.

The Perth system is versatile and can be adapted to fit a wide range of aneurysm configurations including ectatic proximal necks and dilated iliac arteries. This avoids the limitations of being confined to standard graft dimensions. Being a bifurcated system, it does not require a distal aneurysm neck to seat the graft. A 20-Fr delivery sheath is relatively small and reduces the likelihood of difficulties with iliac arteries of smaller calibre. The main disadvantage of a custom-made system is that it is labour intensive. Clinically apparent embolization has not been encountered and this may represent an advantage of self-expanding stents over balloon-expandable stents. However, by far the most important consideration when comparing the merits of one system to another will be the long-term results; these remain to be established.

Acknowledgement

We wish to acknowledge the enormous contribution to the conception design and production of the Perth System made by David Hartley.

References

1. Parodi JC, Palmaz JC, Barone HD. Transfemoral intraluminal graft implantation for abdominal aortic aneurysms. *Ann Vasc Surg* 1991; **5**: 491–9.
2. Chuter TAM, Green RM, Ouriel K, Deweese JA. Infrarenal aortic aneurysm structure: implications for endovascular repair. *J Vasc Surg* 1994; **20**: 44–50.
3. Andrews SM, Cuming R, MacSweeney ST, Barrett NK, Greenhalgh RM, Nott DM. Assessment of feasibility for endovascular prosthetic tube correction of aortic aneurysm. *Br J Surg* 1995; **82**: 917–19.
4. May J, White G, Waugh R, Yu W, Harris J. Treatment of complex abdominal aortic aneurysms by a combination of endoluminal and extraluminal aortofemoral grafts. *J Vasc Surg* 1994; **19**: 924–33.
5. Yusuf SW, Baker DM, Hing RE *et al.* Endoluminal transfemoral abdominal aortic aneurysm repair with aorto-uni-iliac graft and femorofemoral bypass. *Br J Surg* 1995; **82**: 916.
6. Chuter TA, Wendt G, Hopkinson BR *et al.* Transfemoral insertion of a bifurcated endovascular graft for aortic aneurysm repair: the first 22 patients. *Cardiovasc Surg* 1995; **3**: 121–8.
7. Lawrence-Brown MMD, Hartley D, MacSweeney STR *et al.* A self expanding short leg endoluminal bifurcate graft system – development and early experience. *J. Cardiovasc Surg* (in press).
8. Parodi JC. Endovascular repair of abdominal aortic aneurysms and other arterial lesions. *J Vasc Surg* 1995; **21**: 549–55.
9. Lumsden AB, Allen RC, Chaikof EL *et al.* Delayed rupture of aortic aneurysms following endovascular stent grafting. *Am J Surg* 1995; **170**: 174–8.

18

The Leicester experience

Matthew M. Thompson, Ahktar Nasim and Peter R.F. Bell

Department of Surgery, Clinical Sciences Building, Leicester Royal Infirmary, Leicester LE2 7LX, UK

Introduction

Endovascular aneurysm repair is a useful addition to the vascular repertoire for treating infrarenal abdominal aortic aneurysms.[1] At present, the group based at the University of Leicester and Leicester Royal Infirmary has gained a representative experience of three forms of endovascular aortic procedures: aortoaortic reconstructions using the Endovascular Technologies EGS system (EVT, Menlo Park, CA, USA), aortobi-iliac procedures with the Stentor system (Mintec, Freeport, Bahamas), and aortouni-iliac reconstructions with an 'in house' device. Both the Mintec and EVT systems have been well described in Chapters 6 and 8, and elsewhere.[2,3] This chapter reviews the initial experience of endovascular aneurysm repair using an endograft that is assembled from commercially available components, and is used for aortouni-iliac procedures. This endograft may be used in a larger proportion of patients than commercially available tube or bifurcated systems, and has the added advantage that the individual components cost far less than available manufactured devices.

Design of the delivery system and endoprosthesis

The endoprosthesis consists of a tapered expanded polytetrafluoroethylene (ePTFE) (Impra, Droitwich, UK) graft, which is attached to a Palmaz balloon-expandable stent (Johnson and Johnson Interventional Systems, Bracknell, UK), in turn mounted on a 3-cm balloon angioplasty catheter (Gambro, Sidcup, UK). This series of coaxial

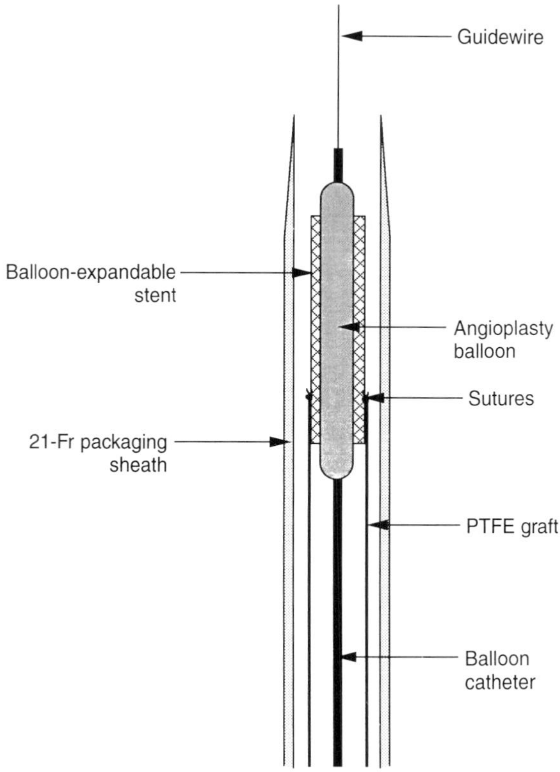

Fig. 18.1 Diagrammatic representation of the endograft, which consists of a series of coaxial components. After Thompson *et al.*[17]

components forms the basis of the endograft, which is packaged inside a 21-Fr sheath (William Cook Europe, Letchworth, UK) (Fig. 18.1). To avoid damage to the endoprosthesis, the packaged device is delivered into the aorta through a 25-Fr introducer sheath. The design of endograft was adapted from the method initially described by Parodi *et al.*[4] in 1991, and has since been used by the Leicester group in a series of experimental models.[5]

The endograft is introduced into the arterial circulation via a temporary iliac conduit, and used to perform an aortouni-iliac reconstruction as previously described by May *et al.*[16] A diagrammatic illustration of this technique is illustrated in Fig. 18.2. In this method, the aneurysm is excluded from the circulation by placement of a long

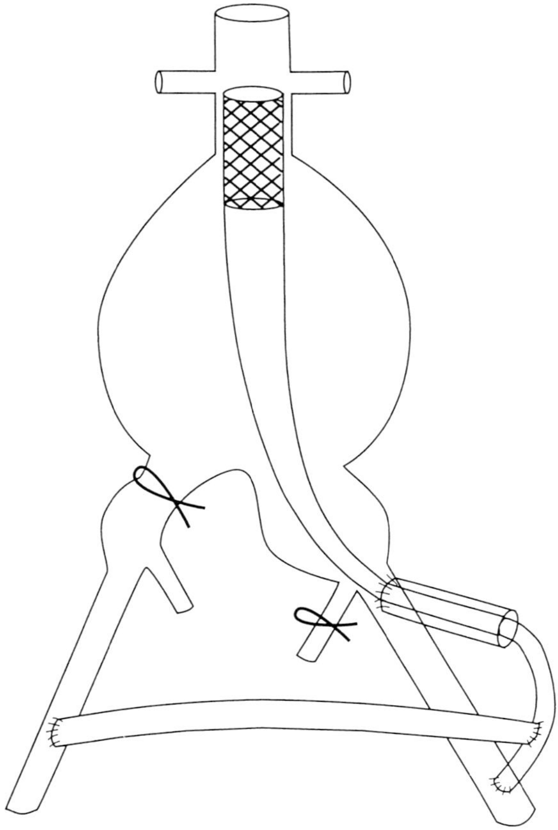

Fig. 18.2 Diagrammatic illustration of a tapered aortouni-iliac graft. The graft is secured at the proximal end by means of a single balloon-expandable stent. The endoprosthesis is then passed through the temporary iliac conduit and anastomosed to the ipsilateral common femoral artery. The procedure is completed by a femorofemoral crossover graft combined with occlusion of the contralateral common iliac artery.

tapered aortouni-iliac graft anchored to the proximal aneurysm neck with a single proximal stent. The device is inserted via a temporary iliac conduit and, after placement of the aortic stent, the tapered graft is passed through this conduit and anastomosed to the ipsilateral common femoral artery by means of standard surgical techniques. The revascularization is completed by a femorofemoral crossover graft combined with occlusion or ligation of the contralateral common iliac artery. This manoeuvre stops blood refluxing into the aneurysm sac and also allows retrograde perfusion of the internal iliac artery.

Components used in the endoprosthesis

The tapered aortoiliac graft is prepared from a commercially available thin-walled 8-mm ePTFE graft (Impra). The graft is prepared by stretching the ePTFE to predetermined dimensions using a graded series of angioplasty balloons.[7] The proximal 7 cm of the graft is dilated over a 60-min period to 35 mm in diameter using progressively larger angioplasty balloons and finally a 35-mm achalasia balloon (Boston Scientific, St Albans, UK) (Fig. 18.3). The graft is then tapered from 35 mm proximally to 12 mm at the distal extent (Fig. 18.4) and secured to a 5-cm long Palmaz stent (Johnson and Johnson Interventional Systems) with two diametrically opposed 2/0 polypropylene sutures. The graft–stent combination is then mounted on a 30-mm balloon angioplasty catheter (Gambro) and the entire device is then backloaded into a 21-Fr packaging sheath (William Cook Europe) (Fig. 18.5) before use. The proximal graft is initially stretched to 35 mm to compensate for a degree of recoil that occurs following the dilation procedure.

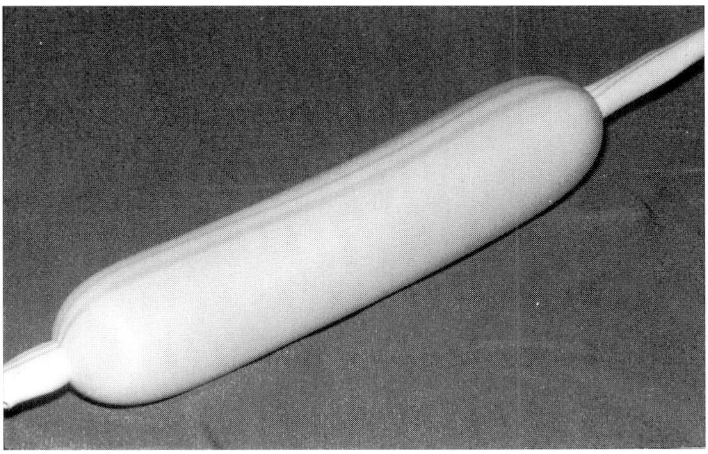

Fig. 18.3 An 8-mm thin-walled ePTFE graft being gradually stretched with a 30-mm balloon angioplasty catheter.

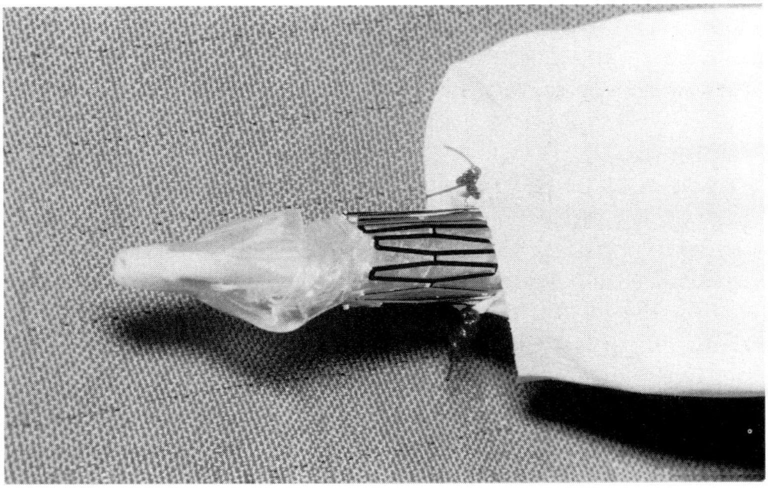

Fig. 18.4 Final appearance of tapered ePTFE graft.

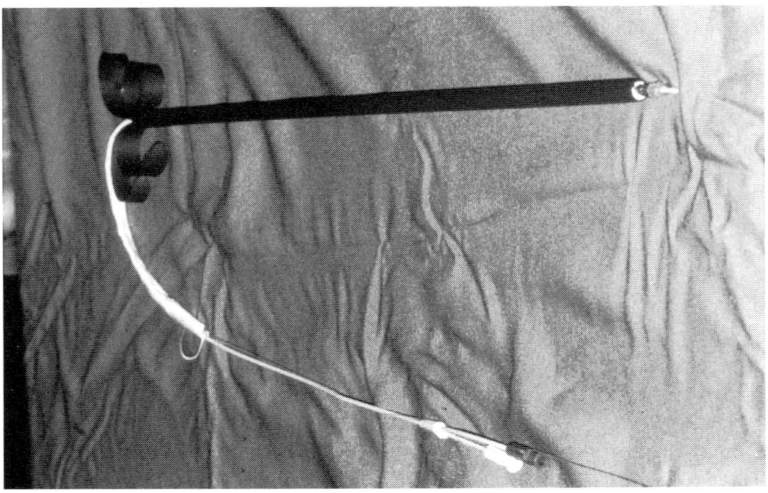

Fig. 18.5 Completed endoprosthesis packaged inside a 21-Fr packaging sheath.

Patient selection procedure

All patients with non-ruptured abdominal aortic aneurysms are assessed with a combination of colour duplex, contrast-enhanced computed tomography (CT) with conventional axial slices and magnetic resonance angiography (MRA).[8,9] Patients who are considered suitable for endovascular aneurysm repair then undergo intra-arterial digital subtraction angiography with a marker catheter. Aneurysms are assessed from the cross-sectional images, and aneurysm morphology is defined. In a series of 82 consecutive patients, MRA proved significantly better at defining aneurysmal morphology than either colour duplex scanning or conventional transaxial CT, although arteriography is mandatory before endovascular repair. In our current series approximately 40% of patients with aneurysms greater than 5.5 cm are suitable for endoluminal procedures.

The main criteria for selection for an aortouni-iliac graft in our centre is a proximal aneurysm neck greater than 1.8 cm in length and less than 26 mm in diameter. The morphology of the aortic bifurcation and iliac arteries does not preclude patients from endovascular aneurysm repair if they have one segment of non-aneurysmal common iliac artery. This segment, however, is essential to allow revascularization of the internal iliac artery contralateral to the graft insertion site following ligation or occlusion of the common iliac system. Excessive iliac tortuosity is not considered a contraindication to endovascular repair as a temporary iliac conduit may be used to overcome this problem.

Procedure

All endovascular procedures are performed in a standard surgical operating theatre under balanced general anaesthesia. The patient is prepared and draped as for conventional aneurysm surgery, and both common femoral arteries are exposed. The endograft is inserted on the side that represents the straightest route to the aortic neck. On the chosen side, a retroperitoneal approach is made to the iliac bifurcation, and the internal iliac artery is ligated and divided. Following heparinization (5000 units), the common iliac artery is partially mobilized and a 10-mm Dacron graft is anastomosed end to side to the external iliac artery. This graft is then tunnelled beneath the inguinal ligament into the groin wound to provide a temporary iliac conduit for graft placement as described by Parodi.[10] In our initial experience it has proved easier to use a temporary conduit for passage of the endograft than to pass large sheaths up a diseased segment of femoral artery. In addition to providing a larger-diameter artery for access, this technique allows any iliac tortuosity to be corrected, and may also minimize the extent of arterial trauma during passage of the 25-Fr introducer sheath. The 25-Fr sheath fits snugly within the 10-mm conduit with minimal blood leakage.

Following release of the iliac clamps, the Dacron conduit is clamped at its distal end and a guidewire (0.89 mm; Meadox, Caddington, UK) is then manipulated through the conduit into the suprarenal aorta under fluoroscopic control. A tapered Van Andel dilation catheter (5-Fr; William Cook Europe) is passed over the guidewire into the aorta, and the guidewire is subsequently removed. To prevent kinking of the vasculature, and to straighten the arterial system before introduction of the endograft, a J-curved Lunderquist guidewire (0.89 mm; Meadox) is passed through the Van Andel dilation catheter, which is then removed. The Dacron conduit is incised longitudinally, and a 25-Fr Teflon sheath with its mandril is passed over the Lunderquist wire into the suprarenal aorta (Fig. 18.6). The Lunderquist wire is removed at this stage, and a 260-cm exchange wire (0.89 mm; Meadox) is passed through the channel in the mandril.

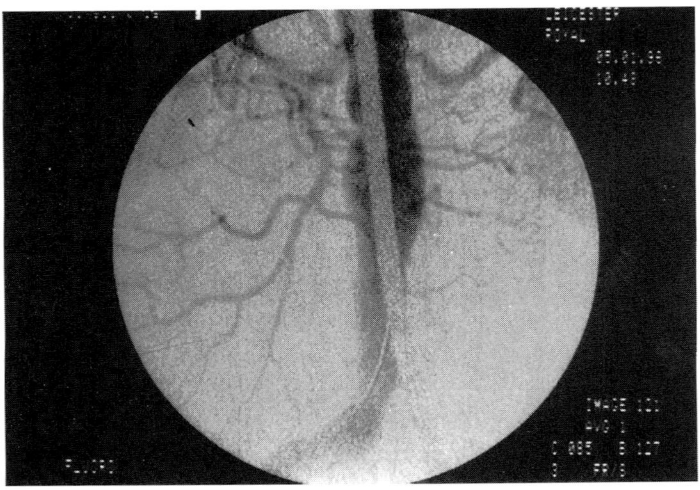

Fig. 18.6 A 25-Fr introducer sheath passed into the suprarenal aorta.

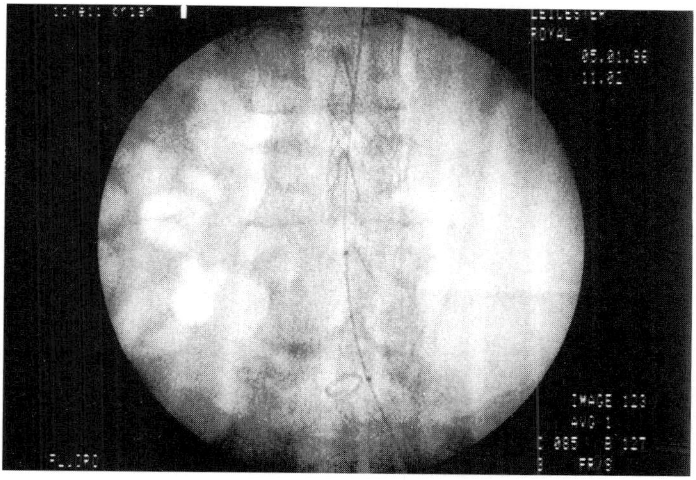

Fig. 18.7 Expanded Palmaz stent at the proximal aneurysm neck. The markers on the angioplasty balloon are visualized.

Following passage of the 25-Fr introducer sheath and mandril, retrograde arteriography is performed via the contralateral common femoral artery. The position of the renal arteries is clearly identified and marked on the image intensifier. The mandril is removed, and the endograft, contained within the 21-Fr packaging sheath, is passed into the aorta within the 25-Fr introducer sheath. The proximal stent is manoeuvred 2–3 cm above the renal arteries, and the 25-Fr sheath is removed. The packaging sheath is then carefully withdrawn to expose the endograft and the upper limit of the stent is positioned 0.5 cm above the lowest renal orifice to allow for shortening of the stent during expansion. The mean arterial pressure is lowered to 70 mmHg and the stent is deployed by inflating the angioplasty balloon to 2 atmospheres pressure for two periods of 60 s (Fig. 18.7). The stent position is adjusted during expansion, with the aim of placing the stent immediately distal to the renal artery origins. The angioplasty balloon is subsequently deflated and removed from the graft lumen. Constant radiological screening is required at this stage to ensure that the angioplasty balloon is removed smoothly without dislodging the expanded stent. A pigtail catheter (5 Fr; Mallinckrodt Medical, St Louis, MO, USA) is passed over the exchange wire, and an arteriogram performed to confirm deployment of the endograft and patency of the renal arteries (Fig. 18.8).

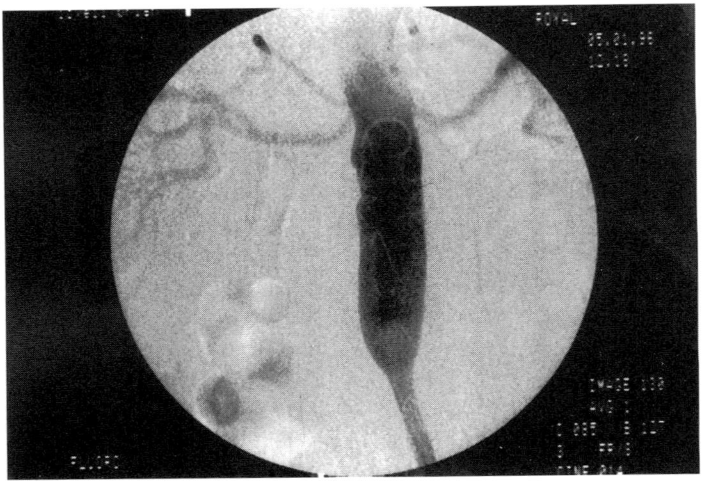

Fig. 18.8 Completion arteriogram illustrating patent renal arteries and the tapered endograft.

The ePTFE graft is anastomosed to the ipsilateral common femoral artery, and a crossover graft performed. Finally, the contralateral comon iliac artery is occluded to prevent reflux into the aneurysm sac and to allow perfusion of the internal iliac artery. This may be achieved by radiological (coil embolization, detachable balloon occlusion) or direct surgical techniques. At present we have experience of all methods, but prefer surgical ligation if the arterial diameter exceeds 14 mm, as this appears to be more reliable in larger vessels.

Complications and management

To date we have performed 14 tapered endovascular procedures. The median age of the patients was 70 years and the median aneurysm diameter 5.8 cm. Four patients had Americal Society of Anesthesiologists grade 3 or 4, and were tertiary referrals specifically for endvascular repair. Two other patients had coexistent abdominal pathology that would have increased the difficulty of conventional surgery; one patient had hereditary haemorrhagic telangectasia affecting the parietal peritoneum with dense peritoneal adhesions, and the other had non-Hodgkin's lymphoma affecting the periaortic nodes which had been treated with periaortic radiotherapy. In addition, a further patient had a 7-cm inflammatory aneurysm with involvement of the right ureter with consequent hydronephrosis. Overall, in the cases performed, there was no mortality and no perioperative systemic complications. There were, however, several procedural complications, with two immediate and one early procedural failure. There have been no late complications.

There were two initial failures in cases where the balloon-expandable stent was deployed too low in the proximal aneurysm neck, with extravasation of blood into the aneurysm sac (proximal perigraft leakage). In both of these cases, the leak was considered to be of sufficient magnitude to warrant immediate conversion to conventional surgery. Both patients underwent uneventful bifurcated graft replacement with no postoperative complications. Both of these immediate procedural failures occurred in the early part of the series and may be attributed partly to the steep learning curve associated with endovascular aneurysm repair. Low deployment of the stent in these two cases occurred partly as a result of uncompensated stent shortening, and also as a result of poor visualization of the stent when the angioplasty balloon was inflated with dilute contrast medium. To overcome this problem, we now use saline to expand the balloon under strict manometric control. The modification provides excellent visualization of the stent as it expands and allows fine adjustment of position to be made during stent deployment. Since adopting this technique, all stents have been positioned correctly.

One patient had a perforation of the common iliac artery during introduction of the 25-Fr introducer sheath, although the endograft was successfully placed. During some of the early cases, passage of the introducer sheath was accompanied by excessive manipulation within the aneurysm sac in attempts to negotiate the aneurysmal tortuosity and to pass the introducer into the suprarenal aorta. This problem has been resolved by using a super-stiff Lunderquist wire to straighten the aneurysmal tortuosity. The Lunderquist wire cannot be directly manipulated within the aneurysm sac because of its relative inflexibility, but may be placed through a tapered catheter. The use of this technique has overcome any problem with arterial tortuosity, and has reduced endoluminal manipulation within the aneurysm sac.

The early procedural failure occurred in a patient who developed a proximal perigraft leak 10 days after graft deployment. The leak was detected on a predischarge duplex scan and confirmed by contrast-enhanced CT. Findings at subsequent transperitoneal revision surgery confirmed that the stent had slipped into the aneurysm sac with complete failure of aneurysm exclusion. Review of the preprocedure magnetic resonance angiograms demonstrated that the proximal aneurysm neck contained a significant quantity of thrombus, and that the true neck diameter was 28 mm, which was not suitable for repair with a 30-mm balloon-expandable stent–graft. This complication, therefore, could be attributed to poor interpretation of the preoperative investigations.

Three patients demonstrated evidence of mid 'trash foot', which resolved spontaneously. This complication appears to be related to lower limb microembolization during the procedure. In a separate study, microembolization during conventional and endovascular aneurysm repair has been quantified by insonating the superficial femoral artery with a 2-MHz Doppler probe during both procedures.[11] This investigation has demonstrated that both particulate and gaseous embolization is increased in endovascular procedures, and that the number of particulate emboli correlates with the development of clinical sequelae. Particulate embolization during endovascular procedures is most apparent during endoluminal manipulations within the aneurysm sac, and it would appear that the number of emboli may be reduced by experience and by strategies to minimize manipulation of large instruments within the aneurysm. Early results from this study suggest that the number of particulate emboli is related to the experience of the operator. There have been no cases of massive microembolization in this series.

Follow-up

Eleven patients were entered into the endovascular follow-up programme. This consists of clinical and colour duplex examinations at 7 days, 6 weeks and 3, 6, 9 and 12 months following the procedure, with contrast-enhanced CT at 7 days and at 3 and 6 months. To date no patients have developed any late clinical complication, and examinations have confirmed that all aneurysms remain completely excluded from the circulation. All excluded aneurysms are completely thrombosed and diminishing in size.

Interestingly, the patient with an endovascularly repaired inflammatory aneurysm has demonstrated a reduction in plasma viscosity and C-reactive protein along with reduction of the diameter of the aneurysm sac. This perhaps is the first circumstantial evidence that endovascular aneurysm repair may reduce periaortic inflammation associated with inflammatory aneurysms.

Summary

This chapter presents our initial clinical experience of endovascular aortouni-iliac bypass grafting with a balloon-expandable stent with a tapered ePTFE endograft. Like many procedures in their infancy, there are many unanswered questions surrounding endovascular aneurysm repair. Our initial experience highlights two particular questions, namely the role of aortouni-iliac grafting and the choice of stent for the procedure.

The advantage of aortouni-iliac procedures is that there is less morphological restriction to their use except for an adequate proximal aneurysm neck. Most tube or bifurcated endografts[3,12,13] have significant morphological requirements that necessitate an adequate length of distal aneurysm neck or iliac arteries less than 14 mm in diameter to allow effective distal fixation. These restrictions obviously reduce the number of patients suitable for endovascular repair. These constraints are largely overcome by the technique described in this chapter, although obviously the procedure relies on a mixture of endovascular techniques and standard surgery. One of the potential attractions of endovascular procedures may be the ability to treat ruptured aneurysms with minimally invasive techniques.[14] Most currently available commercial endografts are custom-made and so could not be used for this purpose. However, the endograft described in this article may be used to treat any patient with a reasonable proximal aneurysm neck and so may be employed in the emergency situation.

One feature of the procedure described above is that the distal anastomoses are sutured, and should therefore not permit perigraft leakage. There have been preliminary reports in the literature of patients developing late perigraft leaks following initially successful endograft placement. Abdominal aortic aneurysms are typified by a complex series of biochemical changes within the arterial wall,[15] and there is no evidence as yet to suggest that endovascular grafting will reverse the dilating process that accompanies aneurysmal disease. It is possible, therefore, that continued expansion of the aortic bifurcation and iliac arteries may jeopardize the success of endovascular repair based solely on stented distal anastomosis. Clearly, long-term follow-up is required to resolve this issue, but we suggest that sutured anastomoses will not be affected by perianastomotic arterial dilatation.

One of the greatest drawbacks to the use of aortouni-iliac procedures is the reliance on femorofemoral crossover grafts to revascularize the contralateral limb. The patency of femoral crossover grafts is reasonable when performed for occlusive arterial disease, but these procedures are often complicated by the development of false aneurysms, infections or seromas in the groin.[16] It is possible that patency and graft-related complications may be reduced, as many patients with abdominal aneurysms do not have associated occlusive disease, but again further follow-up will determine the natural history of these grafts.

The two principal advantages of endovascular aortic surgery in comparison to conventional procedures are the absence of intraperitoneal manipulation and a reduction in aortic occlusion time. Aortouni-iliac grafting avoids transperitoneal exposure even though there is a retroperitoneal incision, and mobilization after operation appears to be similar to patients having EVT or Mintec grafts. One potential disadvantage of the 'home-made' aortouni-iliac grafts is that, although the aorta is not clamped, the aortic flow passes into a blind-ended graft until the femoral anastomoses have been completed. This results in a 30-min period of ischaemia affecting the legs and pelvis. Studies are currently in progress to determine the metabolic consequences of this technique.

References

1. Sayers RD, Thompson MM, Bell PR. Endovascular stenting of abdominal aortic aneurysms. *Eur J Vasc Surg* 1993; **7**: 225–7.
2. Nasim A, Sayers RD, Thompson MM, Bell PR, Bolia A. Endovascular repair of abdominal aortic aneurysms. *Lancet* 1994; **343**: 1230–1.
3. Mialhe C, Amicabile C. Experience with the Stentor system for AAA treatment. *J Endovasc Surg* 1995; **2**: 405.
4. Parodi JC, Palmaz JC, Barone HD. Transfemoral intraluminal graft implantation for abdominal aortic aneurysms. *Ann Vasc Surg* 1991; **5**: 491–9.
5. Sayers RD, Thompson MM, Nasim A, Bell PRF. Endovascular repair of abdominal aortic aneurysms: limitations of the proximal stent technique. *Br J Surg* 1994; **81**: 1107–10.
6. May J, White G, Waugh R, Yu W, Harris J. Treatment of complex abdominal aortic aneurysms by a combination of endoluminal and extraluminal aortofemoral grafts. *J Vasc Surg* 1994; **19**: 924–33.
7. Richter GM, Palmaz JC, Allenberg JR, Kauffmann GW. Die transluminale stentprosthese beim bauchaortenaneurysma. *Radiologie* 1994; **34**: 511–18.
8. Nasim A, Thompson MM, Sayers RD, Hartshorne T, Bell PRF. Comparison of magnetic resonance angiography, computed tomography, colour duplex and arteriography for assessing abdominal aortic aneurysms before endoluminal repair. *Br J Surg* 1996; **83**: 559.
9. Cherryman GR, Moody AR, Rodgers P. New imaging techniques and arterial disease. *Vasc Med Rev* 1994; **5**: 107–20.

10. Parodi JC. Endovascular repair of abdominal aortic aneurysms. In: *Advances in Vascular Surgery*, Vol. 1. St Louis, MO: Moseby, 1993: 85–106.
11. Thompson MM, Smith J, Naylor AR, Nasim A, Sayers RD, Boyle JR, Thompson J, Tinkler K, Evans DH, Smith PRF, Bell PRF. Microembolization during endovascular aneurysm repair. *Br J Surg* 1996 (in press).
12. Chuter TA, Donayre C, Wendt G. Bifurcated stent–grafts for endovascular repair of abdominal aortic aneurysm. Preliminary case reports. *Surg Endosc* 1994; **8**: 800–2.
13. Moore WS, Vescera CL. Repair of abdominal aortic aneurysm by transfemoral endovascular graft placement. *Ann Surg* 1994; **220**: 231–41.
14. Yusuf SW, Whitaker SC, Chuter TAM, Wenham PW, Hopkinson BR. Emergency endovascular abdominal aortic aneurysm repair. *Lancet* 1995; **344**: 645.
15. MacSweeney STR, Powell JT, Greenhalgh RM. Pathogenesis of abdominal aortic aneurysm. *Br J Surg* 1994; **81**: 935–41.
16. Ng RLH, Gillies TE, Davies AH, Baird RN, Horrocks M. Iliofemoral versus femorofemoral bypass: a 6-year audit. *Br J Surg* 1992; **79**: 1011–13.
17. Thompson MM, Nasim A, Sayers RD, Bell PRF. Endovascular aneurysm repair. *Curr Surg Pract* 1995; 7: 21–7.

19

Renal damage

Daryll M. Baker and Peter W. Wenham

Department of Vascular Surgery, Royal Free Hospital, London, UK

Department of Vascular Surgery, University Hospital, Queen's Medical Centre, Nottingham NG7 2UH, UK

Renal failure during open abdominal aortic aneurysm repair

Renal failure following abdominal aortic aneurysm repair, although relatively rare, is associated with high morbidity and mortality rates.[1] Renal damage may occur before, during or after surgery. Patients with pre-existing renal disease are particularly vulnerable to perioperative renal injury.

In addition to more general causes of renal failure in an ageing population, patients with abdominal aortic aneurysms may have preoperative problems more directly related to the underlying vascular disease; for example, they frequently have renal artery atheromatous disease that reduces renal function. Hypertension, sometimes secondary to renovascular disease, or diabetes mellitus is commonly present and may be complicated by nephropathy. Perianeurysmal fibrosis causing an obstructive uropathy can also contribute to renal insufficiency. Patients with ruptured aortic aneurysms face an additional risk with an ill-defined period of preoperative hypovolaemia and peripheral vasoconstriction before surgery, at a time when resuscitation with intravenous fluids is ill advised. Patients with preoperative renal failure may require perioperative and postoperative dialysis support.

During open aortic aneurysm surgery, renal injury may occur whilst placing the proximal aortic clamp, either by a direct clamp injury to the renal artery or by dislodging an atheromatous plaque leading to renal embolization. Aortic cross-clamping also causes major haemodynamic changes, with an acute rise in systemic blood pressure,[2] leading to renal vasoconstriction which causes a 75% increase in vascular resistance, a 38% fall in blood flow[3] and changes in renin–angiotensin mechanisms.[4] Ruptured aortic aneurysm repairs are often associated with intraoperative periods of hypovolaemia, which can precipitate pre-renal renal failure and substantial blood loss that necessitates major blood transfusions with additional risks. When the aortic clamps are removed, further haemodynamic changes occur,[2] with a fall in systemic vascular resistance necessitating fluid replacement to correct hypotension. At the same time, the relatively ischaemic legs and pelvic viscera are reperfused, leading to lactic acidosis,[2] release of oxygen-free radicals and other metabolites associated with reperfusion injury affecting a wide variety of tissues including the kidneys and lungs.[5]

In the postoperative period, cardiac insufficiency and relative hypovolaemia may cause or exacerbate renal failure. These problems may be complicated by assisted ventilation and the use of vasoactive drugs. Optimal management during this time limits the damage done to already compromised kidneys.

Renal failure during endovascular abdominal aortic aneurysm repair

Although endovascular aortic aneurysm repair minimizes haemodynamic changes and limits ischaemic reperfusion injury,[2,6] both of which are believed to be principal causes of renal damage in conventional surgery, an endovascular approach potentially carries its own renal morbidity. These relate to radiographic contrast media and their effects on renal function, intraluminal catheter and graft–stent manipulations, and the risk of graft malplacement obstructing the renal vessels.

The adverse effects of iodinated contrast media on renal function have been well reported, although the mechanism is poorly understood.[4] The patients most at risk are those with low renal blood flows, pre-existing renal failure and dehydration, conditions that commonly coexist in patients undergoing aortic aneurysm surgery.[7] Patients require preoperative angiography to plan their surgery and, during endovascular stent placement, it is not uncommon to use more than 300 ml of contrast medium. Efforts to limit the amount of contrast are important.

The probability of dislodging atheromatous debris emboli is proportional to the degree to which guidewires, catheters and prostheses are manipulated within the aorta during endovascular aortic aneurysm graft implantation.[8] Instrumentation above or at the level of the renal arteries is hazardous. In systems where the aorta is temporarily occluded below the renal arteries, embolic debris within the aorta may be directed preferentially to the renal arteries. Systems in which the aorta remains unoccluded may have an intrinsic safety. In the Nottingham series of 70 endovascular grafts, there has been a single renal arterial embolus (Fig. 19.1). The renal artery embolus was cleared with a combination of suction and intra-arterial thrombolysis.

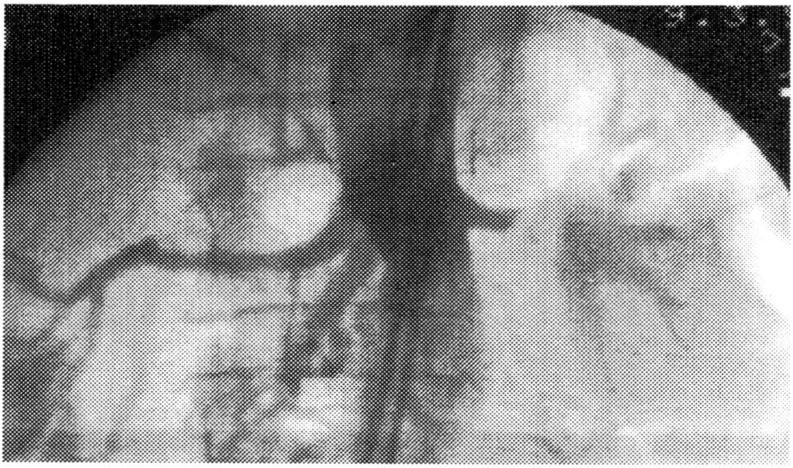

(a)

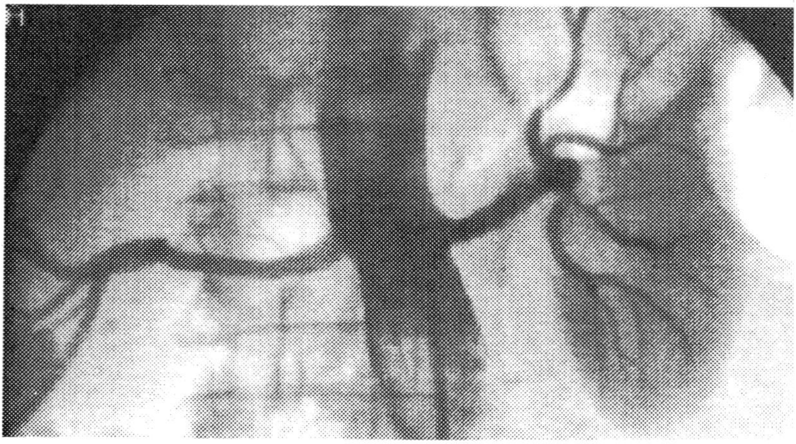

(b)

Fig. 19.1 (a) Embolus occluding renal artery during endovascular graft deployment. (b) The embolus has been cleared by intra-arterial catheter suction and thrombolysis.

The third risk, peculiar to endovascular grafts, relates to the position of graft–stent combinations in relation to the renal arteries. Animal studies have suggested that the effect of placing stents over the origins of the renal arteries is dependent not only on the method and accuracy of deployment, but also on the shape and composition of the different stent struts.[9–13] The Wallstent, which has smooth rounded struts of knitted spring steel wires (Fig. 19.2a), has little deleterious effect on ostium patency or renal function when placed across porcine renal artery origins[10]. The Palmaz stent consists of large flattened struts of polished stainless steel, between which are large interstices (Fig. 19.2b). Provided a strut does not cross the ostium, renal artery blood flow and renal function also remain unchanged. The struts of Memotherm stents, which are made from nickel titanium alloy (Nitinol), have a roughened laser-etched surface and are thrombogenic, causing ostial occlusion in almost all cases when placed across a renal artery ostium of the porcine model (Fig. 19.2c).[10]

In clinical practice, endovascular abdominal aortic aneurysm repair is currently restricted to patients with relatively long infrarenal necks (greater than 1.5 cm). In cases where renal arteries arise from the aorta at the same level, above an adequate length of normal aorta proximal to the aneurysm, placement of the graft is straightforward. Provided the position of the device is checked with repeated imaging at deployment, the risk of covering the renal artery ostia is minimal. Problems arise where the neck is too short for safe graft placement. In patients where this is related to variants in the anatomical configuration of renal arteries, it may on occasions be necessary to sacrifice a lower polar vessel (Fig. 19.3) that is making only a minor contribution to renal function, if a graft is to be deployed. In that case an isotope renography is performed before operation to confirm the proportion of renal function attributed to each kidney before an accessory artery supplying a portion of one kidney is sacrificed during stent deployment. Where the neck is too short for satisfactory placement distal to the renal vessels, the Perth experience (see Chapter 17) has suggested that it may still be possible to deploy an endovascular prosthesis with a Gianturco stent in which the proximal portion is uncovered and deployed across the renal artery origins, while the graft-bearing part of the stent is positioned within the short infrarenal neck making an effective seal.

Irrespective of the risk of early thrombosis, there remains the long-term risk of red cell fragmentation and microembolization from platelet aggregates in relation to the stent over a renal artery origin,

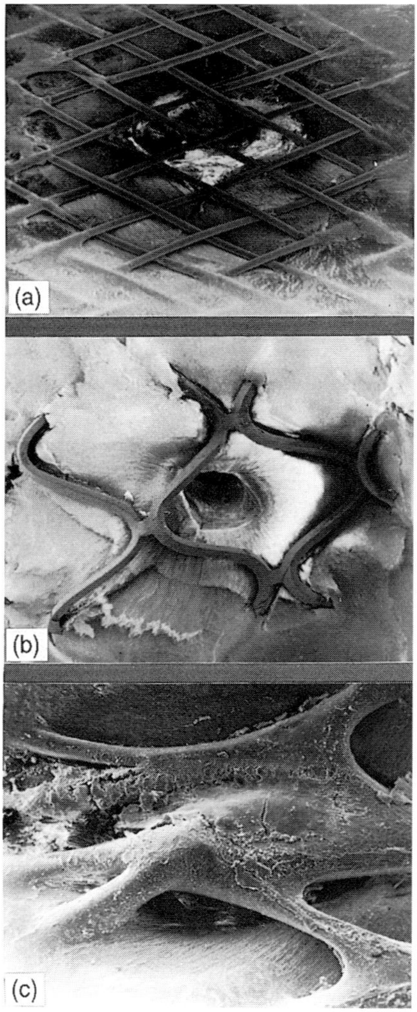

Fig. 19.2 Stents over renal artery ostia (scanning electron microscopy; original magnification $\times 10$). (a) Wallstent. The struts are round and smooth, having no thrombus attached. The ostium is fully patent. (b) Palmaz stent. The struts are flat and large, but with large interstices. The ostium is patent. (c) Memotherm stent. The struts have rough laser-etched surfaces and are very thrombogenic, resulting here in almost complete occlusion of the ostium. By courtesy of Mr P. Birch, Vascular Institute, Sheffield.

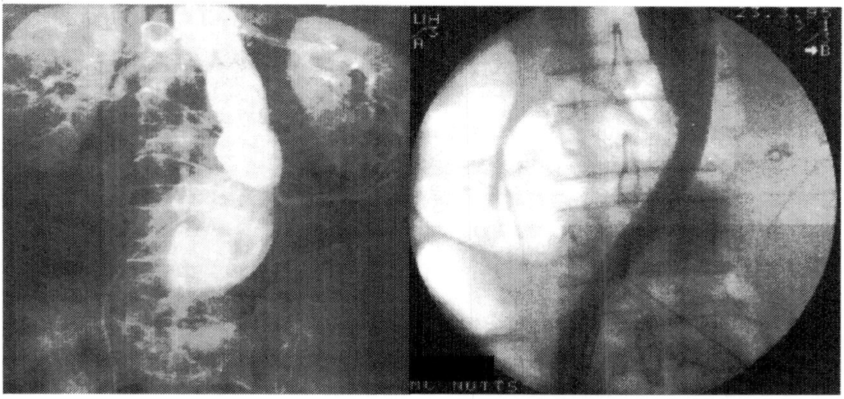

Fig. 19.3 When the aortic neck proximal to the aneurysm below the renal vessels is not long enough, a lower pole marginal branch may be sacrificed.

leading to a progressive reduction in renal function. Despite early animal studies failing to confirm this,[10] should the renal ostium be traversed by a stent, antiplatelet agents may reduce the potential problem.

Is the risk of renal failure during aortic aneurysm repair reduced by an endovascular approach?

Assessment of renal function

Renal failure is relatively uncommon after elective aneurysm surgery and its occurrence is a crude measure of the renal damage that can occur. Biochemical tests used in clinical practice are relatively insensitive as large changes in renal function are needed before these parameters change significantly. For example, serum creatinine concentration rises above the upper limit of normal only when more than half of the functioning kidney tissue has been lost.[14] Albuminuria is a more sensitive measure of renal glomerular damage.[15] Albumin excretion has been shown to rise rapidly during aortic surgery and appears to be a useful marker of endothelial damage and a predictor of the development of multiorgan complications.[5,16] *N*-acetyl glucosaminidase (NAG) is a proximal tubular cell lysosomal enzyme and its urinary excretion provides an early indication of tubular damage.[17]

Urinary NAG measurements have been shown to be a sensitive indicator of subclinical renal impairment in obstructive jaundice[16] and diabetic nephropathy.[18] Both urinary albumin and NAG excretion rates provide sensitive markers of subclinical renal damage, allowing comparison between groups when more advanced changes are relatively uncommon.

Renal function during open and endovascular surgery

Urinary excretion of albumin and NAG rises early in the postoperative period in patients undergoing conventional surgery for aortic aneurysms[5,19], even when blood urea, serum creatinine and creatinine clearance levels remain unchanged. Figures 19.4 and 19.5 confirm that, in a series of ten patients undergoing uncomplicated conventional aneurysm repairs, both these subclinical markers of renal impairment returned to normal over a few days.

In the Nottingham series of 70 endovascular aneurysm grafts, three of the four patients who died within 30 days of surgery suffered renal failure. One patient, an 84-year-old woman with a ruptured aortic aneurysm, underwent aneurysm repair but developed progressive renal failure related to myoglobinuria. Renal failure in the other two cases was part of multiorgan failure, and not the precipitating cause. At

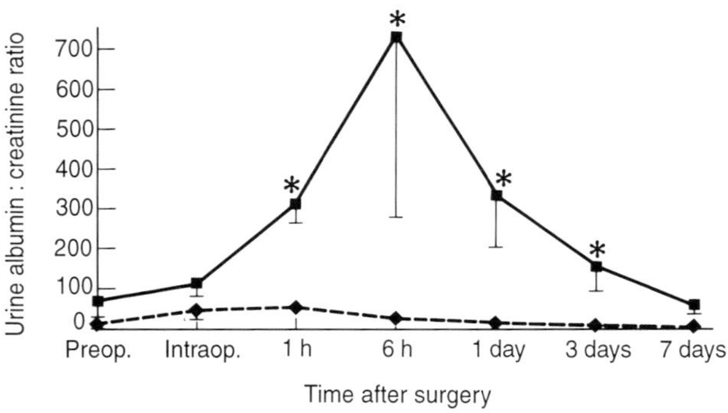

Fig. 19.4 Microalbumin urinary excretion rates at various times before and after aortic aneurysm surgery. Values are expressed as a ratio of the urinary creatinine concentration so as to correct for variation in urinary flow rates and dilution effects. ■——■, Mean values from ten patients undergoing uncomplicated open aortic aneurysm surgery; ◆– – –◆, mean values from ten patients undergoing endovascular aneurysm repair. Error bars are standard error of the mean. $*P < 0.05$ (open versus endovascular surgery).

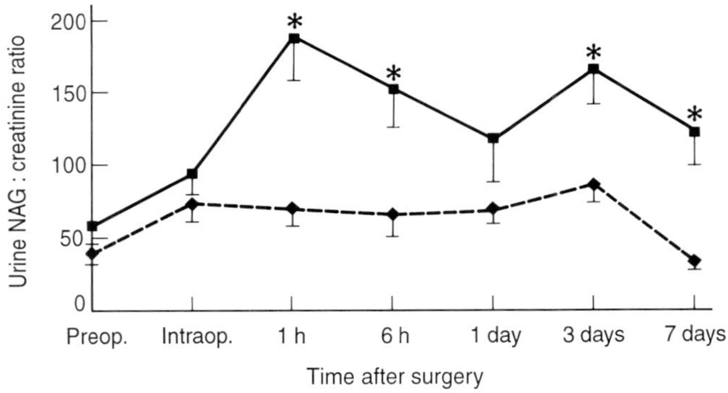

Fig. 19.5 *N*-acetyl glucosaminidase (NAG) excretion rates at various times before and after aortic aneurysm surgery. Values are expressed as a ratio of urinary creatinine concentration so as to correct for variation in urinary flow rates and dilution effects. ■——■, Mean values from ten patients undergoing uncomplicated open aortic aneurysm surgery; ◆– – –◆, mean values from ten patients undergoing endovascular aneurysm repair. Error bars are standard error of the mean. $*P < 0.05$ (open versus endovascular surgery).

a subclinical level, in a small study[20] the albumin and NAG urinary excretion rates were measured in ten patients undergoing endovascular aortic aneurysm repair (seven aorto-biiliac Chuter graft–stents and three aorto-uniiliac graft–stents with a conventional femorofemoral crossover graft). Figures 19.4 and 19.5 show that there was no significant change in postoperative compared with preoperative levels. Thus, even using sensitive markers of renal damage, no deleterious effects of endovascular surgery were detected.

Conclusions

Renal failure during aortic aneurysm repair is associated with high morbidity and mortality rates. Although chronic renal failure is unusual, some form of renal impairment, usually subclinical, is common in conventional open aortic aneurysm surgery.

It is a sensible assumption that measures shown to reduce subclinical renal injury will also be beneficial in reducing more significant problems. Early studies suggest that, despite the specific potential hazards of endovascular repair, the risks of renal injury are substantially reduced when open procedures can be avoided.

References

1. Gornick CC, Kjellstrand CM. Acute renal failure complicating aortic aneurysm surgery. *Nephron* 1983; **35**: 145–57.
2. Baxendale B, Baker DM, Hird RE *et al.* Haemodynamic changes during endovascular graft insertion for aortic aneurysms. *Int Angiol* 1995; **14** (Suppl 1): 247.
3. Gamulin Z, Foster A, Murel D, Simonel F, Aymon E, Faure H. Effect of infra-renal aortic cross-clamping on renal haemodynamics in humans. *J Anaesthesiol* 1984; **61**: 349–59.
4. Miller DC, Myers BD. Pathophysiology and prevention of acute renal failure associated with thoracoabdominal or abdominal aortic surgery. *J Vasc Surg* 1987; **5**: 518–23.
5. Khaira HS, Maxwell SR, Thomason H, Thomason CHG, Shearman CP. Antioxidant depletion during aortic aneurysm repair. *Br J Surg* 1996; **83**: 401–3.
6. Nasim A, Thompson MM, Sayers RD, Smith G, Lunec J. Bell PRF. Endovascular aneurysm repair attenuates the ischaemic reperfusion injury of conventional aortic surgery. Ninth annual meeting of the European Society for Vascular Surgery, October 1995. Abstract 64.
7. Barry KG, Cohen A, Knochel JP *et al.* Mannitol infusion II: the prevention of acute functional renal failure during resection of an aneurysm of the abdominal aorta. *N Engl J Med* 1961; **264**: 967–71.
8. Thompson MM, Smith J, Nasim A *et al.* Microembolisation during endovascular aneurysm repair. Ninth International Congress on Endovascular Interventions, Arizona, 1996. Abstract V-2.
9. Birch PC, Whitbread T, Rogers S, Start R, Beard J, Gaines P. A comparative study on the effects of covering porcine renal artery origins with stents differing in size of strut and interstices. *Br J Surg* 1996 (in press).
10. Birch PC, Start RD, Whitbread T, Palmer I, Beard J, Gaines P. The effects of crossing porcine renal arteries with endovascular stents of differing strut/interstice size. Poster, Pathological Society Meeting, London, 1996.
11. Malina M, Lind M, Brunkwall J, Ivancev K, Lindbald B. Can aortic endovascular stents be placed over renal arteries? VIII Annual meeting of the European Society for Vascular Surgery, September 1994. Abstract 28.
12. Whitbread T, Birch P, Majeed A, Rochester J, Beard JD, Gaines P. A new model for abdominal aortic aneurysms: initial results using a multiple-wire stent. *Eur J Vasc Endovasc Surg* 1996; **11**: 90–7.
13. Nasim A, Thompson MM, Sayers RD, Bell PRF. Investigation of the relationship between aortic stent position and renal function. *Br J Surg* 1995; **82**: 561 (Abstract).
14. Gabriel R. Time to scrap creatinine clearance. *BMJ* 1986; **293**: 1119–20.
15. Mogensen CE. Microalbuminuria as a predictor of clinical diabetic nephropathy. *Kidney Int* 1987; **31**: 637–89.
16. Gawley WF, Corley TF, Johnson AH *et al.* Improved monitoring of renal impairment in obstructive jaundice. *Br J Surg* 1987; **74**: 541.
17. Lauwerys RR, Bernard A. Early detection of nephrotoxic effects of industrial chemicals: state of the art and future prospects. *Am J Ind Med* 1987; **11**: 275–85.
18. Jung K, Pergande M, Schimke E, Ratzmann KP, Illus A. Urinary enzymes and low-molecular-mass proteins as indicators of diabetic nephropathy. *Clin Chem* 1988; **34**: 544–7.

19. Nicholson ML, Baker DM, Hopkinson BR, Wenham PW. A randomized controlled trial of the effects of mannitol on renal reperfusion injury during aortic aneurysm surgery. *Br J Surg* 1996; **83**: 1230–3.
20. Baker DM, Baxendale B, Hind RE *et al.* Renal function during endovascular and open aortic aneurysm surgery. Annual meeting of the Association of Surgeons, London, 1995.

20

Ischaemia–reperfusion injury

Ahktar Nasim, Matthew M. Thompson, Robert D. Sayers and Peter R.F. Bell

Department of Surgery, Clinical Sciences Building, Leicester Royal Infirmary, Leicester LE2 7LX, UK

Introduction

Abdominal aortic aneurysm (AAA) repair is a good model of ischaemia–reperfusion injury.[1–3] During aortic clamping, the lower limbs and the gut may become ischaemic and initiate a series of chemical events that can lead to local and systemic organ damage.[4]

There is now increasing evidence to suggest that tissue injury occurs upon reperfusion. This was shown dramatically by Parks and Granger[5] in a feline model of intestinal ischaemia. They found that the histological changes of injury after 3 hours of ischaemia followed by 1 hour of reperfusion were far worse than those observed after 4 hours of ischaemia without reperfusion. During ischaemia, xanthine dehydrogenase is converted to xanthine oxidase with subsequent build-up of hypoxanthine in the tissues. On reperfusion, this enzyme catalyses the formation of xanthine from hypoxanthine, with the production of reactive oxygen free radicals (OFRs) in the process.[6] It has been postulated that OFRs may generate chemotactive activity leading to directed migration of activated neutrophils into the reperfused tissue.[7,8] Increased levels of cytokines interleukin (IL) 1β, IL-6 and tumour necrosis factor (TNF) α have also been observed following elective AAA repair.[3] These inflammatory mediators may initiate local and systemic organ damage, and account for the multiorgan failure seen in some patients following AAA repair.[9,10]

Endovascular AAA repair avoids intra-abdominal manipulation and aortic clamping. There may be a temporary occlusion of the aorta during deployment of some of the intraluminal prostheses,[11] but this is considerably less than the aortic occlusion during conventional open aneurysm surgery. Endovascular techniques, therefore, have the potential to diminish the severity of ischaemia–reperfusion injury. We have undertaken a study to assess the metabolic response to both conventional and endovascular AAA repair by quantifying oxygen free radical and cytokine production in a non-randomized cohort of patients.

Patients and methods

This study comprised a cohort of 12 patients undergoing AAA repair, six by conventional transperitoneal inlay replacement[12] and six by endovascular techniques. Patient details are recorded in Table 20.1. All operations were performed under general anaesthesia, without epidural opiates or local anaesthetic agents. Intravenous thiopentone was used for induction, and anaesthesia was maintained with a combination of nitrous oxide, oxygen, isoflurane and morphine. Sodium nitroprusside was used to control the cardiac afterload during the procedure. Substances with known antioxidative properties[13] were avoided during the perioperative period.

All patients underwent tube graft repair. Endovascular repair was undertaken with the Endovascular Grafting System (EndoVascular Technologies, Menlo Park, CA, USA).[14] Stent deployment was aided by balloon inflation for 1 min at two atmospheres intraluminal pressure. Two inflations were used both at the proximal and distal stent sites. Deployment of the device was undertaken via the common femoral artery in two cases and via a temporary iliac conduit in the remaining four cases.

Table 20.1 Demographic data of the study patients.

	Endovascular group (n = 6)	*Conventional group (n = 6)*
Median (range) age (years)	72.5 (64–76)	71 (64–85)
Sex ratio (M : F)	6 : 0	3 : 3
Hypertension	3	1
Ischaemic heart disease	4	0
Peripheral vascular disease	3	1
Current smokers	1	3
Median (range) AAA diameter (cm)	5.5 (5–6.2)	5.8 (4.4–7.6)
Median (range) aortic clamp time (min)	—	35 (20–60)

Blood samples were collected from the common femoral vein before aortic clamping or balloon occlusion, during completion of the proximal and distal anastomosis (sutured or stented), and at 5 and 30 min following reperfusion. The samples were centrifuged immediately at 3000 rpm for 5 min and the serum separated. The serum samples were snap-frozen and stored in liquid nitrogen until analysis. In the endovascular group, samples were obtained from the common femoral vein contralateral to the device insertion site.

Determination of oxygen free radical and cytokine production

Generation of OFRs was measured indirectly by determination of immunoglobulin (Ig) G oxidation in plasma using the method of Lunec *et al.*,[15] a method previously used to determine IgG oxidation in rheumatoid sera and synovial fluid. IL-1β, IL-6 and TNF-α were measured with commercially available radioimmunoassays (Amersham International, Amersham, UK).

Results

All metabolites, with the exception of IL-6, showed an increase during the ischaemic and reperfusion periods. The proportional change from baseline values for both cytokines and OFR activity is illustrated in Fig. 20.1. The changes in IL-1β, TNF-α and OFR activity were reduced by endovascular aneurysm repair when compared with conventional procedures. The peak change from baseline values for OFR activity, IL-1β and TNF-α is given in Table 20.2. The reduction in IL-1β and TNF-α was significant at the 95% confidence level using two-way

Table 20.2 Changes in OFR, IL-1β and TNF-α levels during conventional open and endovascular AAA repair.

	Peak level (change from baseline)		
	OFR	*IL-1β*	*TNF-α*
Conventional repair	1.93 (1.4–2.0)	1.42 (0.74–2.03)	1.23 (0.39–1.34)
Endovascular repair	1.55 (1.33–1.92)	1.02 (0.56–1.1)*	0.81 (0.66–0.96)*

*$P < 0.05$ (endovascular versus conventional repair, two-way analysis of variance). Values are medians with interquartile ranges.

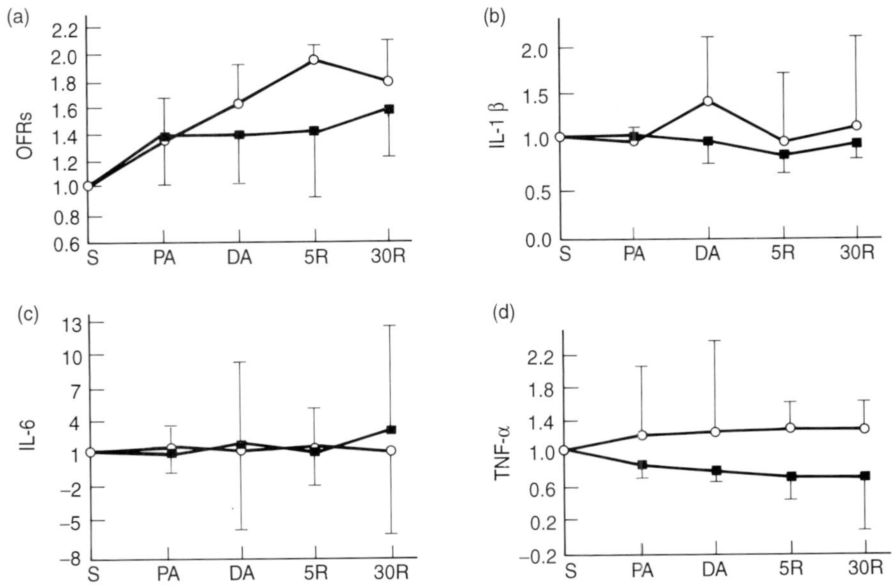

Fig. 20.1 Change from baseline value in (a) oxygen free radical (OFR) and cytokine (b) IL-1β, (c) IL-6, (d) TNF-α generation during endovascular (■) and conventional (○) AAA repair. Samples were collected at the start of the procedure (S), during proximal anastomosis (PA), during distal anastomosis (DA), 5 min (5R) and 30 min (30R) following reperfusion. After Thompson *et al.*[36]

analysis of variance. The fall in OFR activity was not statistically significant.

Discussion and conclusions

The cell damage following ischaemia is now recognized as a biphasic phenomenon, with injury being initiated during ischaemia and exacerbated during reperfusion. During ischaemia, the cell is deprived of the energy needed to maintain ionic gradients and homoeostasis, and failure of enzyme systems leads to cell death. Reperfusion injury is thought to be mediated by an interaction of free radicals, endothelial factors and neutrophils. The resulting injury is similar in most states of tissue hypoperfusion, including AAA surgery, limb ischaemia, organ transplantation, stroke and hypovolaemic shock.

The mechanisms underlying ischaemia–reperfusion injury have been reviewed extensively by several authors.[4,16] The enzyme xanthine oxidase is a major source of free radicals in post-ischaemic tissue.[6] During ischaemia, xanthine oxidase, produced by the conversion of xanthine dehydrogenase, accumulates in the tissues. As a consequence the tissue levels of hypoxanthine, a substrate for xanthine oxidase, increase. During reperfusion, xanthine oxidase uses molecular oxygen to convert hypoxanthine to xanthine, resulting in the production of highly reactive OFRs.[17] The most damaging effect of OFRs is lipid peroxidation, which results in structural and functional cell damage.[18] However, oxygen metabolites produced through plasmalemmal and intracellular sources in ischaemic tissues are unlikely to be responsible for the systemic organ damage, as they are very reactive and short lived.[19] It has been proposed that OFRs may react with endothelial cells to promote formation of inflammatory mediators such as platelet-activating factor (PAF)[20] and leukotriene B_4,[21] which may be responsible for neutrophil activation and adhesion observed in non-ischaemic areas of tissue following ischaemia–reperfusion.[22] Therefore, activated neutrophils are thought to play a pivotal role in cellular injury in organs and tissues that are some distance from the reperfused tissue through release of OFRs, proteolytic enzymes (collagenase, elastase, cathepsin G) and peroxidase.[4,23]

In our study, the largest rise in OFR activity was observed during the revascularization phase, which is in agreement with other human revascularization models.[1,24,25] During infrarenal aortic clamping all structures supplied by the inferior mesenteric, iliac and femoral arteries are predisposed to the ischaemia–reperfusion insult.[26] Murphy *et al.*[25] measured antioxidant compounds (α-tocopherol, ascorbic acid and protein thiols), oxidation products (α-tocopherol quinone) and lipid peroxidation products (lipid-derived malondialdehyde) in patients undergoing thoracoabdominal aneurysm repair. They found that, during ischaemia, the level of antioxidant compounds decreased, whereas that of α-tocopheryl quinone doubled. On reperfusion, the antioxidant activity remained low whilst the levels of lipid peroxidation products increased significantly. These findings suggest that oxidative stress occurs during aortic clamping, and also during the reperfusion phase. Our results showed a slight rise in OFR activity during aortic clamping, which was also observed by Ward *et al.*[1] This may be due to the collateral blood flow via lumbar arteries to the lower limbs whilst the aorta is clamped.[1]

Cytokines are polypeptides produced by cells of the immune system that act as mediators of both the immune response and the response of other tissues in the body to injury. TNF-α and IL-1β are considered to be primarily responsible for the non-hepatic manifestations of the acute-phase response such as fever, raised levels of prostaglandins, tachycardia and accelerated catabolism.[27] IL-6 is primarily responsible for the hepatic component of the acute-phase response, resulting in synthesis of acute-phase proteins.[28,29] There is some evidence to suggest that high levels of IL-1β, IL-6 and TNF-α are associated with increased incidence of adult respiratory distress syndrome and multiorgan failure, and a higher mortality rate in patients after major trauma and AAA surgery.[3,30,31] Previous studies have shown the colon to be a major source of IL-6 response in AAA surgery.[2] Baigrie *et al.*[2] undertook portal and systemic cytokine analysis and found IL-1 levels to be similar in the two compartments but the portal IL-6 levels greatly exceeded systemic levels. Our study has quantified cytokine production from the lower limbs, which may account for the lack of IL-6 response observed. Also the systemic IL-6 levels have been found to peak between 4 and 48 hours after abdominal incision,[31] which is considerably later than our sampling times. IL-6 levels in portal blood may reflect occult cellular injury in the colon, arising during surgery, and further studies including use of intraluminal tonometry to assess colonic ischaemia are required to determine whether exaggerated IL-6 responses are associated with subsequent development of major postoperative complications.[32]

IL-1β and TNF-α are produced primarily by blood monocytes and tissue macrophages, although other cells may produce them in smaller quantities under certain circumstances.[33] In our study, conventional AAA repair was associated with an increase in levels of IL-1β and TNF-α, which is consistent with findings of other investigators.[3] The levels of these cytokines have been found to peak within 1–4 hours of the abdominal incision, preceding the peak in IL-6 levels.[3,34] Their levels remained diminished in the endovascular group throughout the procedure. Norgren *et al.*[35] have also undertaken a similar study in a small series of patients and found TNF-α levels to be significantly higher in the endovascular group. They concluded that the catheter manoeuvres into the aneurysmal thrombotic content may cause extensive cellular activation in the endovascular group. However, further studies are required to evaluate whether there are any differences in patients undergoing tube or bifurcated graft endoluminal repair, as the latter involve greater guidewire and catheter manipulation.

In conclusion, our findings suggest that the ischaemia–reperfusion response associated with conventional aneurysm surgery may be largely negated by endovascular techniques. This may have the potential to decrease the remote organ failure following aneurysm repair, and this idea is worthy of further evaluation.

References

1. Ward A, McBurney A, Lunec J. Evidence for the involvement of oxygen-derived free radicals in ischaemia–reperfusion injury. *Free Rad Res* 1994; **20**: 21–8.
2. Baigrie RJ, Lamont PM, Whiting S, Morris PJ. Portal endotoxin and cytokine responses during abdominal aortic surgery. *Am J Surg* 1993; **166**: 248–51.
3. Roumen RMH, Hendriks T, van der Ven-Jongekrijg J *et al.* Cytokine patterns in patients after major vascular surgery, hemorrhagic shock, and severe blunt trauma. Relation with subsequent adult respiratory distress syndrome and multiple organ failure. *Ann Surg* 1993; **218**: 769–76.
4. Welbourn CRB, Goldman G, Paterson IS, Valeri CR, Shepro D, Hechtman HB. Pathophysiology of ischaemia–reperfusion injury: central role of the neutrophil. *Br J Surg* 1991; **78**: 651–5.
5. Parks DA, Granger DN. Contributions of ischaemia and reperfusion to mucosal lesion formation. *Am J Physiol* 1986; **250**: G749–53.
6. McCord JM. Oxygen-derived free radicals in post-ischaemic tissue injury. *N Engl J Med* 1985; **312**: 159–63.
7. McCord JM. Oxygen-derived radicals: a link between reperfusion injury and inflammation. *Fed Proc* 1987; **46**: 2402–6.
8. Repine JE, Cheronis JC, Rodell TC, Linas SL, Patt A. Pulmonary oxygen toxicity and ischaemia reperfusion injury. A mechanism in common involving xanthine oxidase and neutrophils. *Am Rev Respir Dis* 1987; **136**: 483–5.
9. Soreide O, Grimsgaard CHR, Myhre HO, Solheim K, Trippestad A. Time and cause of death for 301 patients operated on for abdominal aortic aneurysm. *Age Ageing* 1982; **11**: 256–60.
10. Gefke K, Schroeder TV, Thisted B *et al.* Abdominal aortic aneurysm surgery: survival and quality of life in patients requiring prolonged post-operative intensive therapy. *Ann Vasc Surg* 1994; **8**: 137–43.
11. Nasim A, Thompson MM, Sayers RD, Bell PRF. Endoluminal exclusion of abdominal aortic aneurysms. *Vasc Med Rev* 1995; **6**: 269–81.
12. Crawford ES, Crawford JL. *Diseases of the Aorta: Including an Atlas of Angiographic and Surgical Technique*. Baltimore, MD: Williams and Williams, 1985.
13. Crozier TA, Muller JE, Quittkat D, Sydow M, Wuttke W, Ketter D. Effect of anaesthesia on the cytokine responses to abdominal surgery. *Br J Anaesth* 1994; **72**: 280–5.
14. Nasim A, Thompson MM, Sayers RD, Bolia A, Bell PRF. Endovascular repair of abdominal aortic aneurysm: an initial experience. *Br J Surg* 1996; **83**: 516–19.
15. Lunec J, Blake DR, McCleary SJ, Bacon PA. Self-perpetuating mechanisms of immunoglobulin G aggregation in rheumatoid inflammation. *J Clin Invest* 1985; **76**: 2084–90.

16. Grace PA. Ischaemia–reperfusion injury. *Br J Surg* 1994; **81**: 637–47.
17. Sinclair AJ, Barnett AH, Lunec J. Free radicals and antioxidant systems in health and disease. *Br J Hosp Med* 1990; **43**: 334–44.
18. Kellog EW. Superoxide, hydrogen peroxide and singlet oxygen in lipid peroxidation by a xanthine oxidase system. *J Biol Chem* 1975; **250**: 8812–17.
19. Pryor WA. Oxy-radicals and related species: their formation, lifetimes and reactions. *Annu Rev Physiol* 1986; **48**: 657–67.
20. Lewis MS, Whatley RE, Cain P, McIntyre TM, Prescott SM, Zimmerman GA. Hydrogen peroxide stimulates the synthesis of platelet activating factor by endothelium and induces endothelial cell dependent neutrophil adhesion. *J Clin Invest* 1988; **82**: 2045–55.
21. Plamblad J, Malmstein CL, Uden AM, Radmark O, Engstedt L, Samuelsson B. Leukotriene B_4 is a potent and stereospecific stimulator of neutrophil chemotaxis and adherence. *Blood* 1981; **58**: 658–61.
22. Ferrante RJ, Silva MB, Resnikoff M *et al.* Inhibition of leucocyte adhesion at reperfusion decreases tissue damage in post-ischaemic skeletal muscle. *Surg Forum* 1993; **44**: 367 (Abstract).
23. Windsor ACJ, Mullen PG, Fowler AA, Sugerman HJ. Role of the neutrophil in adult respiratory distress syndrome. *Br J Surg* 1993; **80**: 10–17.
24. Rabl H, Khoschsorur G, Colombo T, Tatzber F, Esterbauer H. Human plasma lipid peroxide levels show a strong transient increase after successful revascularization operations. *Free Radic Biol and Med* 1992; **13**: 281–8.
25. Murphy ME, Kolvenbach R, Aleksis M, Hansen R, Sies H. Antioxidant depletion in aortic cross clamping ischaemia: increase of the plasma alpha-tocopheryl quinone/alphatocopherol ratio. *Free Radic Biol Med* 1992; **13**: 95–100.
26. Smeets HJ, Camps J, van Milligen de Witt AWM *et al.* Influence of low dose allopurinol on ischaemia–reperfusion injury during abdominal aortic surgery. *Eur J Vasc Endovasc Surg* 1995; **9**: 162–9.
27. Dinarello CA. Interleukin-1. *Rev Infect Dis* 1984; **6**: 51–95.
28. Castell JV, Andus T, Kunz D, Heinrich PC. Interleukin-6. The major regulator of acute-phase protein synthesis in man and rat. *Ann NY Acad Sci* 1989; **557**: 87–99.
29. Gauldie J, Richards C, Harnish D, Lansdorp P, Baumann H. Interferon B2/B cell stimulatory factor 2 shares identity with monocyte-derived hepatocyte-stimulating factor and regulates the major acute phase protein response in liver cells. *Proc Natl Acad Sci USA* 1987; **84**: 7251–5.
30. Cruickshank AM, Fraser WD, Burns HJG, van Damme J, Shenkin A. Response of serum interleukin-6 in patients undergoing elective surgery of varying severity. *Clin Sci* 1990; **79**: 161–5.
31. Baigrie RJ, Lamont PM, Kwiatkowski D, Dallman MJ, Morris PM. The cytokine response to major surgery. *Br J Surg* 1992; **79**: 757–60.
32. Soong CV, Blair PHB, Halliday MI *et al.* Endotoxaemia, the generation of the cytokines and their relationship to intramucosal acidosis of the sigmoid colon in elective abdominal aortic aneurysm repair. *Eur J Vasc Surg* 1993; **7**: 534–9.
33. Dinarello CA. Interleukin-1 and its biologically related cytokines. *Adv Immunol* 1989; **44**: 153–205.
34. Parry-Billings M, Baigrie RJ, Lamont PM, Morris PJ, Newsholme EA. Effects of major and minor surgery on plasma glutamine and cytokine levels. *Arch Surg* 1992; **127**: 1237–40.

35. Norgren L, Swartbol P, Albrechtsson L. Clinical findings and cellular responses during endoluminal treatment of abdominal aortic aneurysms. *J Endovasc Surg* 1995; **2**: 398–9 (Abstract).
36. Thompson MM, Nasim A, Sayers RD, Thompson J, Smith G, Lunec J, Bell PRF. Oxygen free radical and cytokine generation during endovascular and conventional aneurysm repair. *Eur J Vasc Endovasc Surg* 1996; **12**: 70–5.

21

Quality of life

Daryll M. Baker

Department of Vascular Surgery, Royal Free Hospital, London, UK

Introduction

Elective aortic aneurysm surgery is undertaken as a prophylaxis against rupture and possible death in patients who are usually asymptomatic. After successful surgery, the aim is to return patients to their preoperative quality of life as quickly as possible. Open aneurysm repair subjects the patient to a large abdominal incision, major haemodynamic changes that are likely to increase cardiac complications, as well as a period of pelvic and lower limb ischaemia with resultant reperfusion injury. All these factors are likely to reduce the speed with which patients return to their preoperative quality of life. Other chapters in this book have demonstrated that endovascular aneurysm repair appears to reduce the physical stress the patient is subjected to by reducing haemodynamic changes (Chapter 23), the degree of metabolic trauma (Chapter 20), and renal (Chapter 19) and colonic (Chapter 22) damage. Following endovascular aneurysm repair most investigators report quick recovery times, sometimes with patients up and about and eating within 12 hours, and with a markedly reduced analgesia requirement after operation. Few studies, however, have considered objectively how quickly patients return to their preoperative quality of life following any form of aneurysm surgery,[1–5] let alone after endovascular aneurysm repair. This chapter considers which health-related quality-of-life measure is most appropriate to use in studying vascular procedures and then assesses how the quality of life of patients with asymptomatic aortic aneurysms before surgery changes following elective endovascular as opposed to open abdominal aortic aneurysm repair.

Selecting a health-related quality-of-life measure

To allow comparison with others, it is preferable to use one of the available generic health-related quality-of-life (HRQL) measures, examples of which include the Nottingham Health Profile, the Sickness Impact Profile, the Medical Outcomes Short-Form 36 (SF-36), the EuroQol, the Dartmouth COOP Charts and the World Health Organization Quality of Life measure. Appropriate selection of an HRQL measure is important. It needs to take into account the dimensions of emotional, physical, social functioning and global perception of health and well-being. The HRQL measure has to have proven validity (i.e. to measure what it purports to measure), reliability (i.e. reproducibility) and responsiveness (i.e. sensitivity to change). Measures need to have been adapted successfully to the country of use and, if possible, standard age- and sex-related controls for the given population should have been determined. In practical terms the questionnaire needs to be quick and easy to use by both the patient and the researcher. Preferably it should be suitable to both direct interview and postal follow-up, as well as being inexpensive to implement. For some HRQL measures, use requires written permission and a copyright fee, but this is not universal.

The 36-item Short-Form Health Survey measure (SF-36) fulfils most of these criteria.[6] It consists of 36 questions divided into eight health domains: physical function (ten items); role limitations due to physical (four items) and emotional (three items) problems; pain (two items); general health perceptions (five items); vitality (four items); social functioning (two items); emotional well-being (five items); and a single item on change in health. Each domain is presented as a percentage, with 100% being most healthy and 0% being the worst quality of life. The validity of the SF-36 has been established against clinically defined criterion, performing favourably in discriminating between symptomatic and asymptomatic patient groups, stages and severity of disease, and treatment effects of moderate size.[6] The SF-36 has been adapted successfully from the original American version to a UK form.[7,8] Standard population controls have been published for different British age and sex groups.[7,9,10] It is easy to use, taking the patient less than 10 min to fill in, and the researcher less than 5 min to analyse. The SF-36 is appropriate for administration by self, telephone and face-to-face modes.

Quality of life of patients with asymptomatic aortic aneurysms

Knowledge of the quality of life of patients with asymptomatic aortic aneurysms is important in determining the risk–benefit of surgery. It has previously been determined when comparing an operative with a 'watchful waiting' management plan for small abdominal aneurysms.[11] Using the SF-36 HRQL questionnaire, we have assessed the quality of life of 47 patients who were reported to be well and had asymptomatic aortic aneurysms. The results (Fig. 21.1) have been compared with those of an age-matched healthy population.

'Healthy' was used to describe a person who had no long-standing disability, who had not seen their general practitioner in the last 2 weeks and who had not attended hospital (either as an inpatient or an outpatient) in the last year. The healthiest control group was selected as a 'gold standard' quality of health with which to compare patients with presumed asymptomatic aneurysm. The study group with aortic aneurysms had the usual atherosclerosis-associated risk factors (20% had ischaemic heart disease, 29% hypertension and 2% diabetes) and general age-related health problems (5% had chronic lung disease, 25% arthritis, 13% poor sight and 22% poor hearing).

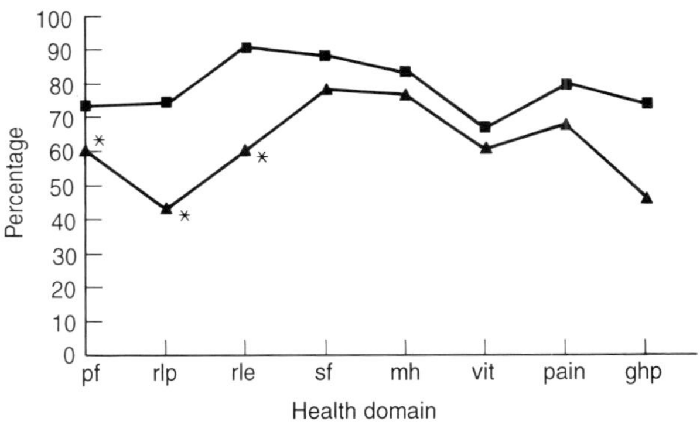

Fig. 21.1 Quality of life of people with asymptomatic aortic aneurysms (▲) compared with age-matched healthy controls (■), determined by means of the SF-36 health-related questionnaire. The eight health domains are: pf, physical function; rlp, role limited physically; rle, role limited emotionally; sf, social functioning; mh, mental health; vit, vitality or energy; pain; ghp, general health perception. The *y*-axis shows the percentage of each domain is significantly different.

Their quality of life was similar to that of a general healthy age-matched population for several SF-36 domains, including social functioning, emotional well-being, energy and vitality, pain and general health perception. The quality of life, however, was significantly reduced in people with aneurysm in the three SF-36 domains of physical function, and role limitation as a result of physical and emotional problems. It was therefore concluded that the person with an asymptomatic aneurysm has a reduced quality of life when compared with an age-matched healthy UK population.

Quality of life after endovascular and open aortic aneurysm repair

The quality of life of 20 patients undergoing successful open operation and of 20 having successful endovascular aneurysm repair was assessed before operation and at 1 and 3 months after surgery using the SF-36 HRQL assessment form. Assessment was made after 1 month, as any immediate postoperative complication (30-day morbidity) would have presented, and such patients were excluded from analysis in this study.

There was no difference in preoperative quality of life in the two treatment groups. When compared with preoperative values, at 1 month there was a marked decline in several quality-of-life dimensions for both treatment groups (Fig. 21.2), in particular physical

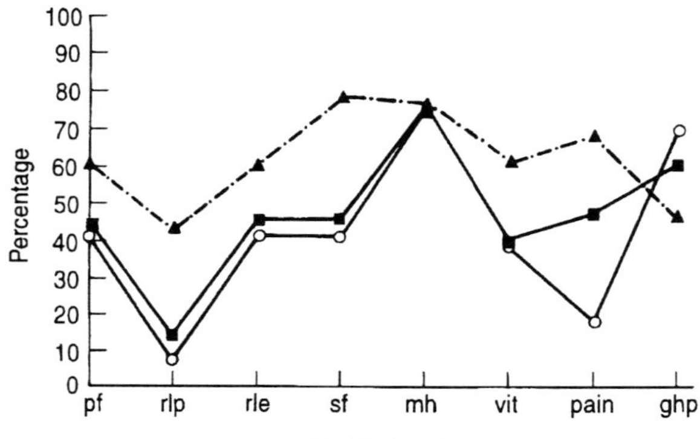

Fig. 21.2 Quality of life 1 month after endovascular (■) and open (○) aortic aneurysm repair compared with preoperative values (▲). The eight health domains are: pf, physical function; rlp, role limited physically; rle, role limited emotionally; sf, social functioning; mh, mental health; vit, vitality or energy; pain; ghp, general health perception. The *y*-axis shows the percentage of each domain.

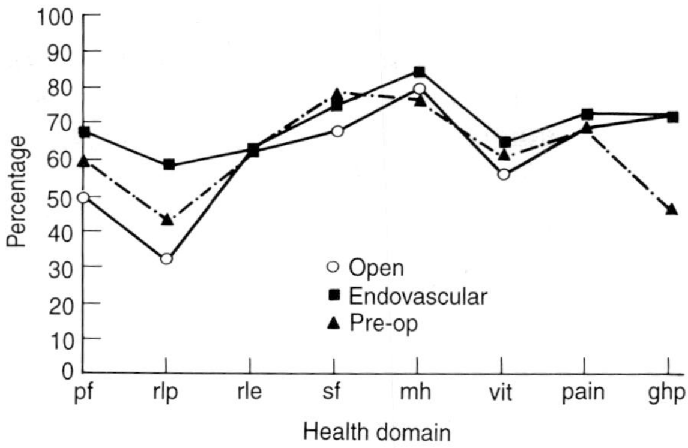

Fig. 21.3 Quality of life 3 months after endovascular (■) and open (○) aortic aneurysm repair compared with preoperative values (▲). The eight health domains are: pf, physical function; rlp, role limited physically; rle, role limited emotionally; sf, social functioning; mh, mental health; vit, vitality or energy; pain; ghp, general health perception. The *y*-axis shows the percentage of each domain.

function, role limited physically, social function, vitality and pain. The two treatment groups showed a similar decline in their quality of life, with the exception being perceived pain, which was greater for open aneurysm repair at 1 month than for endovascular repair.

By 3 months (Fig. 21.3) the quality of life of patients in both groups had returned towards preoperative values, with no significant difference existing for any health dimension except for general health perception, which was greater in both groups after than before operation. As a general trend, the quality of life of patients who have had endovascular repair is better for most domains than it was before operation; for those who had an open repair it remains slightly worse.

Conclusions

The quality of life of people with asymptomatic aortic aneurysm is not as good as that of the healthiest age-matched general population (Fig. 21.1). Despite the fact that an endovascular approach reduces the physical stress during aneurysm repair, the quality of life at 1 month after operation is reduced as much as that suffered by patients undergoing open repair (Fig. 21.2). By 3 months (Fig. 21.3), patients who have undergone either type of repair have regained their preoperative quality of life.

The advantages of endovascular surgery may be associated with offering the procedure to patients whose medical condition would otherwise have prevented an open repair but, when considering patients who are healthy enough to undergo open repair and who suffer no major postoperative morbidity, there is no improvement in the rate of return to preoperative quality of life when compared with open procedures.

References

1. Baker DM, Smith C, Yoeman P, Wenham PW, Hopkinson BR. Aortic aneurysm surgery success: an outcome study using SF36 questionnaire to compare ruptured with asymptomatic cases. *Int Angiol* 1995; **14**(Suppl 1): 158.
2. Magee TR, Scott DJ, Dunkley A *et al.* Quality of life following surgery for abdominal aortic aneurysm. *Br J Surg* 1992; **79:** 1014–16.
3. van Ramshorst B, van der Griend R, Eikelboom BC. Survival and quality of life after surgery for ruptured abdominal aortic aneurysm. In: Greenhalgh RM, Mannick JA, Powel JT, eds. *The Cause and Management of Aneurysms.* London: WB Saunders, 1990: 433–40.
4. Rohrer MJ, Cutler BS, Wheeler HB. Long-term survival and quality of life following ruptured abdominal aortic aneurysm. *Arch Surg* 1988; **123:** 1213–17.
5. Currie IA, Robson AK, Scott DJA, Horrocks M. Quality of life of octogenarians after aneurysm surgery. *Ann R Coll Surg Engl* 1992; **74:** 269–73.
6. Anderson RT, Aaronson NK, Wilkin D. Critical review of the international assessment of health related quality of life. *Qual Life Res* 1993; **2:** 369–95.
7. Jenkinson C, Coulter A, Wright L. Short form 36 (SF36) health survey questionnaire: normative data for adults of working age. *BMJ* 1993; **306:** 1437–40.
8. Garratt AM, Ruta DA, Abdalla MI, Buckingham JK, Russell IT. The SF36 health survey questionnaire: an outcome measure suitable for routine use within the NHS. *BMJ* 1993; **306:** 1440–4.
9. Lyons RA, Perry HM, Littlepage BNC. Evidence for the validity of the Short-form 36 questionnaire (SF-36) in an elderly population. *Age Ageing* 1994; **23:** 182–4.
10. Brazier JE, Harper R, Jones NMB *et al.* Validating the SF-36 health survey questionnaire: new outcome measure for primary care. *BMJ* 1992; **305:** 160–4.
11. Katz DA, Littenberg B, Cronenwett JL. Management of small abdominal aortic aneurysms. Early surgery vs watchful waiting. *JAMA* 1992; **268:** 2678–86.

22

Colonic perfusion

Nabil M. Elmarasy and Waquar Yusuf

Department of Vascular Surgery, University Hospital, Queen's Medical Centre, Nottingham, NG7 2UH, UK

Introduction

Colonic ischaemia is a well-recognized complication of conventional abdominal aortic aneurysm (AAA) repair and contributes significantly to postoperative morbidity and mortality.[1–3] The aetiology of colonic ischaemia is multifactorial (Fig. 22.1), but changes associated with aortic clamping play an important role. In contrast, endovascular repair avoids laparotomy, retroperitoneal dissection and aortoiliac clamping, thereby causing minimal haemodynamic derangement,[4] and has the potential for reducing this complication. The effects of endovascular and conventional AAA surgery on colonic perfusion are presented in this chapter.

Patients and methods

A total of 27 patients undergoing elective infrarenal aortic aneurysm repair were studied; 16 undergoing endovascular repair and 11 having open repair. The patients were divided into two groups depending mainly on the anatomical suitability of the aortic aneurysms for endovascular repair, determined by preoperative spiral computed tomography and/or calibrated angiography in all patients. The two groups were well matched for age, sex, smoking and diabetes. There was a slightly higher incidence of cardiopulmonary problems in the endovascular group but the two groups were well matched for aneurysm diameter and patency of coeliac axis, superior mesenteric, iliacs and hypogastric arteries (Table 22.1). The main differences between the two groups during the operation were the aortic occlusion time and blood loss (Table 22.2). The inferior mesenteric artery (IMA) was not

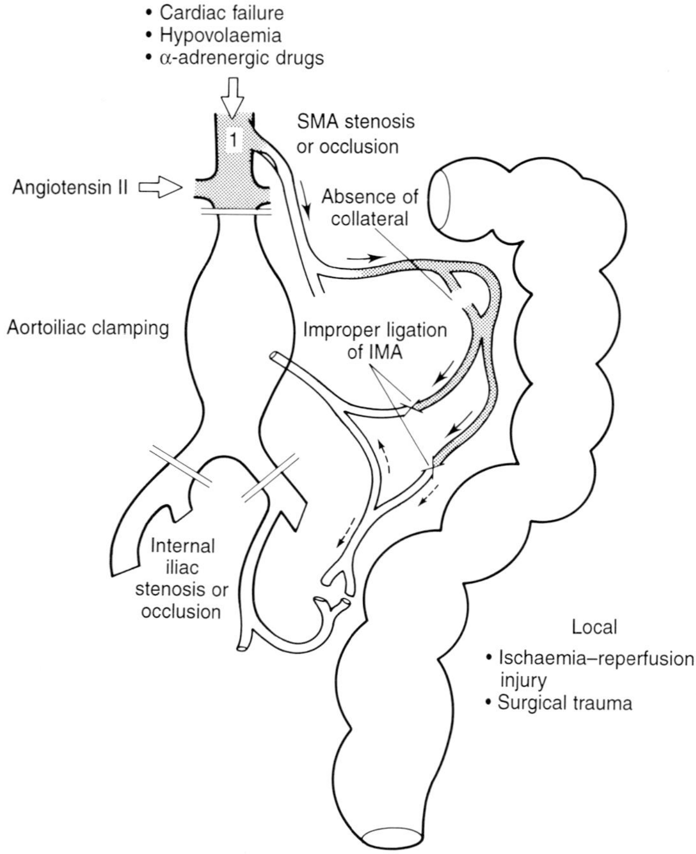

Fig. 22.1 Factors contributing to colonic ischaemia during aortic surgery.

reimplanted in any patient in the open group and was excluded in all cases in the endovascular group. Preoperative and postoperative stool analysis for faecal occult blood was performed and a stool chart was maintained for 5 days. All procedures were performed under general anaesthesia. Standard aortic aneurysm repair with an inlay technique was used for open repair. Endovascular repair was carried out with a bifurcated graft in three patients, aortoaortic in two patients and aortouni-iliac grafting in 11.

Sigmoid intramucosal pH (pH_{im}) was measured using a sigmoid silicone balloon tonometer (Actamed, UK). This was introduced after double phosphate enema immediately after the induction of general

Table 22.1 Patient demographic data, co-morbid conditions and morphology of gastrointestinal aortic branches

	Open surgery ($n = 11$)	*Endovascular surgery* ($n = 16$)
Sex ratio (M : F)	10 : 1	15 : 1
Mean (range) age (years)	69.9 (55–81)	69.6 (54–80)
Smoking		
Current	3	3
Ex-smoker	4	6
Non-smoker	4	7
Diabetes	1	1
Hypertension	7	10
Cardiac disease		
Myocardial infarction	1	3
Angina	1	3
Pulmonary disease	1	2
Renal disease	0	1
Liver disease	0	0
Gastrointestinal disease	1 (partial gastrectomy)	1 (jejunal resection)
Aneurysm diameter (cm)	6.3 (4.5–8.5)	6.2 (4.6–8.5)
Coeliac axis		
Patent	11	16
Stenosed	0	0
Superior mesenteric artery		
Patent	11	15
Stenosed	0	1 (>70% stenosis)
Inferior mesenteric artery	9 (patent ligated) 2 (occluded)	16 (excluded by stent)
Common iliac artery		
Patent	11	16
Internal iliac artery		
Left		
Patent	9	16
Occluded	2	0
Right		
Patent	11	16

anaesthesia using a flexible sigmoidoscope (Fujinon Pyser-SGI Edenbridge, UK).

The tonometer balloon was positioned between 40 and 50 cm from the anal verge, and an assessment of the colonic mucosa was carried out for any pre-existing abnormality. The position of the balloon was

Table 22.2 Operative details

	Open surgery ($n = 11$)	*Endovascular surgery* ($n = 16$)
Type of repair	8 Straight graft 2 Aortobi-iliac 1 Aortobifemoral	11 Aortouni-iliac 3 Aortobi-iliac 2 Aortoaortic
Mean (range) clamping time (min)	61.7 (33–95)	Not applicable
Mean (range) deployment time (min)	Not applicable	2.6 (1–5)
Mean (range) blood loss (ml)	2043 (500–4270)	667 (500–1500)
Faecal occult blood		
Preoperative	11 −ve	16 −ve
Postoperative	2 +ve	16 −ve
First postoperative bowel movement	Watery motion × 1 (5 patients)	Watery motion × 1 (1 patient)

checked by manual examination of the sigmoid colon in the open group after initial laparotomy and by radiological imaging in endovascular group. The position of the balloon was checked again on the first postoperative day with plain abdominal radiography.

The principle of tonometry is based on the free permeability of a silicone balloon to carbon dioxide (Fig. 22.2). Measurement of sigmoid pH_{im} in the most superficial layer of the mucosa is obtained by measuring arterial partial pressure of carbon dioxide (P_{aCO_2}) in the lumen of the gut with a silicone balloon tonometer and the bicarbonate concentration in arterial blood at the same time, and substituting these two values in the Henderson–Hasselbalch equation.[5]

This indirect measurement is based on the assumption that P_{aCO_2} in the most superficial layers of the mucosa is in equilibrium with that in the luminal contents, with which it is in contact. It is further based on the assumption that the bicarbonate concentration in the tissue is the same as that being delivered to it in the arterial blood.[6] It is well known that acid–base balance is intimately related to the adequacy of tissue oxygenation in so far as it relates to the balance between the protons released by adenosine triphosphate (ATP) hydrolysis and consumed by ATP synthesis from oxidative phosphorylation. Tissue pH appears to be determined largely by the P_{aCO_2} attained following buffering of the volatile and fixed acid loads entering the intramucosal extracellular fluid (ECF) and the bicarbonate concentration in the ECF at the time ('buffer hypothesis'). pH_{im} appears to be related to blood flow only in

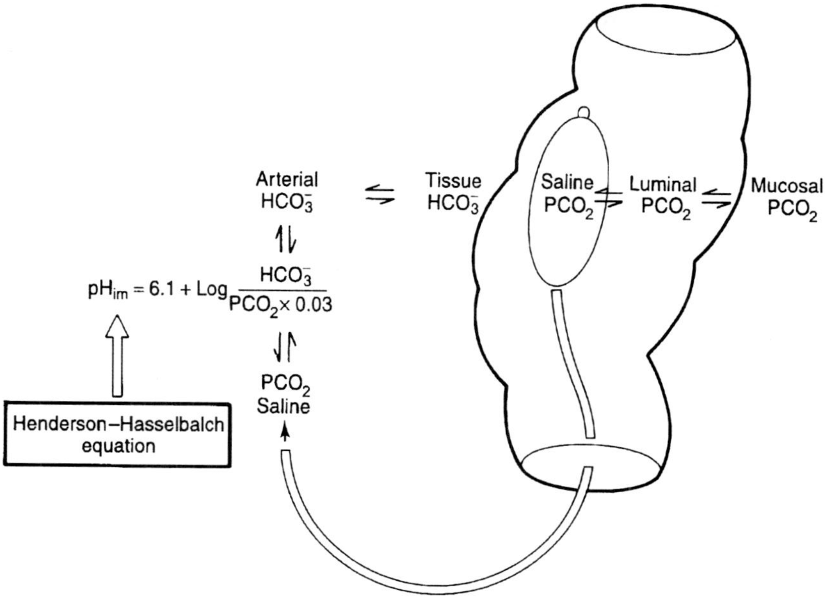

Fig. 22.2 Principle of sigmoid pH_{im} measurement with a silicone balloon tonometer.

so far as it relates to the adequacy of tissue oxygenation. The assumption that colonic intramucosal bicarbonate levels are the same as arterial bicarbonate levels is valid in normal, low, and no-flow states[7]. The indirect measurement of actual colonic pH_{im} is the sum of the effect of two determinants of intramucosal acidosis, including systemic acid–base balance and the degree of unreversed ATP hydrolysis present.[7]

Technique

Once the balloon tonometer had been satisfactorily placed, 2.5 ml normal saline was introduced into the tonometer balloon and left for equilibration of luminal P_{aCO_2} over 30 min. This saline was then withdrawn and analysed for P_{aCO_2} using a blood gas analyser (CIBA CORNING 278). At the same time an arterial blood sample was obtained for analysis of bicarbonate (HCO_3^-) concentration. With these values, the sigmoid pH_{im} was calculated with the help of a slide calculator (Tonometrics, Hopkinton, MA, USA), that allows estimation of the steady-state saline P_{aCO_2}, which is the corrected concentration for the equilibration period.

Sampling time

The baseline sigmoid pH_{im} was measured immediately after induction of general anaesthesia and the second reading was taken 30 min after either clamping of the aorta in the open group or deployment of the stent in the endovascular group. The third reading was taken 30 min after reperfusion in both groups, and subsequent readings were taken at 2-hourly intervals for 8 hours and at 4-hourly intervals for a further 16 hours.

The mean sigmoid pH_{im} in the open and endovascular groups at individual sampling times were compared with the unpaired t test.

Results

The results are shown in Fig. 22.3, in which sigmoid pH_{im} is plotted against time. The line at the pH of 6.86 represents the level below which patients have been found to develop colonic ischaemia in previous studies.[8,9] In our study the lowest mean sigmoid pH remained above this level in both groups, and no patient showed any clinical evidence of colonic ischaemia. However, in the open group, the mean sigmoid pH_{im} fell progressively to a minimum of 7.01 6 hours after reperfusion

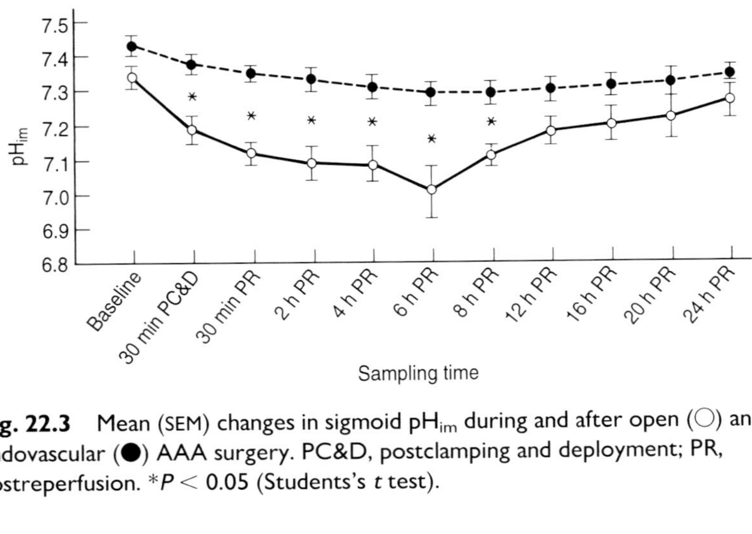

Fig. 22.3 Mean (SEM) changes in sigmoid pH_{im} during and after open (○) and endovascular (●) AAA surgery. PC&D, postclamping and deployment; PR, postreperfusion. $^{*}P < 0.05$ (Students's t test).

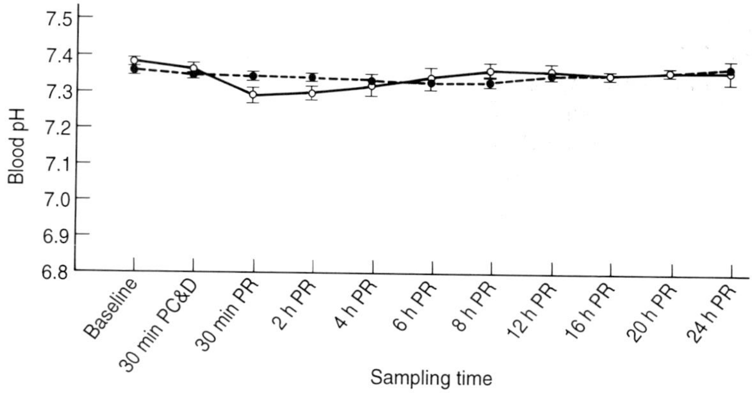

Fig. 22.4 Mean (SEM) changes in blood pH during and after open (○) and endovascular (●) AAA surgery. PC&D, postclamping; PR, postreperfusion.

before gradually returning towards normal after 24 hours. In the endovascular group, a similar but smaller fall was obtained. The difference between the groups from 30-min postclamping and deployment to 8 hours postreperfusion were statistically significant.

In both groups the blood pH was similar and remained within normal limits (Fig. 22.4).

Discussion

Colonic ischaemia is considered to be one of the major complications after AAA reconstructive surgery. The incidence of colonic ischaemia following conventional elective AAA repair has been reported as 1–2% in most retrospective studies, based on clinical criteria.[2,10–12] However, in prospective studies based on preoperative and postoperative colonoscopic examination, the incidence has been reported as 7.4%,[13,14] and as 18–24% when colonic mucosal acidosis measured by sigmoid silicone balloon tonometer was used as an indicator of colonic ischaemia.[8,15] So far, no report has been published on the incidence of colonic ischaemia with endovascular repair. When colonic ischaemia is apparent, the mortality rate is between 40 and 70%.[2,8] The aetiology of colonic ischaemia is multifactorial[2,3,9–12] and for it to occur, a variety of physiological, anatomical and pharmacological factors conspire (Fig. 22.1). From the surgical point of view, the avoidable causes of colonic ischaemia are ligation of the IMA, cross-clamping of the aorta and direct trauma to the colon and/or its collateral blood supply during retroperitoneal dissection. Endovascular technique does not allow reimplantation of the IMA, but the results of IMA reimplantation following open aortic aneurysm repair have been at best equivocal[13,16–19]. However, aortic cross-clamping and retroperitoneal dissection can be avoided by endovascular repair. The results of our study show that ligation of patent IMA in the open group or exclusion of IMA in the endovascular group, either alone or in combination with the internal iliac artery, provided the superior mesenteric artery was patent, did not affect the level of sigmoid pH_{im}, nor did it cause the development of clinically apparent colonic ischaemia. As far as the open group is concerned, a similar observation has been reported by Klok *et al.*[20]

The diagnosis of colonic ischaemia by clinical criteria is inaccurate and liable to delay diagnosis, which makes surgical intervention relatively unsuccessful. However, repeated colonoscopy is unacceptable to patients, and other methods such as direct measurement of colonic perfusion are unsuitable for routine clinical use.[21] The diagnosis of colonic ischaemia can now be made within minutes of its occurrence, before irreversible changes have taken place by indirect measurement of the acidosis that develops in the superficial mucosal layer of the wall of the colon due to a fall in oxygen delivery below tissue requirements.[7] This method appears to be a sensitive indicator of tissue oxygenation, because it mirrors tissue oxygen consumption.[22] Sigmoid tonometry is not only a simple and safe method for detecting colonic ischaemia, but is also very sensitive and specific. The predictive value of this method has been well assessed and validated in previous animal[6] and human studies, with a sensitivity of 100% and specificity of 87–92%.[9,19] It has been shown that a relationship exists between the level and duration of intermucosal acidosis on the day of surgery and the development of colonic ischaemia and death after elective AAA surgery.[8] It is therefore possible that morbidity and mortality following aortic surgery might be reduced if sigmoid ischaemia could be prevented from occurring on the day of surgery or limited to a shorter duration.

Studies in our unit have shown that, in contrast to open repair, patients undergoing endovascular repair remain haemodynamically stable (Chapter 23); this may be due partly to the difference in blood loss and/or to the effect of cross-clamping. Other investigators have also found that the ischaemia–reperfusion response associated with conventional aneurysm surgery may be largely negated by endovascular techniques (Chapter 20). Similarly, the endovascular technique appears to reduce the degree of renal injury during aneurysm surgery (see Chapter 19). These studies suggest that avoidance of aortic clamping during endovascular repair prevents these physiological derangements. The present study shows that colonic ischaemia that occurs during open procedures is related to the effects of aortic clamping and declamping, and provides additional support to the hypothesis that endovascular aortic aneurysm may confer some protection against these changes.

It can therefore be concluded that the degree of colonic ischaemia, as judged by sigmoid pH_{im} measurement, is significantly less during and after endovascular repair than with open surgery. However, results in more patients are required to show whether this observation is supported by a lower incidence of colonic ischaemia and multiple organ failure in those undergoing endovascular repair compared with open surgery.

References

1. Crowson M, Fielding JWL, Black J *et al.* Acute gastrointestinal complications of infrarenal aortic aneurysm repair. *Br J Surg* 1984; **71:** 825–8.
2. Johnson WC, Nabseth DC. Visceral infarction following aortic surgery. *Ann Surg* 1974; **180:** 312–18.
3. Smith RF, Szilagyi DE. Ischaemia of the colon as a complication in the surgery of the abdominal aorta. *Arch Surg* 1960; **80:** 806–21.
4. Yusuf SW, Hopkinson BR. Endovascular repair of aortic aneurysm. *Br J Surg* 1995; **82:** 289–91.
5. Fiddian-Green RG. Assessment of the adequacy of mucosal oxygenation in patients with intraluminally located silicone tonometers. In: Manabe H, Zweifach BW, Messener K, eds. *Microcirculation in Circulatory Disorders.* Tokyo: Springer, 1988: 481–7.
6. Antonsson JB, Boyle CC, Kruithoff KL *et al.* Validation of tonometric measurement of gut intramucosal pH during endotoxaemia and mesenteric occlusion in pigs. *Am J Physiol* 1990; **259:** 519–32.
7. Fiddian-Green RG. Gastric intramucosal pH, tissue oxygenation and acid–base balance. *Br J Anaesth* 1995; **74:** 591–606.
8. Fiddian-Green RG, Amelin P, Herrman JB *et al.* Prediction of the development of sigmoid ischaemia on the day of operation from indirect measurement of intramucosal pH in the colon. *Arch Surg* 1986; **85:** 654–60.
9. Schiedler MG, Cutler BS, Fiddian-Green RG. Sigmoid intramucosal pH for prediction of ischaemic colitis during aortic surgery. A comparison with risk factors and inferior mesenteric artery stump pressure. *Arch Surg* 1987; **122:** 881–6.

10. Ottinger LW, Darling RC, Nathan MJ *et al.* Left colon ischaemia complicating aorto-iliac reconstruction. *Arch Surg* 1972; **105:** 841–6.
11. Ochsner JL, Cooley DA, DeBakey ME. Associated intra-abdominal lesions encountered during resection of aortic aneurysms. *Dis Colon Rectum* 1960; **3:** 485–91.
12. Young JR, Humphries AW, de Wolfe VG *et al.* Complications of abdominal aortic surgery. II. Intestinal ischaemia. *Arch Surg* 1963; **86:** 51–9.
13. Ernst CB, Hagihara PF, Daugherty ME *et al.* Ischaemic colitis incidence following abdominal aortic reconstruction: a prospective study. *Surgery* 1976; **80:** 417–21.
14. Hagihara PF, Ernst CB, Griffen WO. Incidence of ischaemic colitis following abdominal aortic reconstruction. *Surg Gynecol Obstet* 1979; **149:** 571–3.
15. Fiddian-Green RG, Gantz NM. Transient episodes of sigmoid ischaemia and their relation to infection from intestinal organisms after abdominal aortic operation. *Crit Care Med* 1987; **15:** 835–9.
16. Zelenock GB, Strodel WE, Knol JA *et al.* A prospective study of clinically and endoscopically documented colonic ischaemia in 100 patients undergoing aortic reconstructive surgery with aggressive colonic and direct pelvic revascularization, compared with historic controls. *Surgery* 1989; **106**(4): 771–80.
17. Brewster DC, Franklin DP, Cambria RP *et al.* Intestinal ischaemia complicating abdominal aortic surgery. *Surgery* 1991; **109:** 447–54.
18. Bast TJ, van der Biezen JJ, Scherpenisse J *et al.* Ischaemic disease of the colon and rectum after surgery for abdominal aortic aneurysm. A prospective study of the incidence and risk factors. *Eur J Vasc Surg* 1990; **4:** 253–7.
19. Bjorck M, Hedberg B. Early detection of major complications after abdominal aortic surgery: predictive value of sigmoid colon and gastric intramucosal pH monitoring. *Br J Surg* 1994; **81:** 25–30.
20. Klok T, Moll FL, Leusink JA *et al.* The relationship between sigmoidal intramucosal pH and intestinal arterial occlusion during aortic reconstructive surgery. *Eur J Vasc Endovasc Surg* 1996; **11:** 304–7.
21. Crissinger KD, Granger DN. Techniques for measuring blood flow in the splanchnic circulation. In: Marston A, Bulkley GB, Fiddian-Green RG, Haglund U, eds. *Splanchnic Ischaemia and Multiple Organ Failure.* London: Edward Arnold, CV Mosby, 1989: 41–7.
22. Grum CM, Fiddian-Green RG, Pittenger GL *et al.* Adequacy of tissue oxygenation in intact dog intestine. *J Appl Physiol* 1984; **56:** 1065–9.

23

Anaesthetic implications

Bryn R. Baxendale

Department of Anaesthesia, University Hospital, Queen's Medical Centre, Nottingham NG7 2UH, UK

The advent of reliable endovascular techniques to exclude aortic aneurysms from the circulation may represent an important advance in the management of this condition and must now undergo careful evaluation to establish its place in clinical practice. The areas that have a major influence on the anaesthetist's role include the use of a transfemoral approach rather than laparotomy, the absence of a significant period of aortic cross-clamping, thus potentially reducing the intraoperative physiological stress imposed on the patient, and finally the need for less intensive postoperative care. Consequently, endovascular repair of aortic aneurysms has implications for anaesthetic practice throughout the perioperative period, which will be discussed in sequence.

Preoperative assessment

Patients presenting for major vascular surgery have a high incidence of significant coexisting systemic disease. Most frequently this will involve the cardiovascular system,[1] although respiratory and renal pathologies are also important. The resulting physiological impairment must be interpreted in terms of the possible perioperative morbidity or mortality to which it may lead.[2] Many studies have examined the relationship between preoperative myocardial disease and the likelihood of perioperative cardiac complications.[3–6] Multivariate risk factor analyses have been used to try to stratify patients into a number of categories on this basis, but the lack of sensitivity and specificity of the preoperative investigations reduces the overall predictive power of these indices. Some investigators recommend more specialized testing, such as ambulatory electrocardiography and echocardiography, or dipyridamole–thallium scintigraphy. Other authors have documented the incidence of coexisting respiratory disease and renal impairment, and have attempted to describe their association with specific postoperative complications following conventional major vascular surgery.[7,8]

There are insufficient data available at present to quantify the significance of preoperative systemic disease in patients scheduled to receive endovascular surgery. This problem will be addressed as use of the technique grows, and there are some guidelines concerning the minimum preoperative data that should be collected during prospective studies.[9] In addition, there will be a tendency to offer endovascular surgery to patients who previously would not have been considered suitable for conventional surgery. The likely benefit in these cases will have to be balanced carefully against the conceivable risks, especially considering the possibility that the endovascular approach may have to be converted to open surgery.

Intraoperative management

In general terms, the use of a 'balanced' anaesthetic technique is a safe procedure, provided that appropriate drugs, techniques, monitoring and expertise are employed. One of the aims during vascular surgery is to minimize any physiological disturbance that may result in secondary damage to various organs or tissues, with particular attention paid to the detection and management of myocardial ischaemia or dysfunction. During conventional aneurysm surgery this has relied on the use of extensive intraoperative monitoring and prompt pharmacological intervention in order to deal with any significant haemodynamic and metabolic disturbances caused by aortic clamping and subsequent reperfusion of ischaemic tissues.

One of the major advantages offered by endovascular aneurysm repair is that it obviates the need to manipulate aortic blood flow in this way, as complete aortic occlusion occurs for only a brief period during deployment of the prosthesis. In Nottingham we have compared the haemodynamic profile during endovascular ('Chuter' bifurcated graft) and conventional elective repair of infrarenal aortic aneurysms.[10] Ten patients were selected for insertion of a bifurcated stent by the endovascular technique ('endovascular group'), with another ten undergoing conventional graft insertion ('open group'). All patients received a standard general anaesthetic (oxygen–nitrous oxide–

isoflurane by intermittent positive pressure ventilation (IPPV), and low-dose increments of fentanyl 1–3 μg kg^{-1}), avoiding the use of any regional techniques during the intraoperative period. Monitoring included direct measurement of mean arterial pressure (MAP), and a pulmonary artery catheter to measure or calculate central venous and pulmonary artery pressures, cardiac output (CO) and systemic vascular resistance (SVR). In addition, arterial blood samples were taken for lactate concentration. Baseline values were recorded following induction of anaesthesia. Parameters were noted immediately before and after certain critical events, namely occlusion of aortic blood flow (by cross-clamping or proximal endoluminal deployment of the prosthesis), and on sequential reperfusion of the distal tissues when the prosthesis was in place.

The following results are given as mean (SEM) values. On cross-clamping the aorta in the open group there were significant increases in MAP from 98 (6) to 115 (9) mmHg and in SVR from 2303 (259) to 2544 (278) dyn s cm^{-5} with CO decreasing from 3.8 (0.4) to 3.0 (0.5) l min^{-1}. In the endovascular group there were no clinically significant changes related to positioning the proximal end of the prosthesis. On reperfusing the first limb, the open group demonstrated marked decreases in MAP from 89 (4) to 61 (3) mmHg, and in SVR from 2231 (213) to 1578 (216) dyn s cm^{-5}. Blood lactate concentration increased from 1.6 (0.2) to 2.4 (0.4) mmol l^{-1}. By comparison, the endovascular group demonstrated haemodynamic stability at this stage, and there was not any significant alteration in blood lactate concentration. When reperfusing the second limb a further drop in SVR occurred in the open group, from 1803 (251) to 1449 (232) dyn s cm^{-5}, and blood lactate levels increased from 2.2 (0.3) to 2.9 (0.4) mmol l^{-1}. On this occasion the endovascular group showed a similar decrease in SVR from 2039 (227) to 1673 (209) dyn s cm^{-5}, which was not associated with any significant change in MAP, CO or blood lactate concentration. These results are represented in Fig. 23.1, which shows the percentage change in each parameter relative to values immediately preceding each event, and in Fig. 23.2, which provides comparison with baseline values before the commencement of surgery.

This study demonstrates that endovascular infrarenal aortic repair offers a more stable haemodynamic profile, and presents less of a metabolic insult as judged by blood lactate measurements. Although patients undergoing endovascular repair have both femoral arteries clamped for the majority of the operation, there is comparatively little

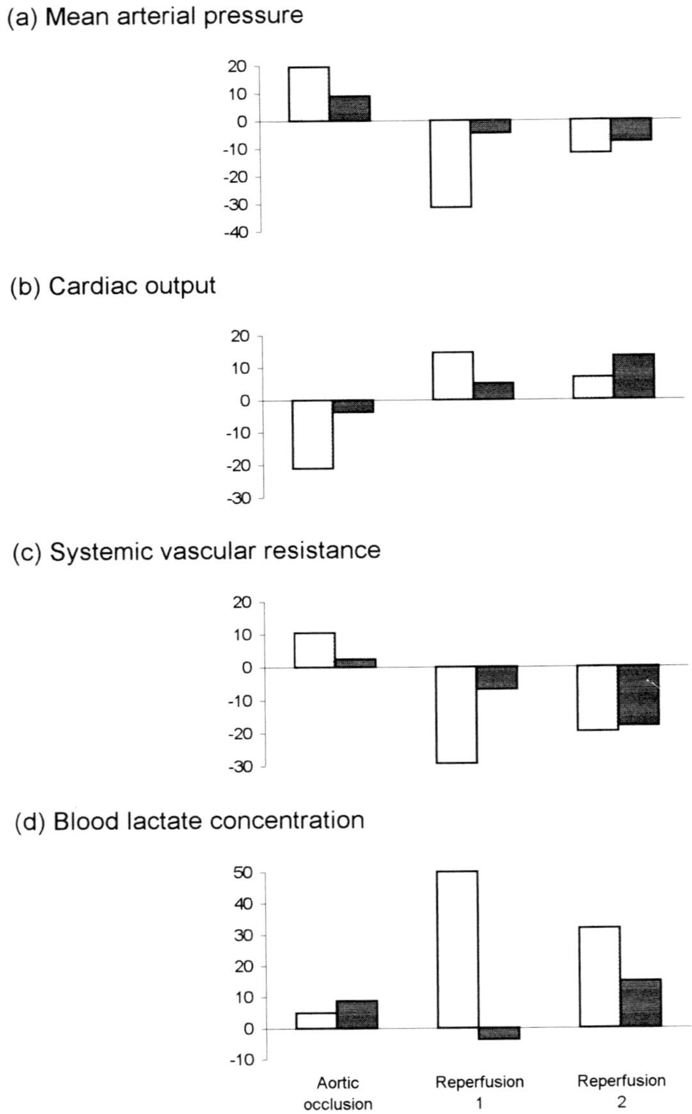

Fig. 23.1 Percentage change in haemodynamic parameters and blood lactate concentration following aortic occlusion and distal reperfusion of the first and second limb. Values are compared immediately before and after each event. □, Open group; ■, endovascular group.

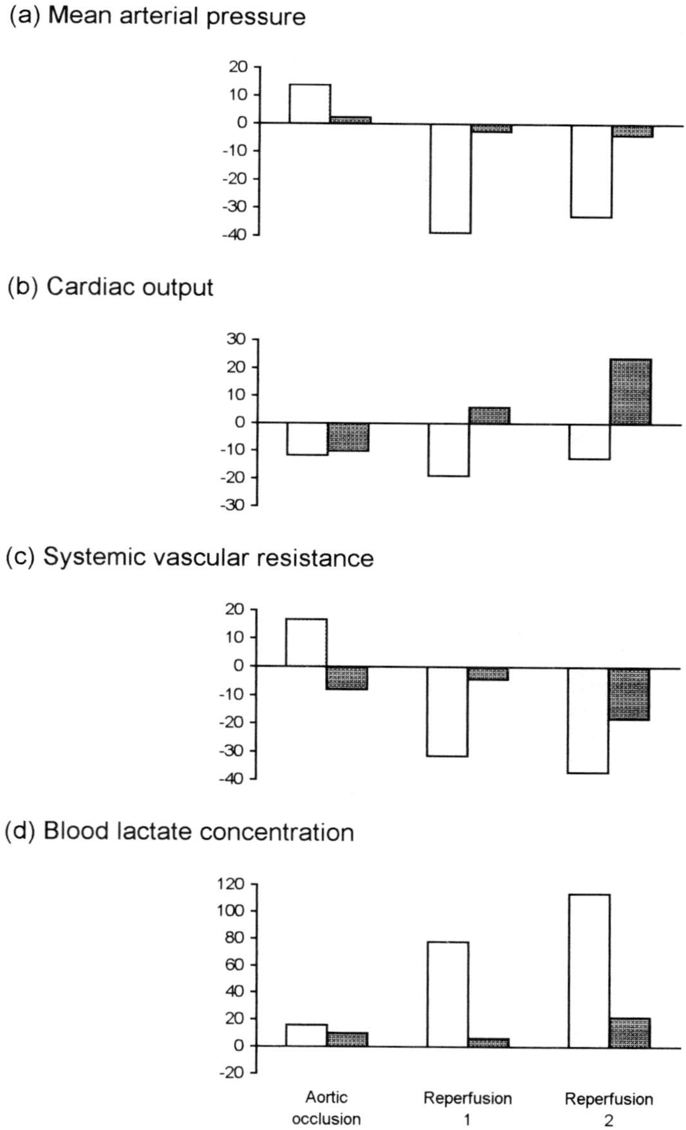

Fig. 23.2 Percentage change in haemodynamic parameters and blood lactate concentration following aortic occlusion and distal reperfusion of the first and second limb. Values are expressed relative to baseline values. □, Open group; ▩, endovascular group.

interference with pelvic visceral perfusion compared with aortic cross-clamping, and some perfusion of the lower limbs will also continue via more proximal arterial branches.

Some endovascular techniques, notably those employing a balloon to expand the proximal stent, require a transient period of relative hypotension in order to reduce the risk of any movement of the prosthesis at this critical point.[11,12] In some patients this may be undesirable because of the potential for causing myocardial ischaemia, cerebral ischaemia, and renal or bowel hypoperfusion. Although specific pharmacological agents (e.g. sodium nitroprusside) can produce this effect, their use is quite specialized because of their profound effect on arterial pressure. It remains to be seen whether this brief period of hypotension produces any significant organ damage. In the study described above, self-expanding stents were employed, thus obviating the need for any such intense pharmacological intervention.

Comprehensive monitoring during aortic aneurysm repair is mandatory owing to the severity of the surgical condition and its association with significant coexisting systemic disease. However, an endovascular technique avoids the need for laparotomy and retroperitoneal dissection, and should result in significantly less blood loss and 'third space' fluid loss. There will be significantly less opportunity for heat loss during surgery, and, combined with the reduction in haemodynamic fluctuation discussed above, the extent of monitoring required during surgery is worthy of reappraisal. This will require all the advantages mentioned above to be balanced against the risk and nature of intraoperative complications.[13] These include physical damage to the femoral or iliac arteries during manipulation of the deployment device, inaccurate site of deployment, or prosthetic obstruction due to kinking. These complications may require more extensive surgery or even conversion to an open procedure, in which case the anaesthetist must be in a position to adjust both the anaesthetic technique and level of monitoring accordingly.

Many centres advocate the use of pulmonary artery (PA) catheters during conventional aortic aneurysm repair in order to monitor left ventricular preload and to estimate cardiac output and systemic vascular resistance. Except when dictated by preoperative cardiac dysfunction, it may be reasonable to use transoesophageal Doppler or echocardiographic monitoring in place of the PA catheter during endovascular repair. Transoesophageal Doppler monitoring of blood flow in the descending thoracic aorta is able to provide a continuous estimate of stroke volume and cardiac output, and has been used effectively to detect and guide management of acute hypovolaemia or myocardial failure.[14] The lack of aortic cross-clamping during endovascular surgery means that the Doppler waveform will maintain its morphology throughout surgery, and allow trend changes to be interpreted relative to alteration of ventricular preload, contractility or afterload. Clinicians experienced with this type of monitoring suggest that it is safe and simple to institute, and can be more sensitive at detecting acute changes in ventricular muscle performance compared with the information provided by an indwelling PA catheter.[15]

Postoperative care

Anaesthetic management of the patient continues into the immediate postoperative period. Conventional aneurysm repair usually necessitates intensive postoperative care, aimed at maintaining satisfactory oxygenation of the blood, providing sufficient analgesia to permit spontaneous breathing without unacceptable sedation or other complications, and restoring any fluid imbalance inherited from the intraoperative period whilst replacing ongoing 'third space' losses. Frequently these goals demand the use of specialized skills, techniques and equipment for the purpose of patient monitoring and management, for example analgesia provided via the epidural route, frequent arterial blood gas monitoring, and in some cases a period of ventilatory or renal support which require patient admission to an Intensive Care Unit.

Endovascular surgery has clear advantages during this period. The lack of an extensive abdominal wound avoids direct impairment of spontaneous breathing due to local pain, and will not necessitate ventilatory support unless demanded by poor preoperative lung function or secondary to some intraoperative complication. The majority of cases suffice with supplementary oxygen by face mask alone. Analgesic requirement for transfemoral wounds are easily managed by administering systemic opioids, and patient-controlled devices are usually acceptable to the patient and nursing staff. Fluid prescription also tends to be more straightforward, as the patient does not have the same degree of intraoperative fluid shifts, not the same likelihood of postoperative losses. Hourly assessment of urine output combined with early measurement of postoperative plasma urea, electrolytes, creatinine and osmolality will detect renal dysfunction promptly. After a short period in the Postoperative Care Unit to confirm satisfactory recovery from surgery and anaesthesia, the majority of patients can safely be transferred back to the surgical ward.

Conclusions

The development of endovascular techniques for aortic aneurysm repair offers distinct advantages to the patient and clinician. Preoperative assessment must be as thorough as that for conventional aneurysm surgery, because the patient population is known to have a high incidence of significant coexisting systemic disease. There is also the possibility that intraoperative complications will demand more extensive surgery. From the anaesthetist's viewpoint, real advantages become apparent during the intraoperative and immediate postoperative period. Studies performed in Nottingham have demonstrated that the intraoperative haemodynamic and metabolic stress imposed on the patient is significantly less than that during conventional aneurysm repair, although no data exist yet to confirm that this results in fewer cardiac complications. The benefit in the Postoperative Care Unit includes easier management of postoperative oxygen requirements, analgesic regimens and fluid balance.

This discussion has concentrated on elective procedures, but those gaining experience with the technique are assessing the feasibility of managing symptomatic aortic aneurysms in a similar manner.[16] This has implications for the anaesthetist that are beyond the remit of this article, related particularly to the patient's preoperative management. There will also be an increasing demand to operate on high-risk asymptomatic patients who have been refused conventional surgery because of the associated morbidity and mortality. However, careful evaluation and controlled study will be required in a few specialist centres before widespread use of this technique becomes possible.

References

1. Hertzer NR. Basic data concerning associated coronary disease in peripheral vascular patients. *Ann Vasc Surg* 1987; **1:** 616–20.
2. Johnston KW. Multicenter prospective study of non-ruptured abdominal aortic aneurysm. Part II. Variables predicting morbidity and mortality. *J Vasc Surg* 1989; **9:** 437–47.
3. Mangano DT. Perioperative cardiac morbidity. *Anesthesiology* 1990; **72:** 153–84.
4. Mangano DT, Goldman L. Preoperative assessment of patients with known or suspected coronary disease. *N Engl J Med* 1995; **333:** 1750–6.

5. Goldman L, Caldera DL, Nussbaum SR *et al.* Multifactorial index of cardiac risk in non-cardiac surgical procedure. *N Engl J Med* 1977; **297:** 845–50.
6. Detsky AS, Abrams AB, Forbath N, Scott JG, Hilliard JR. Cardiac assessment for patients undergoing non-cardiac surgery: a multifactorial clinical risk index. *Arch Intern Med* 1986; **146:** 2131–4.
7. Currie IC, Robson AK, Scott DJA, Horrocks M. Quality of life of octogenarians after aneurysm surgery. *Ann R Coll Surg Engl* 1992; **74:** 269–73.
8. Joseph MG, McCollum PT, Lusby RJ. Abnormal pre-operative creatinine levels and renal failure following abdominal aortic aneurysm repair. *Aust NZ J Surg* 1989; **59:** 539–41.
9. Veith FJ, Abbott WM, Yao JST *et al.* Guidelines for development and use of transluminally placed endovascular prosthetic grafts in the arterial system. *J Vasc Surg* 1995; **21:** 670–85.
10. Baxendale BR, Baker DM, Hutchinson A, Chuter TAM, Wenham PW, Hopkinson BR. Haemodynamic and metabolic changes during endovascular stent insertion for repair of infrarenal aortic aneurysm. *Br J Anaesth* 1995; **74:** 38 (Abstract).
11. Greiff JMC, Thompson MM, Langham BT. Anaesthetic implications for aortic stent surgery. *Br J Anaesth* 1995; **75:** 779–81.
12. Parodi JC. Endovascular repair of abdominal aortic aneurysms and other arterial lesions. *J Vasc Surg* 1995; **21:** 549–57.
13. May J, White GH, Yu W *et al.* Surgical management of complications following endovascular grafting of abdominal aortic aneurysms. *Eur J Endovasc Surg* 1995; **10:** 51–9.
14. Singer M, Clarke J, Bennett D. Continuous haemodynamic monitoring by esophageal doppler. *Crit Care Med* 1989; **17:** 447–52.
15. Roizen MF, Beaupre PN, Alpert RA *et al.* Monitoring with two-dimensional transesophageal echocardiography. *J Vasc Surg* 1984; **1:** 300–5.
16. Yusuf SW, Whitaker SC, Chuter TAM, Wenham PW, Hopkinson BR. Emergency endovascular repair of leaking aortic aneurysm. *Lancet* 1994; **344:** 1645.

Index